Pain and palliative Care

Part 2

Dr Pramod Kumar
MD (BHU), FICA, FIAPM
Dean Medical Sciences, TMU
Moraedabad , India

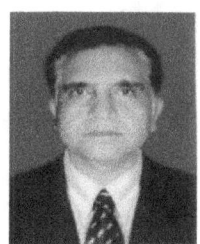

MD (BHU), FICA, FIAPM
Dean Medical Sciences TMU
Formerly Dean PDUMC Rajkot, GAIMS, RMCRCH
About the Author

The author Dr. Pramod Kumar has been a medical teacher in anaesthesiaology since 1975. He has been an ex faculty of IMS, BHD, MGIMS Wardha, SSSIHMS, Prasanthi Nilayam, MP Shah Medical College Jamnagar, PDU Medical College Rajkot & worked as Mdical Superintendent, Dean and Professor of Anaesthesia in eminent Medical Colleges of India. He is a founder member & President of Indian Society for study of Pain, Indian Society of Anaesthesiologists (ISA) – West Zone, Gujarat, Moradbad and Jamanagar branches. He has written more than 80 research papers in National and International journals and is a peer reviewer of IJA, Ind Pain, JACP and Asian Arch Anaesth, IJAA, IJCA. He has written several books e.g. Textbook of Anaesthesia, Textbook of Pain, Clinical Methods in Anaesthesia, MCQ in Anaesthesia, Guide to PNB, Terminal Cancer Care, Veterinary Anaesthesia, Anaesthesia in Dentistry, Pain in Cancer, CPR (in Gujarati) Atlas in PNB and coauthor in Pain Mechanisms and Pain Medicine and Year Book of Anaesthesia. He has received Life Time Achievement Award by ISSP ISA-WZ, ISA Bhopal Award for Academic Excellence, President Silver Medal ISSP, and Founder President SAM ISA and received seven oration awards. His Bio data is listed in American, International, Young Men and Women of achievement, Indo American and Indo European WHO's who. Presently author is working as Dean Academics Medical Sciences, Teerthanker Mahaveer University, Moradabad, UP, India.

PREFACE

The Pain Relief service has taken almost 5 decades since the formation of International Association for study of Pain. In India these services started within a decade after formation of IASP when ISSP was formed in BHU Varanasi. The anaesthesiologist, surgeons & physicians have all joined together in providing pain relief services. However there is still reluctance on the part of medical community to start this service to millions of patients suffering from chronic intractable pain. This book is a further step in creating awareness & trains the pain physicians and postgraduate in South Asia. This book deals with a synopsis of pain mechanisms, various conditions and pain services imparted through peripheral nerve blocks, invasive and non invasive procedures. The second part deals with palliative care in terminal cancer patients which is useful to pain practitioners, UG & PG students and even public at large since the language used is very specific, to the point & simple. This book will be useful to anaesthesiologists since MCI has made Pain Clinic services under anaesthesiology department in a medical college mandatory.

Dr Pramod Kumar

Dedication: **Neha, Brijesh & Anvesha**

Pain and palliative Care

CONTENTS

1.	History of Pain relief	1
2.	Mechanism of Pain	5
3.	Opiate Recetors	15
4.	Dorsal Hornn Receptors	19
5.	Non Steroidal Anti Inflammatory & Muscle Relaxants	22
6.	Opioids	30
7.	Opioid Drug Deliveries	39
8.	Psychotropic Drugs as Analgesics	47
9.	Anti Epileptic and Membrane Stabilizing Drugs as Analgesic	51
10.	Evaluation of Pain and Pain Imaging	53
11.	Peripheral Nerve Blocks	72
12.	Peripheral Nerve Blocks Head and Neck	76
13.	Peripheral Nerve blocks of trunk	80
14.	Lower Limb Peripheral Nerve Blocks	84
15.	Peripheral nerve blocks in Children	92
16.	Post Operative Pain Relief	99
17.	Trigeminal Neuralgia	105
18.	Neuropathic Pain	110
19.	Low Back Pain and Myalgia	116
20.	Labour Analgesia	123
21.	Interventional Pain Management	129
22.	Orofacial Pain and Migraine	140
23.	Pain Clinic	148
24.	Temporomandibular Disorders and Dental Pain	159
25.	Acute Dental and Temporomandibular Pain	164
26.	Pain of Pelvic Origin	169
27.	Ultrasound	177
28.	Pain Imaging	184
29.	Trauma and Pain	188
30.	Palliative Care Magnitude of Cancer Pain	192
31.	Cancer Pain	199
32.	Neuro Psychological Symptoms	213
33.	Psychological Aspects of Cancer Pain Patients	216
34.	Gastro Intestinal Symptoms	220
35.	Urinary Symptoms	227
36.	Management of Cancer Pain	233
37.	Palliative Care Special Problems	238
38.	Children and Elderly Patients	242
39.	Cancer Therapeutics	246
40.	Protocol for Malignant Pain Therapy	251

Annexure

I.	ASA Practice Guidelines for Acute Pain Management in the Perioperative Setting	256
II.	ASA Practice Guidelines for Chronic Pain Management.	258

Chapter 1.

History of pain Relief.

Indian context:
Pain during pregnancy - Valmiki Ramayan- Ashok vatika-
Sita said to Trijata- "whenever Ravan is tourchering me, I feel a pain which is intolerable, similar to the pain which a lady feels when a vaidya is cutting her abdomen to remove a child from her womb".

Fig 1: Rawan pesters Sita   Fig 2: Sushruta operating a patient under herbal fumes

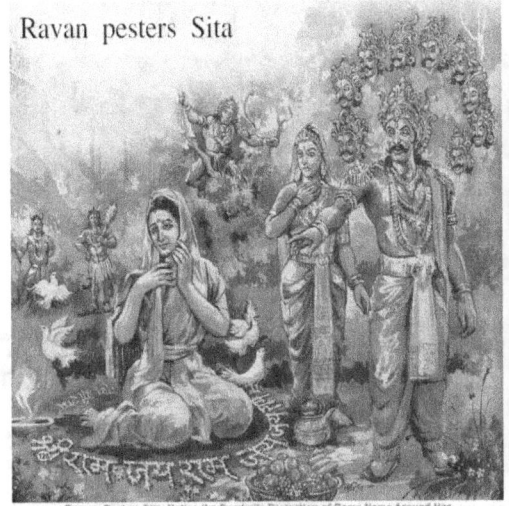
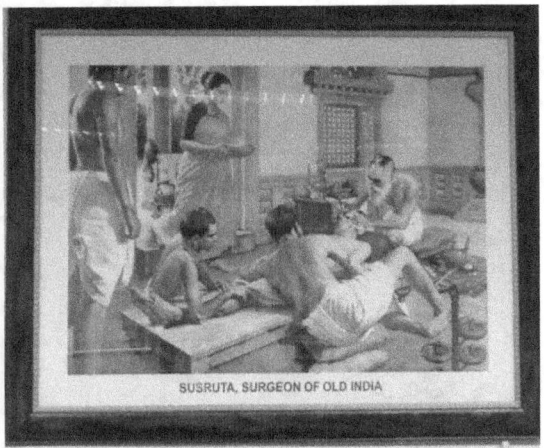

Bible- Old Testament-Genesis-3.16
Garden of Eden – Eve persuades Adam to eat apple. God curses her "Unto women, I will multiply them, sorrow and thy conception, in sorrow though shall bring forth children.

Fig 3: God curses Eve

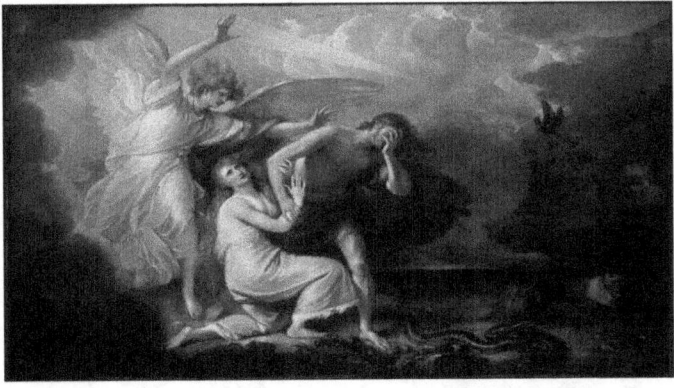

Fig 4: The Chirurgeon's Apprentice 1842.   Fig 5: George Wilson, Edinburgh Amputatio

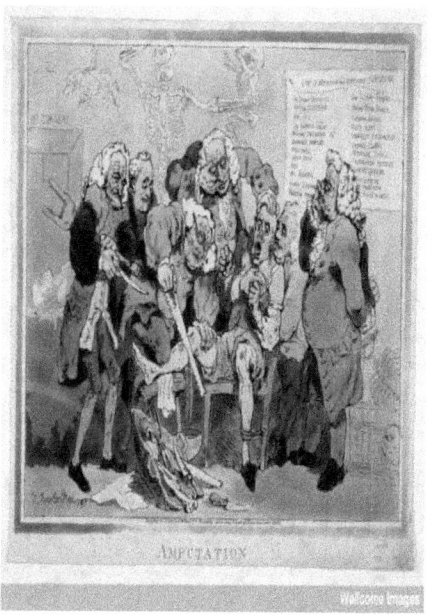
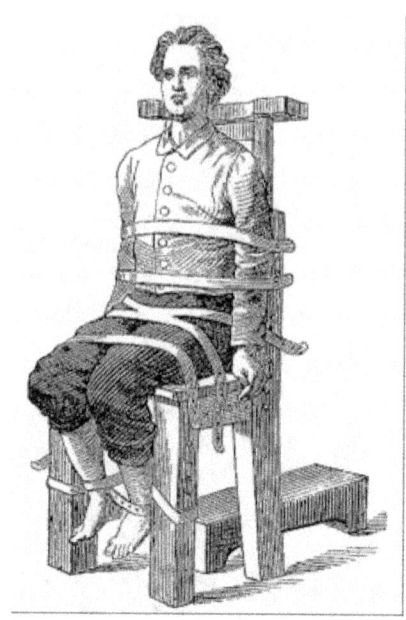

Fig 6: Traditional Chinese medicine/ Acupuncture   Fig 7:   Moxibustion

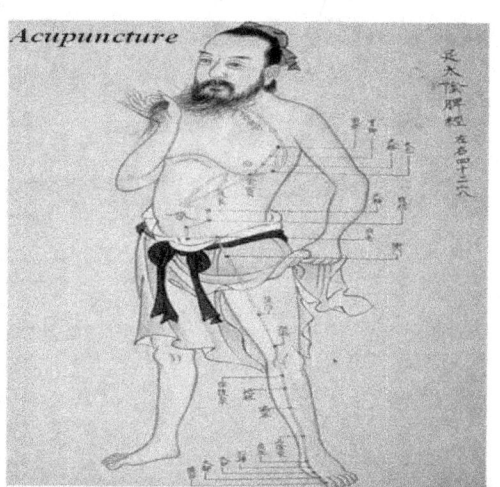
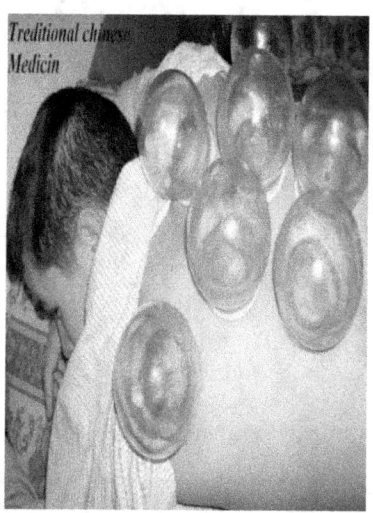

Hippocrates believed that pain was caused by an imbalance in the vital fluids of a human. At this time, neither Aristotle nor Hippocrates believed that the brain had any role to play in pain processing but rather implicated the heart as the central organ for the sensation of pain.[4]

Middle Ages--Methods for labour pain relief: Deep suggestion, Alcohol, Opium, Suspending mother to a tree, Mandrake

Fig 8: Uprooting a Mandrake plant.

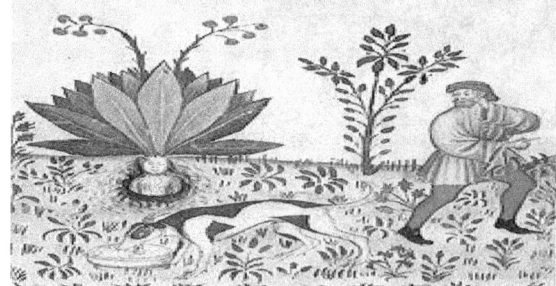

"A BLACK DAY IN THE HISTORY OF MANKIND"

1591 Edinburgh A young woman named Euphanie Macalyane got the punishment for seeking pain relief during labor. She was burnt alive on direct order from King of Scotland James VI.
Sir J.Y.Simpson -Ether –19 Jan 1847, Chloroform –8 Nov 1847
Sir .John Snow 1857- Father of General Anaesthesia. Queen Victoria received Chloroform for labour pain during the birth of prince Leopold. John Snow gave anaesthesia to her at the birth of Prince Leopold (8th child) in 1853 and in 1857 at the birth of Princess Beatrice.

Fig 9: Sir John Snow   Fig 10: Queen Victoria

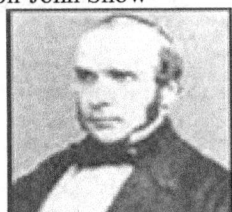
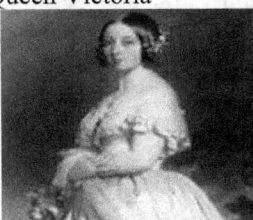

In the 11th century, Avicenna theorized that there were a number of feeling senses including touch, pain and titillation

The advent of Ether inhalation for surgical pain was a revolution in the field of pain relief. Since steam engine was installed within that week the news spread to Europe within a fortnight, the fast speed at which a steam boat crossed the Atlantic Ocean. This idea was fast taken up by the physicians of the continent and Ether anaesthesia was well established. In India, the news reached within a fortnight and Ether was used successfully in surgical pain at Secunderabad. John snow's Chloroform anaesthesia on a handkerchief to Queen Victoria during the birth of prince Leopold lead to its official recognition throughout the world.

Numbing effects of cocaine- Coca leaves were used by aborigine American Indians to relieve stress and it was in 1860; the extract of Coca leaves was purified by Albert Nieman. In 1844, Carl Koller an intern first published the numbing effect of cocaine on mucus membrane on the suggestion of his friend Sigmund Freud, who at the time was away on his honeymoon. This anaesthetic property of cocaine was recognized worldwide leading to local anaesthetic use in eye surgery[3]. The advent of anaesthesia marked a triumph of mankind over pain. However the pain mechanism and anatomy was not much known. The contribution of Professor Bonica, P.D Wall & Tony Yaksha greatly influenced the treatment of pain with their basic & clinical research. Their findings and wisdom guided the medical fraternity, anesthesiologists in particular. Dr. Rowenstein, till his death in 1960, was famous for his research on has special course in anatomy, physiology and therapy of pain. Cancer pain remains a global problem. WHO estimated 3.5 million people suffering from pain (95% in terminal stage) without adequate pain relief? The reasons for inadequate treatment sited were over regulation of opioids and their under use in treating cancer pain.

Research- with the discovery of opiate receptors & endogenous opiates, the knowledge of pain was enhanced. The Gate control theory of pain proposed by Melzack & Wall was a landmark in the advancement of pain research. However delivery of pharmacologically active agents to discreet sites in the nervous system remains a challenge. In 1986 clinical pharmacology of opioid analgesics conference identified controversies like controlled studies, choice, methods of administration tolerance and drug abuse of opioids. The healthcare costs and private & Government agencies' failure to recognize pain management needs of a patients were realized.

International Assoc for Study of Pain: 1973
The Indian Society for Study of Pain (ISSP) :1984. Founder members- Dr. V Rastogi, Dr. Pramod Kumar, Dr K. Pande, Dr A Lal, Dr MT Bhatia, Dr Yajnik.
- The First President Dr.Akram Lal, Secretary: Dr. V Rastogi, Treasurer: Dr. Pramod Kumar.
- First National Conference in Varanasi in1985.
- India chapter of IASP
- Indian J Pain 1984.
- PDCC, Fellowship Program, Diploma in Pain

South Asian Association of Regional Pain Societies (SAARPS)
Started in 2002 with permission taken by ISSP from International Association for Study of Pain (IASP). First conference at Dhaka, Bangladesh 2003
Founders – Dr P. Kumar, Dr P Bajaj, Dr Iqbal (DHAKA),, Dr Shrestha (Nepal), Dr Nelli (Sri Lanka).

References
1. Booth, Martin. Opium a History. London: Simon & Schuster, 1996
2. Meldrum, Marcia. "A History of Pain Management." Opioids: Past, Present and Future. Journal of the American Medical Association. Web. 08 Nov. 2011. <http://opioids.com/pain-management/history.html.
3. Textbook of Pain, 2nd Ed, CBS Pub New Delhi 2008.
4. Kumar Pramod - Terminal cancer care 2nd Edition, CBS Medical Pubs, New Delhi 200
   Kumar Pramod - Guide to Peripheral Nerve Blocks 1st Edition CBS Medical Pubs, New Delhi 2008
5. Kumar Pramod - A Handbook of pain management & related symptoms in cancer, Samvedana, Indraprastha Apollo Hospital New Delhi, 2003
6. Kumar Pramod - Illustrated Atlas on peripheral nerve blocks Anaesthesia Dept. Jamnagar 2002.

Chapter 2.

Mechanism of Pain

Two types of persistent pain:-
Nociceptive / inflammatory pain[1]:- The most peripheral apparatus for pain pathway is nociceptors which is present all over the body. On application of natural stimuli of adequate intensity to the skin, two sequential pain sensations are elicited. They are related to the activation of myelinated A-delta fibers (>2m/sec) and unmyelinated C fibers (<2m/sec). Most Studies used heat and mechanical stimuli to study nociception and therefore nomenclature of CMH and AMH is used to refer to C fiber mechano-heat sensitive receptors and fiber mechano-heat sensitive receptors respectively. Activity in nociceptor induces an increase in sympathetic discharge but the converse is not true under usual circumstances. Sympathetic nervous system pain dependent activity is referred to as sympathetically maintained pain (SMP) which is seen in acute herpes zoster, soft tissue trauma. Tissue damage results in a cascade of events leading to enhanced pain to natural stimulus.
Neuropathic pain: - Examples include post-herpetic neuralgia, complex regional pain syndrome (CRPS) and Phantom limb pain. This type of pain arises from injury to the peripheral / central nervous system. It is burning in quality. It is less responsive to opioids but responds to local anesthetics, anticonvulsants, and tricyclic anti depressants [2].
Mechanism of sensitization at primary afferent nociceptors:- Although there are no pain fibers in peripheral or central nervous system, there are anatomically and physiological specialized peripheral afferent fibers that responds to noxious stimuli. These thinly myelinated A-delta and unmyelinated C-afferents terminate as free unencapsulated peripheral nerve endings.
Physiological specificity of primary afferent is indicated from the following,
1. Nerve compression first blocks large fibers and nonpainful mechanical sensation, then the sensation mediated by small fibers and later the perception of noxious stimuli.
2. Local anesthetics block small diameter fibers first and abolish pain.
3. Electrical stimulation of single primary afferents in the conscious human subject evokes pain only when thresholds for A-delta and C-fibers are reached. The former do not respond to painful stimuli but are necessary for normal quality of pain perception. In the absence of these large fibers all sensations are perceived as burning, indicating the breakdown of specificity when large fibers are blocked. Convergence of large and small diameter afferents at the level of the dorsal horn underlies this phenomenon.

Allodynia: - The stimuli that normally are not painful e.g. movement and light touch become painful. The pain produced by touching sun burnt skin or movement of an arthritic joint [3].
Hyperalgesia: - Hyperalgesia is an exacerbated pain produced by a noxious stimulus e.g. slapping sun burnt skin or reaction to noxious stimuli in a subject whose large fibers in the arm are blocked by compression.
Primary sensitization mechanism: - After a tissue injury, the threshold for firing of A-delta and C nociceptive afferent is lowered to a non-noxious range. Mechanism involves synthesis of arachidonic acid from membrane lipids via steroid sensitive phospholipase A2 enzyme. Arachidonic acid is acted upon by cyclooxygenase enzyme to produce prostaglandins which act directly on the peripheral terminals of A-delta and C fibers, while their electrical activity remains unchanged. Light touch can now activate a C- fiber and produce pain. Aspirin and NSAIDs are effective through cyclooxygenase inhibition. COX-2 enzyme inhibitors, Celecoxib and Rofecoxib have a better utility without GIT side effects of Aspirin and NSAIDs.

Fig. 1: **Mediators produced by injury, inflammation at the terminal neurons.**

Tissue damage
⇊
Inflammation➔ Bradykinin, H+, ATP ➔ Excitation --------------- ➔   N
⇊   O
Lymphocytes   Release   Opioids, Growth factors,   Excitation   C
                                                                                                                        I   N
Platelets   ---------------➔Cytokines, Histamine,   --------------- ➔   C   E

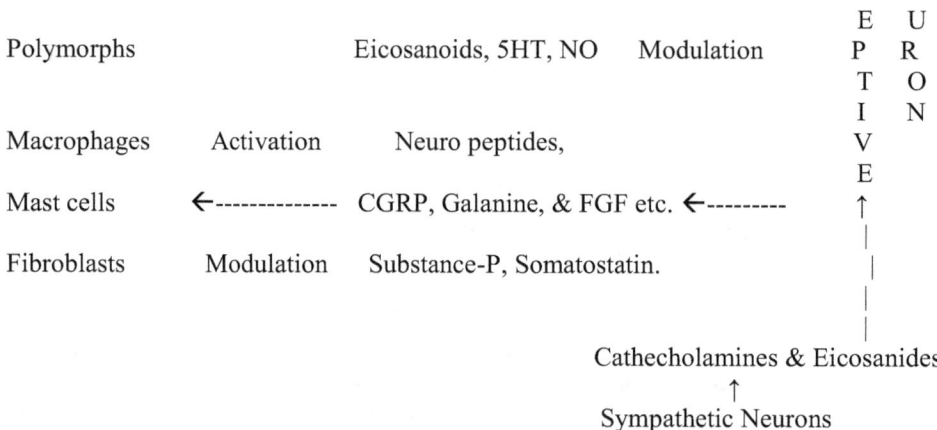

Substance P: - An 11 amino acid peptide neuro transmitter synthesized by primary afferent nociceptors. Substance-P is released in the dorsal horn and activates second order "pain" transmission neuron in the dorsal horn. It is released from the peripheral terminals of C-fibers and contributes to local, neurogenic inflammatory mechanisms, including vasodilatation, warmth, redness and swelling.

Capsaicin, an irritant is the pungent ingredient in the hot pepper. It stimulates C-fibers because they express the venilloid (VR!) / Capsaicin receptor. VR1 receptor also responds to noxious heat and is gated by pH. The acidity of injured tissue may enhance pain via VR1. Topical Capsaicin creams have been introduced to control a variety of pains. Their efficacy remains to be established.

Onward transmission of pain impulse[4]

When the depolarization at the junction of the receptor and the axon to which it is attached reaches threshold level, an impulse is propagated along the surface of the axon. The nociceptive information is relayed by A-delta and C fibers through posterior roots into the spinal cord. The gray matter in the spinal cord is divided in to 10 layers (Laminae). The skin afferents terminate in Laminae- I, II, & V of the dorsal horn, where those from viscera, muscles and the other deep tissues in Laminae- I, V & X. The neurons in the spinal cord are classified as those specific to nociceptive specific neurons and nonspecific or wide dynamic range. These axons pass from dorsal horn to the contra lateral side of the spinal cord. They further travel up with anterolateral region of the cord to form synapse with neurons in Thalamus, Mesencephalon or Reticular formation. N-methyl-D- aspartate receptor is activated in response to tissue damage along with other neuro peptides e.g. substance-P. Dorsal horn is the seat of control, excitatory and inhibitory influences (Fig. 2). These alterations in the functional performance of the cord will alter sensory processing and are likely to account both for failure to react to tissue damage on some occasions and the generation of pain in reaction to low intensity stimuli in others. Understanding the factors controlling or determine which mode the spinal cord is essential in order to understand the pathogenesis of pain. A damage to peripheral or CNS may alter or result in irreversible changes in sensory processing and disorders.

Spinal cord laminar organization (1):- In 1954 Rexed demonstrated that the gray matter of the spinal cord could be divided into distinct laminae or layers. Physiological studies too have demonstrated an analogous, functional laminar organization. An electrode penetrating the gray matter of the dorsal horn records cells in the following sequence,

Lamina-I(Marginal Layer) :- Cells respond primarily and in some cases exclusively to noxious stimuli. Some also respond to innocuous i.e. non-injury stimulation. Many Lamina-1 cells contribute axons to the spino-thalamic tract.

Lamina-II (Substantia Gelatinosa):- contains small interneurons, many of which respond to noxious input. Lamina-II neurons modulate cell of Lamina- I & V. Lamina –I & II receive direct primary afferent input only from small fibers.

Lamina-III & IV: - Cells respond to innocuous, hair brushing and tactile skin stimulation, and do not increase their response when receptive field is pinched i.e. noxious stimulation.

Lamina-V: - Cells respond to noxious and non-noxious stimuli and are wide dynamic range cells (WDR). They also respond to noxious visceral stimuli and receive excitatory input from large small diameter afferent fibers.

Lamina-VI: - Cells respond to joint movement as well as to cutaneous stimulation.

Physiology of Wide Dynamic Range cell:-

In addition to convergence of different modalities of input, WDR neurons in Lamina-V receive inputs from a relatively large area in a phenomenon called Spatial Convergence. The single cells of lamina-V of dorsal horn of spinal cord have a complex receptive field consisting of at least two distinct regions. In the center both innocuous and noxious stimuli are excitatory. In the surrounding regions, non-noxious stimuli (carried by large fibers) are inhibitory. This factor accounts for pain relieving effects of TENS. On the other hand removal of the inhibitory components of the receptive field as in nerve injury might increase the response of a WDR cell to a noxious stimulus. The lesion causing selective damage to sources of inhibitory inputs to WDR neurons can produce pain.

Spinal cord neurons do not transmit pain: - Some cells in dorsal horn responds to noxious stimuli and many of them are at the origin of ascending pathways. Although some of these neurons respond exclusively to noxious stimuli, most also respond to non-noxious mechano-receptive inputs. They may be activated by temperature changes. Thus several modalities are carried by spino thalamic tract axon. There is no specific line for pain, in contrast to neurons in lemniscal system which are more specific.

Fig. 2: Schematic of nociceptive receptors from various part of the body to the brain

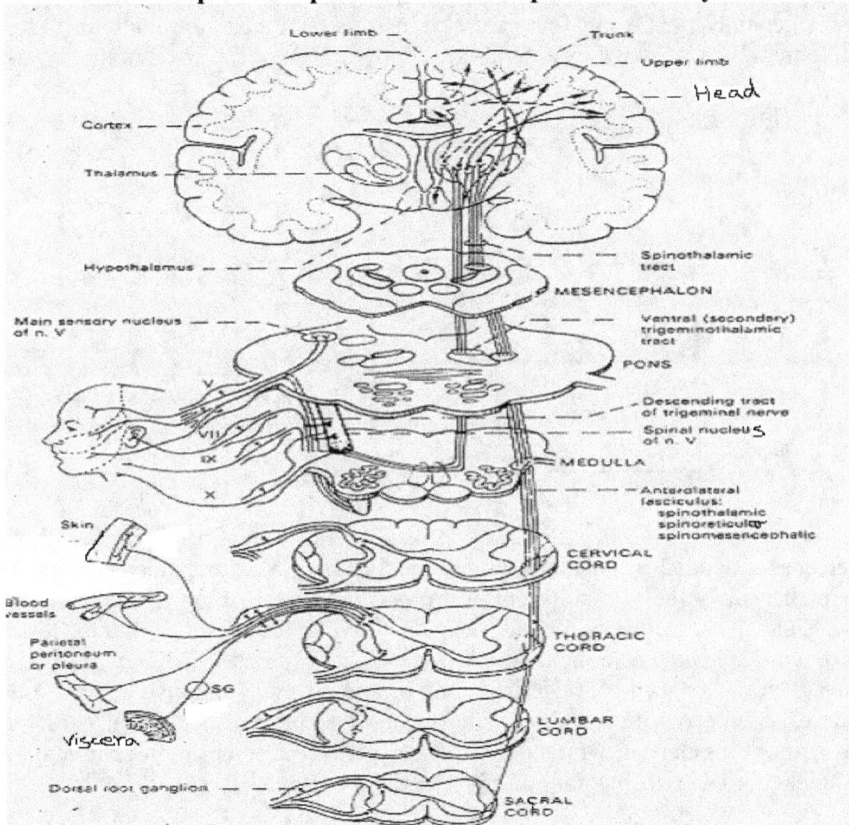

Gate control theory: - Melzack and Wall published their Gate control theory of pain in 1975 that took in to account the evidence of physiological specialization, central summation, patterning and modulation of input and influence of psychological factors. They proposed modulation of afferent fibers input to T cells by spinal gating mechanism in the dorsal horn, stimulation of small fibers keep the gate open while large input by large fibers close the gate. The central control triggers fibers activating selective cognition and modulating and influence through descending fibers [5] (fig. 3)

Fig 3: In 1981, Melzack and Wall modified their theory to take into account information acquired since the original proposal. Their model includes excitatory and inhibitory links from substantia gelatinosa to the transmission cells as well as the descending inhibitors of control from brain stem. These theories have provoked the development of new approaches to pain therapy.[6]

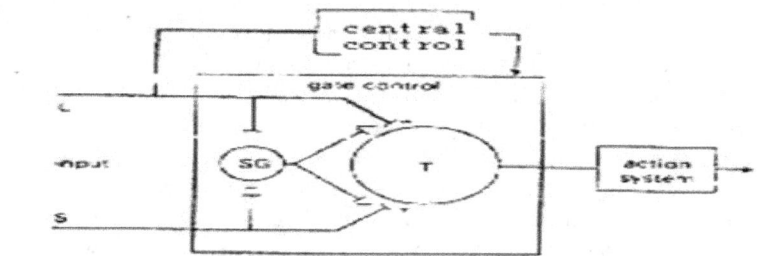

Fig 4: Schematic of the gate control theory of pain. L.Large -diameter fibres. The fibres project to the substancia gelatinosa (SC) and first central transmission T cells the inhibitory effect on the SC on the afferent terminals is increased by activity in L fibres and decreased by activity in S fibres.

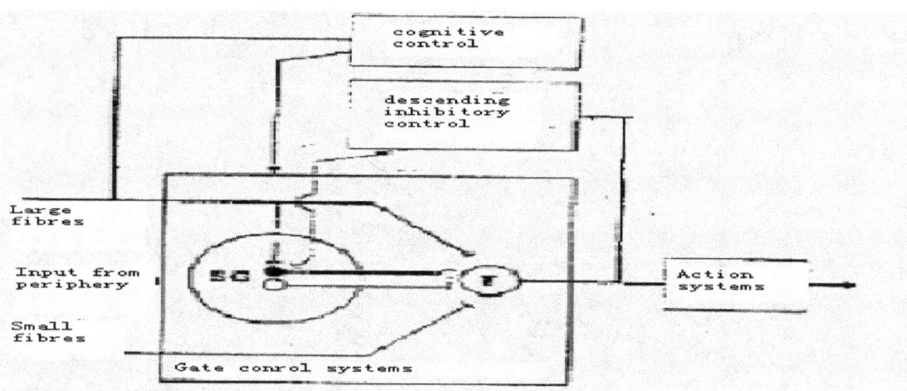

Secondary hyperalgesia (central sensitization):- Acute pain is brief while post operative pain may be considered as extended acute pain. Unfortunately noxious stimuli may sometimes evoke long term, persistent changes in the excitability of dorsal horn neurons leading to a greater response to subsequent impulse. This phenomenon is called secondary hyperalgesia into contrast to primary sensitization described earlier. Glutamate acting via N-methyl-D-aspartate(NMDA) receptor has a role in this condition. The secondary hyperalgesia can be prevented by preemptive analgesia using local anesthetic blockade of afferents from a surgical site, in order to prevent the spinal cord from experiencing the noxious stimulus associated with surgery. Under general anesthesia, patient is unaware of the stimulus but the spinal cord and the memory of injury can still be established.

Referred Pain:- The WDR cells that receive input from somatic nociceptive primary afferents in the skin and deep tissue also receive input from nociceptors in the viscera. This phenomenon presumably underlies the referral of visceral pain to somatic structures. For example, Inflammation of the peritoneal surface of the diaphragm may cause referred pain of right shoulder. The afferents that innervates diaphragm arise from C3-C5 segments and run with phrenic nerve.

Ascending Pathways: - Since surgical section of anterolateral spino thalamic tract relieve pain in the contra lateral side; it has been thought earlier that spino thalamic tract is pain tract. But cutting the antero lateral quadrant does not selectively cut spino thalamic tract. Recently many ascending pathways have been found to transmit nociceptive messages to brain.

Spinothalamic tract (STT):- Cells of origin are located in Rexed's Laminae I & V, majority of these axons cross locally in anterior commissure and ascend in the contra lateral antero lateral column, terminating in ventro posterior thalamic nucleus. From there the axons go to somato sensory cortex in post central gyrus. Some of the spinothalamic tract axons terminate within medial thalamus in the intralaminar nuclei, having large receptive fields with little topographic organization. Firing of neurons in medial thalamus is influenced by behavioral state as reduced pain in humans who are destructed.

The inputs from medial thalamus are projected to many cortical, sub cortical sites including limbic and motor regions. The diversity of these projections may reflect the variety of emotional and motor responses which pain evokes. The posterior nucleus of thalamus where majority of spinothalamic axons terminate, recently has been identified to receive specific information about noxious and temperature stimuli from lamina-I of dorsal horn. This region of thalamus sends projection to the insular cortex.

The spinoreticular tract (SRT);- is located in the antero lateral quadrant. Some SRT axons terminate on cells involved in descending pain modulation pathways so may be involved in phenomenon of counter irritation where the pain reduces the severity of another. Other SRT axons make up spino reticulo thalamic tract, which terminate in the medial thalamus along with STT described above.

Spinomesencephalic tract terminate primarily in superior colliculus and the peri aqueductal gray (PAG). This projection to PAG activates descending pain control networks. PAG neurons are involved in autonomic and somato motor aspect of defense reaction. The superior colliculus part of this tract is involved in multi sensory integration, behavioral reactions and orientation.

Post synaptic dorsal horn column pathways: - Mostly axon collaterals of large diameter primary afferents and some of the Lamina-V axons project axons in this column, terminating in Cuneate and Gracile Nuclei. These may be responsible for transmission of the visceral pain.

Spino- ponto- amygdala system originates in Laminae- I & V of the dorsal horn, ascending in the dorso lateral funiculus. It projects to the para brachial area of the pons and from there to amygdala. This system may be involved in fear and memory of pain, as well as behavioral and autonomic reactions to noxious events e.g. vocalization, flight, pupil dilatation and cardio respiratory responses.

Cortical processing of Pain:- Early observations by Kead and Holmes(1911) in soldiers who had extensive injuries of cerebral cortex continued to perceive pain. Penfield and Boldrey(1937) reached a similar conclusion when patients rarely reported pain sensation after electrical stimulation of their cerebral cortex during surgery for removal of epileptic foci. They concluded that cerebral cortex played only a minimal role in pain perception despite nociceptive information reaching a number of cortical areas.[4]

Recently, Positron Emission Tomography (PET) to measure regional cerebral blood flow and use of functional magnetic resonance imaging (fMRI) to show changes in blood oxygenation showed that several cortical regions are activated during pain. The heat, touch, capsaicin stimulus activated primary and secondary somato sensory cortices (S1, S2), anterior cingulate cortex (ACC) and insular cortex(IC).

This distributed cerebral activation reflects complex nature of pain involving discrimination, affective, autonomic and motor function. The anatomical connectivity to insular cortex suggests integration of somato sensory information with memory and homeostasis. ACC contributes to affective component and modulation of motor and autonomic reactions. S1 & S2 cortices contributes to spatial, temporal and intensity distribution. Due to this high degree of connectivity, a discrete lesion in any of these regions does not produce a precise, permanent deficit in pain perception. It shows functions performed by one region taken over by another, showing plasticity and resiliency showing essential nature of nociception for survival.

Supra spinal mechanisms are inhibitory part of the brain mechanism. Electric stimulation of mid brain PAG produces analgesia in humans along with inhibition of firing of dorsal horn neurons that responds to pain. The descending control is mediated via an excitatory connection from the PAG to Serotonin (5HT) containing neurons of the nucleus Raphe Magnus of Medulla. The 5HT axons from there inhibit the firing of neurons in laminae I, &V. There also exist parallel descending noradrenergic inhibitory controls acted upon by Tricyclic antidepressant. The circuit from PAG to spinal cord constitutes brain's end organ pain control system.

Descending inhibitory pathways (DIP) begins in cerebral cortex and descends to thalamus and peri aqueductal gray (PAG) of mid brain which is rich in opiate receptors responsible for secreting enkephalin and endorphins. Fibers from PAG descend to nucleus Raphe Magnus (NRM) in brain stem, responsible for secretion of 5HT alleviating pain threshold and contributing depression. Then fibers descend to spinal cord, exciting other inhibitory neurons to secrete transmitter gamma amino butyric acid

(GABA). These lower fibers of DIP synapse with inter neurons, communicating pain signals entering spinal cord via A-delta and C fibers as well as second order neurons in lateral spino thalamic tract. Thus DIP acts at all levels where pain signals first enter the CNS. In addition to pain and depression, neuro transmitters also enhance tissue healing, increasing quality of sleep time and in general increasing the quality of life.

Neuromatrix theory proposed by Melzack where brain processes a neural network and it integrates multiple inputs to produce output pattern which produces pain. The synaptic architecture is determined by genetic and sensory influences. The inputs acting of neuromatrix or sensory, cognition and emotional inputs, intrinsic inhibitory and body stress regulation activity e.g. Cytokines, autonomic, immune and opioid system. Glial activation and its associated proinflammatory cytokine release are being implicated in exaggerated pain states, thus linked to acute peripheral inflammation, chronic nerve trauma and infection.

Opiates, opioids and endorphins: - PAG and dorsal horn have high opiate receptor concentration which binds morphine and naloxone and intrinsic endorphin peptides. The latter has been cloned providing future development of newer analgesics. The placebo activates the endorphins and reversed by naloxone. TENS, acupuncture also does the same. Hypnosis does not involve endorphin release. The morphine injection inhibits Lamina-I, V and blocks release of neuro transmitters e.g. Substance-P from small fibers

ACUTE PAIN – PHYSIOLOGICAL RESPONSE
- Tissue damage – actual or potential
- Release of algesics – Prostaglandins, 5 HT, substance P, bradykinins
- Generation of noxious stimuli
- Increased muscle and sympathetic tone
- Increased metabolism and oxygen consumption

PRIMARY AFFERENT MECHANISMS
- Stimulation of Aδ and C fibers in skin and viscera
- Release of peptides – substance P (SP) neurokinin (NKA) and calcitonin gene related peptide (CGRP)

EFFECTS OF PEPTIDES
- INFLAMMATION
- HYPERAEMIA
- PLASMA EXTRAVASATION
- LEUCOCYTE ADHESIONS

AXON REFLEX FLARE
- Contraction of smooth muscles in
  - Airways
  - Urinary bladder
  - Iris and other tissues
- Leads to
  - Increase in blood flow
  - Increase in immune cell response
- Benefits of reflex flare
  - Increased blood flow to local area
- Disadvantages of reflex flare
  - Tissue damage due to persistent inflammation
  - Reduced pH in tissue due to increased H+ ions in stomach and muscles

CALCITONIN GENE RELATED PEPTIDE (CGRP)
- Released from sensory nerve endings by antidromic firing
- Local reflex trigger by increase intracellular Ca^{++} leads to inflammation

Fig 5: Capsaicin receptor

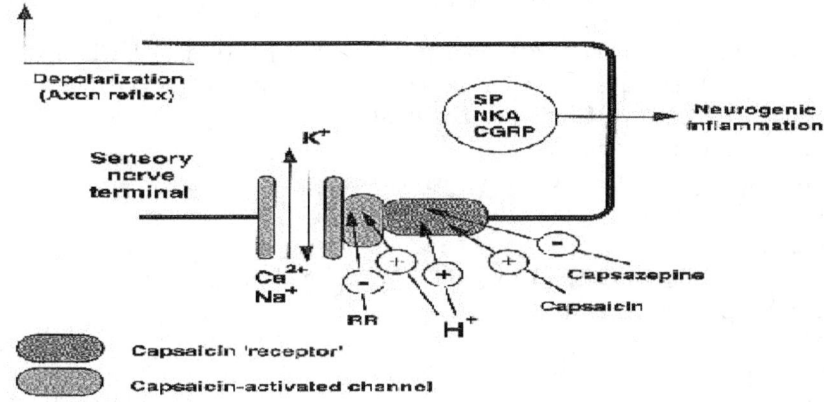

RESPIRATORY EFFECTS
- Acute pain in upper abdomen and thorax
  - Reflex increase in abdominal muscle tone in expiration.
- Leads to muscle splinting
  - Inability to breath, cough deeply
- Hypoxia
- Hypercarbia
- Retention of secretions
- Pneumonia, atelectasis
- Increase O_2 consumption
- Lactic acid production
- Reduced, pulmonary compliance

CARDIOVASCULAR EFFECTS
- Pain stimulates sympathetic neurones
- Tachycardia
- Increased stroke volume
- Increased myocardial oxygen consumption

FEAR OF AGGRAVATION PAIN
- Reduced physical activity
- Venous stasis and platelet aggregation
- It leads to
  - Myocardial ischemia
  - Infarct
- Deep vein thrombosis

GASTROINTESTINAL EFFECTS
- Impulses from viscera and somatic
  - (e.g. Surgical)
  - Nausea and vomiting
  - Ileus
  - Epidural analgesia reduces ileus

URINARY RETENTION IN PAIN
- Reduces motility of urethra
- Reduced motility of bladder

STRESS RESPONSE TO PAIN

- Tissue injury
    - Neuroendocrine
    - immunological
    - Intercellular biochemical

NEUROENDOCRINE RESPONSE TO PAIN
- Hypothalamic pituitary endocrinal and sympathoadrenal interactions leads to
    - Increased sympathetic tone
    - Hypothalamic stimulation
    - Increased catabolic secretion (cortisol, ACTH, ADH, GH, Glucagon, cAMP)
    - Decreased anabolic hormone secretion (e.g. insulin, testosterone)

EFFECTS OF NEUROENDOCRINE RESPONSE
- Sodium and water retention
- Increased blood glucose, ketone bodies
- Increase free fatty acids
- Increase lactate
- Increased metabolism – substrate mobilization from storage depots
- Increased O_2 consumption

PEDIATRIC PATIENTS
- Physiological abnormalities similar to adults
- Assessment of pain difficult due to developmental, cognitive and emotional difference

PHYSIOLOGICAL RESPONSE
- Tissue damage – actual or potential
- Release of algesics – Prostaglandins,
- 5 HT, substance P, bradykinins
- Generation of noxious stimuli
- Increased muscle and sympathetic tone
- Increased metabolism and oxygen consumption
- Inflammation produces prostaglandins at the dorsal horn
- Prostaglandins sensitize primary afferent by
    - Activation of silent nociceptors at Na^+ channels
    - Interfering with glycinergic inhibitors
- NSAIDs inhibits production of prostaglandins
- **EFFECTS OF PEPTIDES-** INFLAMMATION, HYPERAEMIA .PLASMA, EXTRAVASATION, LEUCOCYTE ADHESIONS.
- **AXON REFLEX FLARE-** Contraction of smooth muscles in Airways, Urinary bladder, Iris and other tissues
- Leads to Increase in blood flow, Increase in immune cell response.
- **CALCITONIN GENE RELATED PEPTIDE (CGRP)-** Released from sensory nerve endings by antidromic firing
- Local reflex trigger by increase intracellular Ca^{++} leads to inflammation

CARDIOVASCULAR EFFECTS
- Pain stimulates sympathetic neurones
- Tachycardia
- Increased stroke volume
- Increased myocardial oxygen consumption

ELDERLY PATIENTS
- More systemic disease – e.g. cardiac, pulmonary, endocrine
- Different attitude
- Different expectations about treatment
- Pain is reported less in elderly (Altered pain threshold??)

Inhibition of COX-2 activity
   NSAID on a COX active site
- A hydrophobic channel runs from surface of membrane into interior of the molecule
- Aspirin inactivates both COX-1 & 2 by
    - Acetylating on active site serine

- o   Which interferes with binding of arachidonic acid
- Ibuprofen competes with arachidonic acid for COX active site
- Flurbiprofen and indomethacin – form a salt bridge between carboxylate of the drug and thus inhibits COX-1&2

Opiate receptors
Brain Stem, Spinal Cord, Amygdala, Limbic, Thalamus, S.G.
Types: mu-receptors – Supraspinal Analgesia, gamma-dysphoria. kappa- Spinal Analgesia, Sedation, delta-Selective on leu-enkeph.
Endogenous Opioids:-
  1) Endorphins - Hypothalamus, III ventricle.
  2) Leu-encaphlin - Brain Stem, Spinal Cord.
  3) Met-encaphlin - Dorsal Horn, Morphine like.
Action Reversed by Naloxone
TNS, Acupuncture, Ketamine, Placebo.

Aging and pain

There is a prevalence of muscloskeletal and joint pain of the neck, back, hip and knee and stiff joints on awakening in older (above 75 yrs) as compared to patients with mean age of 40 years, according to National Health Nutritional Survey [epidemiologic follow up study in 1982-1984.[9] even in cases where prevalence of pain was not higher in the older group, the intensity of pain was reported as more severe as were symptoms associated with depression and limitations of activities of daily living. Musculoskeletal pain has more impact in the old age.

 Laboratory studies showed effect of age on psychyphysical of pain sensitivity as below.
1. Thermal
    a. Radiant heat: Response slightly higher pain, sensory and reactionary thresholds in elderly patients.
    b. Contact heat: In sensory threshold no age effects
    c. Cold pressor: Tolerance is lower in males while minimal increase in female with increasing age
2. Electrical shock
    a. Cutaneous: sensory threshold and tolerance is lower in elderly.
    b. Tooth: In sensory thresholds no age effects, lower discrimination accuracy in elderly, and response bias not affected.
3. Pressure on tendoachilles: Tolerance lowers in elderly, sensory threshold higher.

 Osteoarthritis is most common joint disorders in the elderly and has considerable effect on illness behavior and suffering.[3] this is more prevalent in knee joint in the female population due to physiologic, psychological and social factors.
 There are no age differences in pain sensitivity.
Presbyalgos – age in later years of life systematically influencing pain sensitivity and perception is termed presbyalgos. The presbyopia above 55 years of age is loss of visual accommodation, compounded buy lens opaqueness is a frequent problem.
Presbyaccusis – is the progressive loss of higher frequency sounds, decreased speech recognition is due to peripheral changes in the labyrinth.[4]
Causes of presbyalgos –
1. age dependent loss of receptors for pain (nociceptors)
2. changes in primary nociceptors afferents
3. changes in more central mechanisms subserving pain sensation and perception
4. changes in descending pain control mechanisms
5. Birth cohort differences in socio-cultural history that influence the meaning of pain.

Dementia: effect of dementia on pain sensibilities and expression is unclear. Wide distribution of cerebral degenerative, loss of communicative and cognitive skills, as well as failure of basic reflexes (gag reflex) critical to survival in later stages of dementia leads to altered pain sensation. Pain assessment can be improved following newer pharmacological agents for symptomatic treatment of dementia. The pain perception, characterized by indifference leads to misdiagnosis of fracture of major bones simply because of pain is not reported.[5] the cure providers should be more educated, more efficient methods to assess and treat the pain in the older patients in needed.

Psychosocial problems of pain in elderly from family interviews showed the following results:
Loneliness and social isolation
Learned helplessness
Acute stress and anxiety
Maladaptive environment
Autonomous depression
Personality disorder
Organic syndrome
Hypochondriasis

Management
Increased family interactions
Time-limited psychotherapy
Behavior modification through family
Good communication from physician
Benzodiazepines
Antidepressant therapy

Special considerations in geriatric pain assessment:[6]
1. General considerations:
   a. recognize that age itself does not reduce pain sensitivity
   b. recognize that there is no evidence that age per se influences qualitative properties of pain
   c. recognize the importance of encouraging the patient to discussing the pain
2. co-morbidity : illness and symptoms presentations in elderly who is often characterized by multiplicity, duplicity and chronicity
3. Mental status: cognitive impairment assessment eg. dementia
4. Depression : pain as a source of depression
5. Activities of daily living – differentiate between limitations caused by painful or non pain related dysfunction. The former leads to depression.
6. Medications : assess all current and recent medications (check the brown pill bag)
7. Family and social support systems should be maintained.

References:-
1. Basbaum A, Bushnell C. Pain, basic mechanism. In an updated review, refresher course syllabus, Giamberardino MA(Ed), Seattle, IASP Press , 2002, 3-7
2. Basbaum A J, Jessel T. The perception of pain. In Kendel ER, Schwatz J, Jessel T(Ed.) Principles of Neuro science, New York, Appleton & Lange, 2000, 472-491
3. Koltzernburg M, Neural mechanisms of cutaneous nociceptive pain. Clin. J. Pain, 2000, 16: S131-138.
4. Wall P D and Melzack R. Textbook of Pain, 3ed, chapter-3, Edinburgh, Churchill Livingston, 1996, 57-78
5. Renfield W, Boldrey E. Somatic motor and sensory representation in the cerebral cortex of man as studied by electrical stimulation, Brain:1937:60:389-443.
6. Melzack R, Wall PD, Pain mechanism a new theory. Science 1965:150:971-979. Head H, Holms G. Sensory disturbances from cerebral lesions. Brain: 1911:84: 102-254.
7. Woolf CJ, Wall PD. The relative effectiveness of C-primary afferents on facilitation of flexor reflexes in rats. J. Neuro Sci. 1986;1433-7.
8. Iggo A, Guilband G. Tegner R Sensory mechanism in arthritic rat's joints. In: Kruger L, Libokins JC (ed). Advances in pain research and therapy.Volum.6 New York, Raven press, 1984:83-93.
9. National Health nutritional survey (NHA WES) I Epidemiologic follow up study (1982 – 1984), 187 plan and operation of the National Health and Nutritional Survey I epidemiologic follow up study (1982-10\984) Vital Health statistics series I, No. 22, DHSS Pub No. (DHS) 87-1324.

Chapter 3.

OPIATE RECETORS

Family of G-protein coupled receptors
- Opiate receptors
- Muscarinic receptors
- Adenylate cyclase
- Adrenergic
- GABA
- Somatostatin receptors

Opioid receptor mediated G-protein effectors
- Short term effectors – Ca++ - all receptors - K+ -   µ and δ
- Long term effectors – AMP   - Phospatidylinositol
- K+ channel effects
    - Hyper polarization of neuronal membranes
    - Decrease synaptic transmission
- Ca++ channel effects
    - Decrease in neurotransmitter release
    - Reduction in neurotransmission
- Action at peri aqueductal grey area
    - Opiate receptor increase after degree of inhibition of neural pools
    - Decrease transmission of pain impulse from periphery
- Action at spinal level
    - Neuromodulator at presynaptic level
    - Neurotransmitter at post synaptic level

Table 1: CHARACTERISTICS OF OPIATE RECEPTORS:

	µ	δ	κ
Tissue bioassay	Guinea pig ileus	Mouse vas deferens	Rabbit vas deferens
Endogenous ligands	Enkephalin β endorphins(?)	enkephalin	Dynorphin
Exogenous agonist ligand	Morphine phenylpiperidines DAMGO, DAGO	DPDPE DADLE Deltorphin	µ 50488 Butorphenol Bremazocine
Antagonist	Naloxone Naltroxone	Naloxone Naltrindole	Naloxone N or BNI
Cloned (human)	Yes	Yes	Yes
Subtypes	1,2,3	1,2,cx,ncx	1,2,1a,2a,b
G-protein coupled	yes	yes	yes
Adenylate cyclase	Inhibits	Inhibits	Inhibits
Ca++ channels	Inactivates	Inactivates	Inactivates
K+ channels	increases	increases	increases

Table 2: CHARACTERISTICS OF OPIATE RECEPTORS:

Actions	Analgesia, sedation, respiratory depression, miosis, Bradycardia, nausea, vomiting and incr. GI mobility	Supraspinal analgesia, respiratory depression	Diuresis, spinal analgesia, dysphoria, decreased respiration
Site of action Supraspinal	Periductal grey area, median and magnus raphe neuclei, gigantocellular and reticullar	Periductal grey area, pallidus Raphe nucleus, gigantocellular reticular	Periductal grey area, caudal, linear, median magnus and reticular
Spinal cord	yes	yes	yes
Dorsal root ganglion	yes	yes	yes

Newer advances in opiate receptors
- DNA coding
- Molecular biology
- Cloning single receptor types
- To determine Bio-Pharmacological characteristics

µ receptor subtypes
- µ1 and µ2
- Ligands – DAMGO, Phenylpiperidines
- Antagonist of ligands – Naloxone, Naloxonazine
  MOR1 gene disruption in Exon
- Ligand – Heroin, Morphine – 6 - glucuronide

Table 3: δ receptors: decrease in adenyl cyclase activity, increases Ca^{++} ion concentration δ subtypes

Receptors subtypes	Antagonists	
	competitive	Non equilibrium
δ1	DPDPE/DADLE	BNTX DALCE
δ2	Deltorpine T1/DSLET	Naltriben 5'-NTII
DOR 1	DPDPE	Naltriben

δcx complex with µ or κ receptors, δncx – δncx1(synonym – δ1⁻), δncx2(synonym – δ2⁻)

Fig 1: k-receptors:

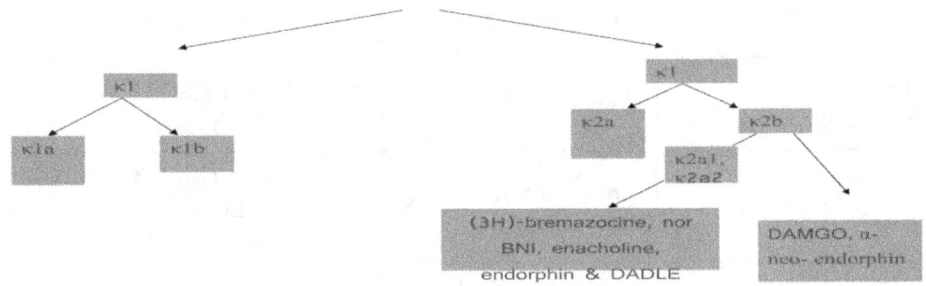

ORPHAN RECEPTOR – ORL1
- Structure homology to μ, δ and κ
- No pharmacological homology
- No endogenous ligand so orphan
- Decrease affinity – benzomorphan, bremazocine
- Disadvantage – increase concentration leads to motor impairment

OTHER OPIATE RECEPTORS
- ε – specific for β endorphins
- ζ –
- λ – 4,5 epoxymorphinans
- ς – affinity for enkephalins

Table 4: SELECTIVE OPIATE LIGANDS

Receptor type	μ receptor	δ receptor	κ receptor	ORL1
Selective agonists	Endomorphin-1 Endomorphin-2 DAMGO	(D-Ala2) deltorphinT (D-Ala2) deltorphinT1 DPDPE,SNC80	Enadoline μ – 50488 μ - 69593	None
Selective antagonists	CTAP	Natrindole TIPP-Ψ ICI-174864	Nor binaltorphimine	None
Radioligand	(3H)-DAMGO	(3H)-natrindole (3H)-PCI-DPDPE (3H)-SNC121	(3H)-enadoline (3H)-46593	(3H)-nociception

Table 5: MAMMALIAN OPIOID LIGANDS

Precursor	Endogenous peptide	Amino acid sequence
Pro-opiomelanocortin	β endorphin	YGGFMYSEKSQTPLVTL FKNAIIKNAYKKGE
Pro-dynorphin	(met) enkephalin (leu) enkephalin	YGGFM,YGGFL,YGGFMKF, YGGFMRLG,YGGFMRRV-NH2, YGGFMRRV-NH2
Pro-enkephalin	Dynorphin- A&B Dynorphin – A(L8) A & β-neoendorphin	YGGFLRRIRPKLKWDNQ YGGFLRRI,YGGFLRKYP YGGFLRRQFKVVT,YGGFLRKYPK
Pro-nociceptin/QFQ	Nociception	FGGFTGARKSARKLANQ
Pro-endomorphin	Endomorphin-1 Endomorphin-2	YPWF-NH2Y PWF-NH2

CLINICAL APPLICATIONS
- EXOGENOUS LIGANDS – Morpine, codeine, thobaine
- Side effects – respiratory depression, tolerance
- Aim – selective analgesic property of drug
- Later
    - epoximorphinans, morphinans
    - Benzomorphine (pentazocine) - dysphoria
    - Phenylpiperidines – Pethidine
- 4-amino-piperidines – Fentanyl

LATER APPLICATIONS
- Morphine simplified to Methadone
- Thebaine somplified to propavines
- Addition of 6 membered ring – etomorphine (1000times > morphine)
- µ receptor drugs – more analgesic
- κ site- ketazocine –potent analgesic
    - Spiradoline, enadoline – dysphoria
    - Asimadoline – inflammation
    - Neuro protective action of κ drugs

δ selective – TAN-67, SB 213698 – better analgesic

References

1. Textbook of Pain, 2nd Ed, CBS Pub New Delhi 2008.
2. Kumar Pramod - Guide to Peripheral Nerve Blocks 1st Edition CBS Medical Pubs, New Delhi 2008

CHAPTER 4.

DORSAL HORN RECEPTORS

Many neurotransmitters and neuro modulators were involved in the dorsal horn. Excitatory amino acid glutamate acts at N-methyl D-aspartate (NMDA) and non-NMDA receptors e.g., AMPA (alpha amino3-hydroxy 5-methyl 4-isoxazdepropionic acid), kainate and metabotropic glutamate receptors [1] (Table 1).

Several peptides released by primary afferents e.g., substance P and neurokinin A (acting through neurokinin receptors) calcitonin gene related peptide, opioid receptors, GABA, serotonin and adenosine receptors are receptors involved in neurotransmission and neuro modulation.[2] These reduce or modify the nociceptive impulse and offer a multimodal choice for pain relief.

The opioids have been used for postoperative pain mainly, also used in malignant and non-malignant pain. Intrathecal or epidural drug delivery is dictated by operative procedure and projected duration of the need for analgesia. Epidural route is preferred following withdrawal of subarachnoid micro catheters following risk of post dural puncture, headache and CSF leakage. Opioid agonists possess different selectivity against different type of pain e.g., Mu against thermal pain, kappa against pressure or visceral pain(Butorphanol, buprenorphine)in case of the later drugs, response difference in sex occurs due to oestrogen-opioid interactions in the dorsal horn[3]. Morphine is used in the range of 1–6 mg and 0.1mg, fentanyl 0.025–0.1mg and 0.005–0.01mg by epidural and intrathecal route respectively. The respiratory depression remains a major side effect with the use of opioids.

Alpha 2 Agonists
Clonidine and adrenaline provide spinal analgesia in acute and chronic patients. It provides dose related anxiolysis, sedation and augments the quality and duration of peripheral nerve block with local anaesthetics. It is taken 2 mg epidurally and 150–450 microgram intrathecally. Side effects include hypotension and bradycardia which is not present with the more potent dexmeditodimine[4]. A dose of 0.35 mg/kg intrathecally provides motor blockade upto 177.2 minutes when used along with sensorcaine (Kumar et al). There was no haemodynamic or other side effects.

Cholinomimetics and Cholinesterase Inhi-bitors
Stimulation of cholinergic receptors is a mechanism of endogenous analgesia. The muscarinic agonists may have a role in producing analgesia e.g., cholinesterase inhibitor neostigmine. However, there is a poor effect to side effect ratio. Intrathecal (100 mg) produced nausea, vomiting and transient lower extremity weakness, which is dose related[5].

Benzodiazepines
Benzodiazepines enhance the effect of GABA upon $GABA_A$ receptors and produce analgesia, which is reversible with benzodiazepine antagonist flumazenil as well as the GABA antagonist bicuculline. Baclofen used for spasticity acts on $GABA_B$ while muscimal acts in $GABA^A$ receptors. In animal studies limited data on intrathecal and epidural midazolam suggests a potential neurotoxicity after a single dose [4].

Ion Channel Blockers
Because spinal nociception depends upon ion flux to trigger postsynaptic depolarization in dorsal horn neurons mu or delta opioid agonist inhibit potassium flux.

Table 1: Dorsal horn receptor and peptides

	Presynaptic	Postsynaptic	Role	Drugs acting
Peptides	Glutamate Substance P	AMPA receptor (Na^+ influx) neurokinin-1 (IP3,DAG) NMDA(Mg^+, Ca^+, Na^+ outflow)	Central sensitization Long–term memory (increased)	Ketamine MK-801
Receptors	Opioid (k,mu,sigma) GABA B, 5HT 3 Benzodiazepines adenosine	GABA B, GABA A 5HT 1B alpha 2 adenosine	Decrease nociceptive input Increase alpha 2 Seratonin	Opioids noradrenaline Clonidine

Fig 1: Dorsal horn receptors and drugs acting on it

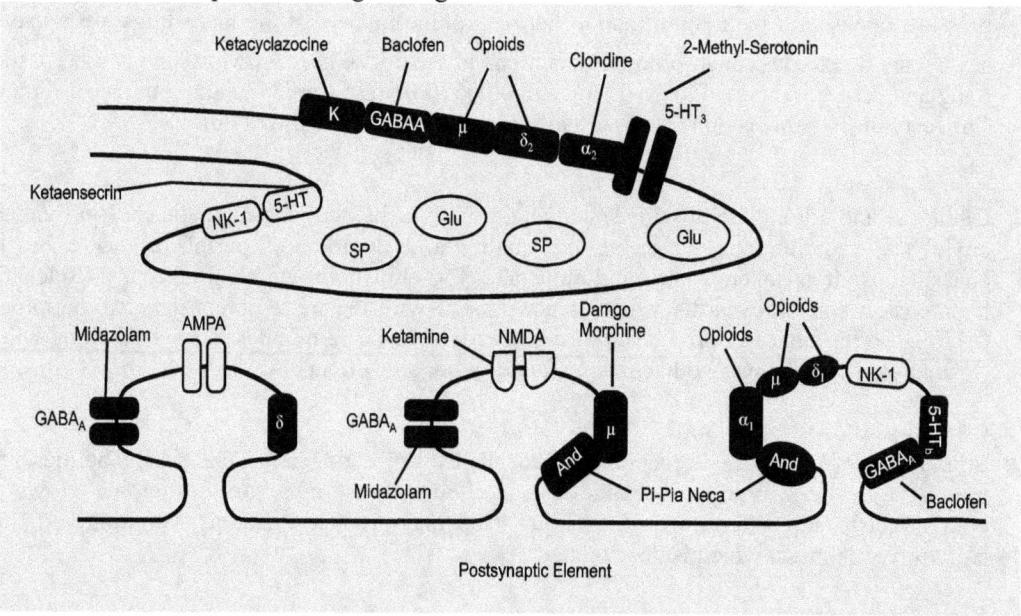

Kappa agonist inhibits calcium flux and local anaesthetics inhibit sodium flux. Calcium influx initiates the intracellular cascade of genetic and biochemical responses to pain. Calcium channel blockade potentiates opioid analgesia while suppressing opioid abstinence syndrome. L-type voltage calcium channel block (L- VSCC) may not provide effective analgesia when given alone but nimodipine potentiates morphine analgesia. However, N–type VSCC abound on neurons and its synthetic analogue SNX– 11 is a potent analgesic for morphine resistant pain of neuropathic or malignant origin. Side effects are nausea, orthostatic hypotension, headache, constipation and confusion. Preclinical data on potassium channel block also points towards analgesic effects[6].

NMDA Agonists

Ketamine blocks the open calcium channels on NMDA receptor complex. It has been used along with local anaesthetics and opioids to prolong postoperative analgesia without any respiratory depression. However, epidural/spinal ketamine produces a shorter duration of analgesia with possibility of psychomimetic effects.

Other NMDA open channel blockers e.g., dextro–metorphan, phencyclidine and glycine binding drugs have been used in experimental stages. Amitriptylline is found to suppress NMDA induced hyperalgesic states intrathecally in animals. It also enhances analgesia by augmenting the effects of noradrenaline and serotonin [4] (Fig. 1).

NSAIDS and Nitric Oxide Synthase Inhibitors

These inhibit intracellular enzymes activated by calcium entry into the postsynaptic cell (nitric oxide synthetase and phospholipase). These in turn generate nitric oxide and arachidonic acid, the latter being a substrate for cyclooxygenase isoenzymes, COX –1 and COX– 2. Spinal injection of NOS inhibitor L-NAME blocks thermal hyperalgesia as well as NMDA induced hyperalgesia. Lysine salicylate intrathecally provides analgesia for refractory cancer pain. Acetaminophen intrathecally provides analgesia and reversal of hyperalgesia [7].

Adenosine and Non Opioid Peptides

Adenosine receptors A1 and A2 are linked to analgesia, through spinal cord adenosine release, which if blocked by intrathecal theophylline producing hyperalgesia. Opioids and serotonin when used intrathecally releases adenosine and produces analgesia [8].

Other peptides are substance P and related tachykinins like somatostatin, produce epidural/spinal analgesia [10,11]. However, histopathological changes in spinal cord may present which is dose related. A dose of 20 microgram may be neurotoxic in rats but doses below 15 microgram are not [9]. Its use was abandoned until its stable analogue octreotide produced analgesia in cancer patients by intrathecal infusion [4].

References

1. Wilcox GL. Excitatory neurotransmitter and pain. In bond MR, Charlton JE and Woolf CJ, Vol 4, pp 97–117, Amsterdam, Elsevier.
2. Bond MR, Charlton JE and Woolf CJ, (eds); Proceedings of 6th world congress on pain, Pain research and management series, Vol 4 pp 97– 117, Amsterdam, Elsevier, 1991.
3. Amandusson A, Hermansion O, Blomquist A, Estrogen receptor like immuno reaction in dorsal spinal horn and medulla of female rat. Neuroscience lett. 196; 25, 1995.
4. Cousins MJ, and Bridenbaugh (Eds) Neural blockade in clinical anaesthesia and management of pain. 3rd edition, pp 946. Philadelphia, Lippincott Raven, 1998.
5. Kumar P, et el Clonidine with lignocaine or bupivacaine intrathecal in spinal analgesia. Ind. Journal of anaesthesia, 1993; 41:240–242.
6. Lauretti GR, Reis, Prado WA and Klampt JG. Dose response study of intrathecal morphine Vs intrathecal neostigmine, their combination or placebo for post op analgesia in patients undergoing anterior and posterior vaginoplasty. Anaesth Analg. 1996; 82–1182.
7. Malmberg AB, Yaksh TL. Antinociceptive actions of spinal NSAIDs on formalin test in rats. J. Pharm. Exp. Therapy, 1992; 163, 136.
8. Delander GE and Wahl JJ. Behaviour induced by putative nociceptive neurotransmitter is inhibited by adenosine or adenosine analogues co–administered intrathecally. J. Pharm. Exp. Therapy, 1988; 246–565
9. Chrubasik J, Meynadier J, Scherpereli P, et al. The effect of epidural somatostatin on post op analgesia, Anaesth,.Analg. 1985; 4:3085–3985.
10. Kumar Pramod. Textbook of Pain. 1st Edn. New Delhi. Modern Publishers, 2005.
11. Kumar P. Drug in Anaesthesia. 1st Edn. New Delhi, Modern Publishers, 2006.

Chapter 5:

Non Steroidal Anti Inflammatory & Muscle Relaxants

1. Classification of Non Steroidal Anti- Inflammatory Drugs-

Salicylates
  1. Aspirin (acetylsalicylic acid)
  2. Diflunisal
  3. Salsalate

Fenamic acid derivatives
  1. Mefenamic acid
  2. Meclofenamic acid
  3. Flufenamic acid
  4. Tolfenamic acid

Propionic acid derivatives
  1. Buprofen
  2. Naproxen
  3. Fenoprofen
  4. Ketoprofen
  5. Flurbiprofen
  6. Oxaprozin
  7. Loxoprofen

Acetic acid derivatives
  1. Indomethacin
  2. Sulindac
  3. Etodolac
  4. Ketorolac
  5. Diclofenac (Safety alert by FDA)
  6. Nabumetone

Enolic acid derivatives
  1. Piroxicam
  2. Meloxicam
  3. Tenoxicam
  4. Droxicam
  5. Lornoxicam
  6. Isoxicam

Selective COX-2 inhibitors (Coxibs)
  1. Celecoxib (FDA alert)[1]
  2. Rofecoxib (withdrawn from market)
  3. Valdecoxib (withdrawn from market)
  4. Parecoxib FDA withdrawn, licenced in the EU
  5. Etoricoxib FDA withdrawn, licenced in the EU
  6. Firocoxib used in dogs and horses

Sulphonanilides
Nimesulide (systemic preparations are banned by several countries for the potential risk of hepatotoxicity)
Others: Licofelone acts by inhibiting LOX & COX and hence known as 5-LOX/COX inhibitor.

2. Anti inflammatory classication based on Acidity –
ASPIRIN (acidic)

- High plasma protein binding
- pKa 3.5-5.5
- High concentration in inflamed tissues, blood, GIT and kidney. Hence side effects
- Block COX-2 locally

PHENAZONES (Non acidic)
- Neutral pKa 4-4.5
- Evenly distributed throughout body

Table 1: Acidic NSAIDs (Brune and Lanz, 1985)

Sub class	pKa (protein binding)	Time to peak plasma concentration	Elimination half life	Single dose range (max. daily dose)
Low potency ➢ Aspirin ➢ Salicylic acid ➢ Ibuprofen	3.5 2.9 4.4	-0.25h 0.5-2h 0.5-2h	20min 2.5-7h 2-4h	0.05-0.1g (6g) 0.5-1g (6g) 0.15-100g (300g)
High potency ➢ Acetyl proprionic acids (ketoprofen, blurbiprofen) ➢ Arylacetic acids (diclofenac) ➢ Indomethacin, ketorolac ➢ oxicams	4.2 4 4.5 4.9	0.5-2h 0.5-24h 0.5-2h 0.5-2h	1.1-4h 1-2h 2.6-11.2h 4-10h	15-100mg (300mg) 25-75mg (200mg) 25-75mg (200mg) 4-12mg (16mg)
Intermediate potency ➢ Salicylates diflunisal ➢ Arylproprionic acid ➢ Arylacetic acids 6MNA	3.8 4.15 2.4	2-3h 2-4h 3-6h	8-12h 13-15h 20-24h	250-500mg (1g) 0.5-1g (2g) 0.5-1g (1.5g)
High potency (slow elimination) ➢ Oxicams ➢ Tenoxicam	5.1 5.0	3-5h 3-5h	14-160h 25-175h	20-40mg (initially 40mg) 20-40mg

CYCLOOXYGENASES
- 1991-gene code
- COX-1&2 discovered, cloned, characterized
- Forma groove/channel opening in membranes
- COX inhibitor enters through this groove

- COX-2 channels larger than COX-1

Patho physiology of COX-1&2

➢ COX-1
  - Iso enzymes inmost tissues
  - Produces prostaglandins
  - Does normal cell functions – "house keeping"
  - Blocked by NSAIDs

➢ COX-2
  - Inducible enzymes – cytokines
  - Acts on inflammatory cells – macrophages
  - Regulated by glucocorticoids
  - Present in macula densa, UG tract, CNS
  - Blocked by NSAIDs

Fig 1: Physio pathogenesis of COX-1 and COX-2 (Kay Bruce)

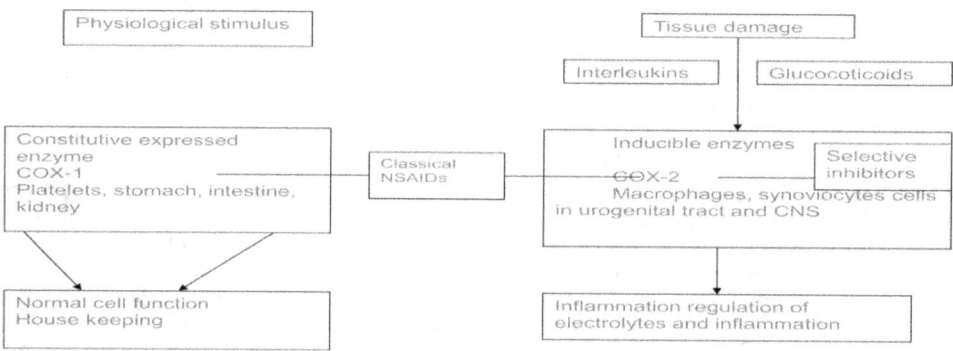

Table 2: Indications of NSAIDs

Indications	High dose	Middle dose	Low dose
Acidic NSAIDs ➢ Spondylitis, gout, arthritis ➢ Cancer pain (bone) ➢ Active arthrosis (inflammation) ➢ Myofascial pain ➢ Trauma(swelling) ➢ Post operative pain	Diclofenac, indomethacin, piroxicam, ibuprofen Diclofenac, ibuprofen, piroxicam, indometha No No No No	Diclofenac, indomethacin, piroxicam Diclofenac, ibuprofen, piroxicam, indomethacin Diclofenac, ibuprofen, piroxicam, indomethacin Diclofenac, ibuprofen, piroxicam, indomethacin Diclofenac, ibuprofen, piroxicam, indomethacin	No Acetyl salicylic ibuprofen Ibuprofen, ketoprofen Ibuprofen, ketoprofen Ibuprofen, ketoprofen Ibuprofen, ketoprofen

		Diclofenac, ibuprofen, piroxicam, indomethacin	
Non acid NSAIDs ➢ Acute pain and fever ➢ Spastic pain (colic) ➢ Associated with fever ➢ Cancer pain ➢ Headache, migraine ➢ Associated viral infections	Coxibs ? ? ? yes ?	Pyrozolinones Yes Yes Yes Yes Yes	Anilines No No Yes Yes yes

Non acidic NSAIDS- Anilines
- Paracetamol
- Weak, indirect inhibitors of cycloexygenases (COX-2)
- Doses 0.5-1gm
- Liver toxicity at high doses 1g/10kg
- Metabolite – benzoquinones binds to DNA in liver and kidney
- Prevention by glutathione, N-acetyl cysteine
- Use – fever, mild pain, viral headache
- Combination with aspirin and caffeine cause nephropathy

Non acidic NSAIDS- Phenazones
- Dipyrone
- Antipyretic analgesics
- Causes agranulocytosis, shock reaction
- Stevens-Johnson's syndrome
- No GIT and renal toxicity

Table 3: NON ACIDIC NSAIDs

Pharmacological subdivision	Plasma protein binding	Time to peak concentration	Elimination half life	Single dose (daily dose)
Acetaminophen paracetamol	5-50%	0.5-1.5hr	1.5-2.5hr	0.5-1g(1-6g)
Phenazone (antipyrine)	<10%	0.5-2hr	5-24hr	0.5-2g(1-6g)
propylphenazone	10%	0.5-1.5hr	1-2.5hr	0.5-2g(1-6g)
Metamizole (depyrone)	20-50%	1-2hr	2-4hr	0.5-2g(1-6g)
Selective COX inhibitors Celecoxib Rofecoxib	>90% >80%	2-4hr 2-4hr	9-15hr 12hr	40-200mg(400mg) 12-25mg(25mg)

Prostaglandins and hyperalgesia
- Inflammation produces prostaglandins at the dorsal horn
- Prostaglandins sensitize primary afferent by
  - Activation of silent nociceptors at Na^+ channels
  - Interfering with glycinerg9ic inhibitors
- NSAIDs inhibits production of prostaglandins

Inhibition of COX-2 activity
- NSAID on a COX active site
- A hydrophobic channel runs fro surface of membrane into interior of the molecule
- Aspirin inactivates both COX-1&2 by
  - Acetylating on active site serine
  - Which interferes with binding of arachidonic acid
- Ibuprofen competes with arachidonic acid for COX active site
- Flurbiprofen and indomethacin – form a salt bridge between carboxylate of the drug and thus inhibits COX-1&2

Fig. 2: Distribution of acidic antipyretic analgesics in the human body. (dark areas show increased concentrations)

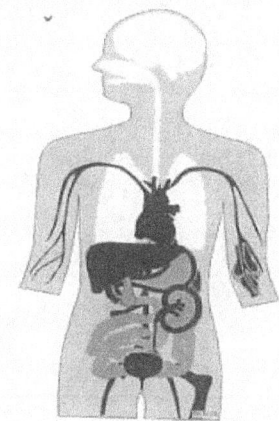

Clinical use of acidic NSAIDs (aspirin)
- Pain, fever, inflammation
- Dose range to 1g
- Inhibits COX-2 at the concentration that does not block COX-1
- Classified according to potency, elimination half life

Selective COX-2 inhibitors
> **Celecoxib and rofecoxib**
- Slow absorption and elimination
- Mild analgesia – not used in acute pain
- Comparable to other NSAIDs
- Use – osteoarthritis, rheumatoid arthritis

COX-2 and GIT
- Prostaglandin protection
- Low GIT side effects – dyspepsia
- May influence peptic ulcer healing due to angiogenesis

COX-2 and kidney
> Immunoreactivity of COX-2 in
- Renal vasculature
- Medullary interstitial cell
- Macula densa s
> **COX-1 immunoreactivity**
- Collecting ducts
- Loop of Henle

- Renal vasculature
- This effects renin-angiotensin system

Renal effects
- Due to renin angiotensin system
- Peripheral edema
- Hypertension
- Preexisting hypertension is exacerbated
    - Inhibiting mechanism of water and Na+ excretion
    - Prostacyclin reduction
- Caution: hypertension, heart failure, fluid retention

COX-2 and cardiovascular system
- COX-2 inhibitors inhibits prostacyclin
- Thromboxane – prostacyclin balance
- Hypercoagulability
- Effects comparable to other NSAIDs

VIGOR study (2000)
- Rofecoxib vs. Naproxen in Rheumatoid Arthritis patients
    - Increased incidence of myocardial infarction
- Class Trial (2000) Celecoxib vs. Diclofenac in osteoarthritis patients
    - No difference in cardiovascular events
    - Reason : rheumatic patients more prone to CVS effects

Conclusion
- COX-2 inhibitors better in GI disorders
- Acetominophen, phenazone are comparable to COX-2 inhibitors

Skeletal Muscle Relaxants
Use to treat 2 different types of conditions
1. Spasticity
2. Muscular pain or spasms

Spasticity
Upper motor neuron syndromes
Exaggerated cutaneous reflexes, autonomic hyper-reflexia, dystonia, contractures, paresis, and fatigability.

Muscular pain or spasms
Peripheral musculoskeletal conditions, fibromyalgia, tension headache, myofascial pain syndrome and mechanical low back or neck pain.

Drugs classified as skeletal muscle relaxants
1. Baclofen,
2. Carisoprodol,
3. Chlorzoxazone,
4. Cyclobenzaprine,
5. Dantrolene,
6. Metaxalone,
7. Methocarbamol,
8. Orphenadrine, and
9. Tizanidine

Drugs approved for the treatment of spasticity
Baclofen: Blocks pre-and post-synaptic GABA B receptors
Dantrolene: centrally acting agonis to fa2 receptors
Tilzanidine: directly inhibits muscle contraction by decrease in g there lease of calcium from skeletal musclesar

Epirisone
4'-ethyl-2-methyl-3-piperidinopropiophenonehydrochloride)
Inhibits gamma-efferent firing and local vasodilatation activity
Potential indications
1. Spastic paralysis in conditions such as cerebrovascular disease
2. Spastic spinal paralysis
3. Cervical spondylosis [1]
4. Postoperativ esequelae (including from cerebrospinal tumour) [2]
5. Sequelae to trauma(e.g. spinal trauma or head injury)[2]
6. Amyotrophic lateral sclerosis
7. Cerebralpalsy
8. Spinocerebellar degeneration
9. Spinalvasculardiseasesandotherencephalomyelopathies
10. Cervical syndrome, periarthritis of the shoulder, and lumbago.

Action of Epirisone
1. Skeletal muscle relaxation
2. Relaxation of hypertonic skeletal muscles
3. Improves intramuscular blood flow
4. Suppression of spinal reflex potentials
5. Reduction of muscle spindle sensitivity via motor neurons
6. Vasodilatation and augmentation of blood flow
7. Analgesic action and inhibition of the pain reflex in the spinal cord.

Table 4: Possible Mechanism of Actionof Muscle Relaxants.

MOA	Result
Inhibitory action on α- and γ- efferent neurons in the spinal cord and supra-spinal structures	Direct muscle relaxant action
Sodium channel blocking, at either Adelta- or C- fibers conducting pain signals to the spinal dorsal horn neurons.	Anti nociception
An elevation of the electrical threshold required for generation of the action potential and a ca^{2+} antagonistic activity in the smooth muscle cells of the basilar artery	Vasodialation and increased Blood flow
Blocks the postjunctional α1- and α2- adrenergic, muscarinic, serotonergic receptors and prejunctional α2- adrenoceptors, and reduce the prostacyclin synthesis via a mechanism other than cyclooxygenase inhibition	Centrally acting. Skeletal muscle relaxant (Tizanidine like action)
Sympatho-suppressive action in resting skeletal muscles, without any effect on the micro-neurographically recorded muscle sympathetic nerve activity in actively contracting muscles	Due to increases local blood flow

Flupirtine
Selective neuronal potassium channel opener.
Ion channels play a vital role in pain signal initiation and conduction.Less attention has been paid to the role of K+ channels in pain.K+ channels play an essential role in setting the resting

membrane potential and in controlling the excitability of neurons. K+ channels represent potentially attractive peripheral targets for the treatment of pain

Probable Mechanism of Action

Site of Action – CNS (Both Spinal and Supra spinal

Involvement of descending adrenergic pathways (Initial studies)

↓

(Indirect) action at N-Methyl-D-aspartate (NMDA) receptors Antagonist action(Subsequent studies)

↓

Activation of a G-protein regulated inwardly rectifying K(+) (GIRK) ion channel(Present)

Action and Indications-
Chronic musculoskeletal pain
Migraine and
Neuralgias
Fibromyalgias
Flupirtin's analgesic and muscle-relaxant properties were comparable to tramadol
Side effect profile
The most common adverse effects-
1. Drowsiness
2. Dizziness
3. Heartburn
4. Drymouth
5. Fatigueand
6. Nausea

References

3. Textbook of Pain, 2nd Ed, CBS Pub New Delhi 2008.
4. Kumar Pramod - Terminal cancer care 2nd Edition, CBS Medical Pubs, New Delhi 2005
5. Kumar Pramod - Guide to Peripheral Nerve Blocks 1st Edition CBS Medical Pubs, New Delhi 2008
6. Kumar Pramod - A Handbook of pain management & related symptoms in cancer, Samvedana, Indraprastha Apollo Hospital New Delhi, 2003
7. Kumar Pramod - Illustrated Atlas on peripheral nerve blocks Anaesthesia Dept. Jamnagar 2002
8. Bresolin N, Zucca C, Pecori. Efficacy and tolerability of eperisone in patients with spastic palsy: a cross-over, placebo-controlled dose-ranging trial. A. Eur Rev Med Pharmacol Sci. 2009 Sep-Oct; 13(5): 365-70.
9. Bresolin N, Zucca C, Pecori A.Efficacy and tolerability of eperisone and baclofen in spastic palsy: a double-blind randomized trial. Adv Ther. 2009 May; 26(5): 563-73. Epub 2009 May20.
10. Sartini S, Guerra L.Open experience with a new myorelaxant agent for low back pain. Adv Ther. 2008 Aug; 99(4): 347-52.
11. Beltrame A, Grangie S, Guerra L.Clinical experience with eperisone in the treatment of acute low back pain.Minerva Med. 2008 Aug; 99(4):347-52.
12. Tariq M, Akhtar N, Ali M, Rao S, Badshah M, Irshad M. Eperisone compared to physiotherapy on muscular tone of stroke patients: a prospective randomized open study. J Pak Med Assoc. 2005 May; 55(5):202-4.
13. J Clin Pharm Ther, 2010 Nov 28. Dol: 10.1111/j. 1365-2710.2010.01233.x (Epub).

Chapter 6.

Opioids

Opioids (agonists and antagonists) bind preferentially to the receptor, morphine and nor-morphine show greatest relative preference for the receptor. Methadone, NMDA receptor blocker shows a significant binding to receptors, while buprenorphine, and naloxone bind to all three receptor types. The binding affinity of buprenorphine to the receptor is smaller than that of naloxone, which explains why the latter only partially reverses buprenorphine toxicity.Codeine and heroin have a poor binding to opioid receptors and are prodrugs while the pharmacologically active species are morphine and 6-monoacetyl morphine[1] respectively.

PHYSICOCHEMICAL PROPERTIES OF OPIOIDS

The physicochemical properties of drugs substantially control their passive transfer across biological membranes. Two factors, their relative lipophilicity, low partition co-efficient and degree of ionization at physiological pH affect the rate and extent of transmembrane flux and binding to critical receptors. For various opioid drugs, there are small differences in their molecular weights, but greater differences in their pKa and lipophilicity. The higher the O/W partition coefficient value, the greater is the lipophilicity.

Table 1 : Binding affinities of various opioids to guinea pig and cloned human opioid receptors [3]

Opioid	Binding affinity		
	Guinea pig		Cloned human
	Delta	Kappa	Mu
Morphine	90	317	1.8
Normorphine	310	149	4.0
Levorphanol	5.6	9.6	0.6
Codeine	>10000	ND	2700
Methadone	15.1	1628	4.2
Fentanyl	151	470	7.0
Pethidine	4345	5140	385
Pentazocine	106	22.2	7.0
Buprenorphine	1.3	2.0	0.6
Naloxone	27	17.2	1.8

Thus, more hydrophilic (e.g., morphine) or lipophilic (e.g., sufentanil) opioids have a lower meningeal permeability[4]. This biphasic relationship is hardly surprising when opioid drugs , like all drugs, must traverse multiple aqueous and lipid bilayers (e.g., membranes) to reach their site of action at the opioid receptor. Consequently, drugs with partition coefficients towards the extremes are disadvantaged with respect to transmembrane permeability compared to opioids with a more well-balanced partition coefficient. Time curve is to manipulate (i.e., delay) , the absorption rate, as in the case of various sustained- release oral morphine, oxycodone, and hydromorphone formulations and transdermal fentanyl..

METABOLISM

The liver is the primary site of biotransformation of most drugs, including opioid drugs. Metabolism also occurs to a variable extent (depending on the opioid) in the organs of the body that come into initial contact with the opioid. For example,during absorption from the gastrointestinal tract (following oral administration) and lung (pulmonary administration). Indeed other organs (e.g., kidney and brain) also metabolize opioid drugs. Although the skin has demonstrable capacity to metabolize a range of drugs, fentanyl is not metabolized during transdermal absorption [5].

The terminal half-life for most opioids varies between 2 and 7 hours, the notable exception being methadone, where the extremes are as short as 6 hours and as long as 150 hours. Most patients will be in a range of 12–60 hours[13] (Table 2).

Morphine is mainly metabolized by conjugation with glucuronic acid to form the 3- and 6-glucuronides (Phase 1 reaction), with a minor route being N-demethylation to produce normorphine (Phase II reaction). Codeine and heroin (3,6-diacetylmorphine or diamorphine) are morphine analogues. Codeine is converted to morphine via hepatic metabolism catalyzed by cytochrome P450 isoform 2D6 [14]. Thus codeine is considered to be a prodrug for morphine in view of its poor binding to the □ - receptor. However, the major metabolite is codeine-6-glucuronide, which, unlike morphine-6-glucuronide (M6G) would not be expected to have significant analgesic activity as it would require conversion to M6G by O-demethylation.

Fentanyl is metabolized in the liver by N-demethylation catalyzed by the 3A4 isoform of cytochrome P450 to form norfentanyl. There are other minor routes of metabolism including amide hydrolysis and hydroxylation [6]. The metabolites are believed to be inactive. The 3A4 isoform is also the major determinant of both alfentanil and sufentanil metabolism [15].

Pharmacogenetic Aspects of Cytochrome P450 Metabolism

Cytochrome P450 2D6 is involved in the metabolism of codeine (and its derivates) to morphine (and corresponding derivates) by O-demethylation. There is a polymorphic distribution of this isoform in Caucasians such that 8–10% of the population lack the capacity to perform this conversion. This variation results in the subdivision of patients into two groups, either extensive or poor metabolizers. Thus, poor metabolizers will not experience analgesia following codeine administration. Further, codeine metabolism could be inhibited in extensive metabolizers by the concurrent administration of other drugs, also metabolized by this isoform. It has been suggested that it is predominantly codeine and not morphine that is responsible for the side effects observed following codeine administration [16].

Renal Excretion

Analgesic and toxic effects observed after morphine administration to patients with poor renal function are probably due to M6G rather than morphine. M6G accumulates[17] and it is not uncommon to be unable to detect morphine in blood samples collected a few hours after morphine administration. Similarly, norpethidine accumulates at a greater rate in patients with renal insufficiency, with a corresponding greater potential for neurotoxicity. Therefore, other opioids such as fentanyl, methadone, or possibly hydromorphone should be considered in lieu of morphine in chronic noncancer pain patients with significantly reduced renal function.

Metabolite Pharmacodynamics Effects

Some opioid metabolites have pharmacological effects that are either positive (i.e., contribute to analgesia) or negative (i.e., contributes to the adverse events profile). Morphine-6-glucuronide and normorphine have intrinsic analgesic activity, particularly the former. The status of morphine-3-glucuronide (M3G), is still controversial with suggestions ranging from it being inactive[18] to being a functional antagonist at other receptors[19] because it does not bind to opioid receptors.

OPIOID USE IN DRUG DEPENDENT PATIENTS

Increasing attention is being given to the relationship between the long-term prescription of opioids to treat chronic noncancer pain and drug-seeking behaviour or frank opioid addiction [20]. Pain is seen by some patients as the vehicle that may be more likely to convince practitioners to prescribe opioids rather than admitting to a drug dependence problem. However, it is essential to recall that opioid dependent individuals can suffer from chronic pain just like any other member of society. Recent evidence suggests that methadone maintenance patients can demonstrate a hyperalgesic response to experimental pain, depending on the pain stimulus employed[21]. These findings only add an additional layer of complexity as they indicate that acute pain should be taken seriously and treated aggressively in opioid dependent patients.

Sex Difference in Reported Pain and Analgesic Response

Special Interest Group of the IASP on Sex, Gender and Pain was established in 1996 at the 8th World Congress on Pain in Vancouver. There are many examples of sex differences; women are likely more than men to report chronic pain conditions, but prevalence rates vary for condition and age[22]. The reasons for this variability are numerous and include hormonal, psychological, neurophysiological, and neuropharmacological factors.

Acute pain studies using various □ –receptor agonists have shown variable results, with some authors indicating that males require more postoperative analgesia than females, but have evidenced no differences in plasma concentrations or minimum effective concentrations of the opioid agonist[23]. Other studies suggest no gender difference in analgesic consumption rates.

A series of studies have shown that k-receptor agonists result in improved analgesic outcomes for females that are not convincingly explained by sex differences in pharmacokinetics [24]. There is also suggestion of a sex difference in the analgesic response to NSAIDs such that only male volunteers reported pain responses to ibuprofen pharmacokinetics between males and females.

Tramadol is administered as a racemate and has a dual mechanism of action; the d-enantiomer exhibits preferential but weak binding activity at m-receptors and is a more potent inhibitor of serotonin re–uptake, while the l-enantiomer is more efficient in blocking nore-pinephrine uptake [25].

The combination of morphine and ketamine may result in improved analgesia in patients with neuropathic pain compared with morphine alone. Ketamine is also an NMDA –receptor blocker and acts at a site different from the NMDA recognition site. However, the d-enantiomer has more potent blocking action at the NMDA receptor than does the l-enantiomer [26].

Morphine, hydromorphone, fentanyl, codeine and naltrexone are devoid of NMDA-receptor antagonist activity, while levorphanol has very weak blocking action compared to dextromethorphan.

SYSTEMIC EFFECTS
1. Cardiovascular System
The effects of opioids on any system are studied with morphine as the prototype.

Morphine causes impairment of compensatory sympathetic nervous system response, and these causes venous pooling, thereby reducing the cardiac output and systemic blood presence.

Morphine causes hypotension by stimulating the vagal nuclei in the medulla oblongata.

It may also exert a direct effect on the sinoatrial node, these causing bradycardia and slow conduction through the atrioventricular node as well. This may, in part explain the decreased vulnerability to ventricula or fibrillation.

Opioid induced histamine release and associated hypotension are both variable in incidence and degree. This can be prevented by using smaller doses of the opioid (morphine < 5 mg/min IV) and optimizing the intravascular fluid volume.

The opioid does not sensitize the heart to catecholamines, nor does it prevent the tachycardia and hypertension associated with painful surgical stimulation. However, it can be attenuated by using large doses of the opioid.

The combination of opioid agonists, such as morphine along with nitrous oxide or inhalational agents, results in cardiac depression, which does not occur with the drug administered alone.

2. Ventilation
Morphine causes depression of the respiratory centre, in the medulla oblongata, and this decrease the responsiveness of the respiratory centre to increased levels of carbondioxide. This is because, morphine actson the neurons of the brain stem and decreases the release of the neurotransmitter, acetylcholine, thereby preventing the hypercarbic response. This results in elevated levels of $PaCO_2$ after morphine administration.

The opioid agonists primarily cause these effects by action on Mu_2 receptor, which is a dose dependent depression of ventilation. Opioids also interfere with pontine and medullary ventilatory centres, and these leading to prolonged pauses between breathes and periodic breathing.

High levels of opioids will result in apnoea, the patient remains conscious, but is able to initiate and breath when asked to do so. The ventilatory depressant action of opioids is more pronounced in elderly patients, and who are sleeping. Opioids cause decrease in the ciliary action, increase in the airway resistance by direct action, and indirectly through release of histamine.

3. Nervous System

Opioids decrease the cerebral blood flow and intracranial pressure. They can cause changes, in EEG, which are similar to those evoked by sleep pattern i.e., the rapid a-waves are replaced by the flow of d-waves.

Opioids should not be given to patient of head injury, because,
(i) It will interfere with wakefulness.
(ii) Causes miosis
(iii) Depress ventilation further thus elevating $PaCO_2$
(iv) Head injury itself causes alteration in blood brain barrier, resulting in increased sensitivity to opioids.

Skeletal muscle rigidity, especially of the thoracic and abdominal muscles, is common with large doses of opioid especially, if administered rapidly. This is due to interaction of opioids with dopaminergic and gamma-aminobutyric acid responsive neurons. Skeletal muscle rigidity, will cause difficulty in ventilation, and if mannual attempts are made to inflate the lung in this condition, will lead to decrease in the venous return. Another cause of inability to ventilater after induction is due to closure of the vocal cords.

Miosis is due to excitatory action of the opioids on the Edinger- Westphal nucleus of the occulomotor nerve.

4. Biliary Tract

Opioids increase the tone of the biliary smooth muscle, resulting in increase in intrabiliary pressure thus leading to biliary colic or epigastric discomfort. The incidence is more with fentanyl. This can be antagonised by administration of naloxone or glucagon (2 mg I.V.) which unlike naloxone, will not severe its analgesic action concentration of smooth muscle of the pancreas, will lead to increases in plasma amylase level and lipase level, which may mimic the picture of acute pancreatitis.

5. Gastrointestinal Tract

Commonly used opioids like morphine and fentanyl cause delayed gastric emptying, by increasing the tone of pyloric sphincters. Also, the propulsive movement in the small and large intestine is reduced, leading to increased water absorption and constipation.

Delay in gastric emptying, increases the chances of aspiration, in anaesthetised patients.

6. Nausea and Vomiting

Opioid induced nausea and vomiting is due to stimulation of chemoreceptor trigger zone in the floor of fourth ventricle, due to its dopamine agonist action.

Morphine

Figure 1 shows the chemical structure of morphine. Morphine is the gold standard against which all other opioids are compared. It is most commonly used for acute pain in adults and children. It is hydrophilic and does not cross blood brain barrier. It has a poor bioavailability of 20 to 30% which necessitates a large oral dose when converted from parenteral to enteral route. It is used as 10 to 15 mg IM orally and also by IV (10 mg) epidural (3 to 5 mg) spinal route (0.1 to 1 mg).

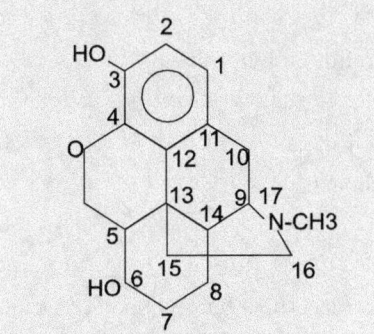

Fig 1: Chemical formula of Morphine

Morphine is metabolised in liver by microsomal mixed function oxygenase that requires P-450 system; metabolising to morphine-6 glucuronide in active form and excreted through kidney. Morphine induces histamine release so used with caution in asthma and allergies. It produces vasodilatation and causes hypotension in hypovolaemic patients. Other side effects are dizziness, constipation, nausea, vomiting, bradycardia, respiration depression, urinaryretention, pruritus, and in high doses myoclonus and seizure. In neonate an immature P-450 enzyme system results in prolonged metabolic rate and higher brain concen-trations and decreased renal clearance seizures [3].

Pethidine

It has one tenth potency of morphine and same drug profile. Its metabolite is normophine with ½ analgesic potency of original base. It interacts with MAO inhibitors in depression. It causes hallucinations, delusions, agitations and seizures. It causes neuroleptic malignant syndrome—hyperpyrexia, acidosis, shock and death.

Butorphanol

Butorphanol is a nitrogen substituted 3, 14 dehydrase morphines. N-cyclo butylmethyl group is responsible far the mixed agonist antagonist activity and lipophilicity, whereas the hydroxyl group at C_{14} for additional antagonist activity. The removal of OH at C_6 position also increases analgesic activity.

Mechanisms of Action

Butorphanol is a synthetic opioid, which is a mixed agonist-antagonist.

Butorphanol and its metabolities are agonist at the k-opioid receptor, thereby producing effects like dyspnoea and sedation. It is mixed agonist-antagonist at mu-opioid receptor, thereby producing effects like euphoria, bradycardia and miosis [2].

Potency

Butorphanol has been found to be 7 times more potent than morphine, 30 to 40 times more than meperidine and 20 times more than pentazocine.

Pharmacokinetics

The onset of action after I.V. administration is within 10 to 15 sec, with a peak of onset at 0.1 to 1 hr and duration of action, lasting for 3 to 4 hours. It has a half-life of 2.1 to 8.8 hours.

After IM administration, the onset starts at < 10 to 15 minutes with a peak action at 0.5 to 1 hour and duration of action lasting 3 to 4 hour.

Butorphanol is metabolized in the liver chiefly to hydroxy butorphanol, whereas nor-butorphanol is produced in small amounts. Since oral bioavailability is only 5 to 17 %, due to high first part metabolism, no oral formulation is available.

The drug binds with plasma proteins, to an extent of 80%. Elimination occurs by urine and faecal route with most (70 to 80%) of the dose is recovered in the urine, and 15% in the faeces. About 5% of the dose is recovered in urine as butorphanol and less than 5% is excreted in urine as norbutorphanol.

The metabolism of the drug through transnasal route is the same as through IM route.

Parenteral butorphanol has been detected in neonatal cord serum with mean neonatal serum concentration, not significantly different from mean maternal serum concentration, following a 1 or 2 mg intramuscular dose. Sedation is the most common side effect and local effects like nasal irritation and metallic taste are infrequent, so it rapidly course cribriform plate into CNS, neurotoxicity is a potential concern with its cause.

Table 1: Onset, duration of butorphanol

Parameter	IV	IM
Onset	Rapid	10 –15 min
Peak	0.5–1 hour	0.5 –1 hour
Duration	3 – 4 hours	3.4 hours
Half–life	2.1– 8.8 hours	

Adverse Effects

(i) Cardiovascular: By its action on the Mu receptors, butorphanol can cause hypotension, as observed in < 1%, of the cases, given 1 mg of the drug, through IV route. Similar adverse effect can occur if large doses are administered.

(ii) CNS: Dizziness, confusion, anxiety, exophoria, floating feeling, somnolance nervousness, paraesthesia, abnormal dreams, agitation, dysphoria, hallucinations, lastily, drug dependence.

(iii) Dermatologic: Sweating, rash.

(iv) GIT: Nausea, vomiting, dry mouth.

(v) Others: Lethargy, headache, impaired urination, blurred vision.

Contraindication

Hyper sensitivity to butorphanol
Drugs interchange.
When Butorphanol is used along with CNS depressants like alcohol, barbiturates, tran-quilizers, it may result in increased central nervous system depressant actions.
Butorphanol should not be used along with MAO inhibitors and 14 days after administration.

Codeine

It is used in oral form in combination with acetaminophen, or aspirin. It causes nausea and allergy. It causes less nausea and vomiting. It has a bioavailability of 60%, following oral route and plasma half-life of 2.5 to 4 hour with onset of action 20 minutes and duration 60 to 120 minutes. Approximately 120% metabolised to morphine and causes analgesia. Dose: 0.5 to 1 mg/kg. APC contain 12 aspirin acetaminophen, paracetamol and 1 mg codeine per 5 mL. IV injection causes, apnoea, hypotension, histamine release.

Fentanyl

Fentanyl is highly lipid soluble equilibrates rapidly on effector side and has no active metabolites. There is increased clearance in children up to 3 to 12 months of age but a prolonged half life. It can be used IV, IM, SC, transmucosal and transdermal (Duragesic). It is used for short procedures under GA and postsurgical and burns pain relief. It is administered in frequent boluses or continuous IV infusion in 0.5 to 1.0 microg/kg.

Side Effects: Tolerance and dependence by continuous infusion especially in children in ICU.

Sufentanyl

Sufentanyl in 0.25 to 1.0 microg/kg dose prevents haemodynamic response to laryngoscopy, if given before induction. Maintenance of anaesthetic is achieved with N_2O (60%) and O_2 and intermittent bolus doses of 0.1 to 0.25. microg/kg. The ED50 of sufentanyl for skin incision is twice as that for intubation is 2.08 mg IV. The ED50 ratios for sufentanyl, fentanyl, and alfentanil in N_2O to O_2 anaesthesia are 1:2:150. Sufentanyl infusions of 1.0 microg/kg /hr are associated with less postoperative problems. For ventilation 0.25 microg/mL is used.

pKa of sufentanyl is as same as that of morphine (8.0). It is twice as lipid soluble as fentanyl and highly bound (30%) to plasma proteins. Its extractions ratio of (0.8) from liver, means changes in liver flow alters its clearance. It is metabolised by dealkylation, oxidative N-dealkylation, oxidative D-demethylation and aromatic hydroxylation. Major metabolite is N-phenyl piper-amide. It is execrated unchanged in urine due to extensive tubular absorption in kidney.

Alfentanil

Alfentanil clearance (4 to 9 mg/kg) is less than that of fentanyl. It has a long elimination half-life and is less lipid soluble than fentanyl. It is bound to plasma protein at pH 7.4 and it is 90% unionized because of low pKa (6.5). Metabolism occurs by N-alkylation-demethylation aromatic hydorxylation and ether glucuronide. Its major metabolitic is norfentanyl. Others are desmethy-lalfentanyl, desmethyl fentanil, with little opioid activity. Patients with P-450 3A enzyme activities have low alfentanl clearance.

Doses: 5 to 50 microg/kg used to supplement sedative hypnotic induction or to prevent response to laryngoscopy. Anaesthesia can be maintained with 60% N_2O and O_2 at dose of 0.5 to 2.0 g/L/min infusion or bolus of 5 to 10 g/kg. Affentanil infusion should be minimized 15 to 30 minutes prior to end of surgery.

Remifentanil

Remifentanil is a synthetic opioid related to fentanyl congeners; with ester structure, making it susceptible to hydrolysis by blood and tissue non specific esterases, resulting in rapid metabolism. It is a weak base with pKa of 7.07, high lipid solubility, highly bound to plasma proteins (70%). It is unstable in solution so prepared just before use. After IV injection there is a extrahepatic hydrolysis. Its metabolism is by de-esterification for a carboxylic acid metabolite; GI 90291, which depend on renal clearance. Other pathway is dealkylation. It is excreted 90% in urine which are inactive metabolites.

It is administered as a bolus of 1 microg/kg in combination with propofol for induction of anaesthesia. It can result in hypotension and bradycardia in 10 to 30% patients. So an infusion of 0.1 to 1.0 microg/kg/min after a bolus is effective, safe, haemodynamically stable, rapid emergence and return.

Table 2: Opioids intravenous equianalgesic ratio

Drug	Relative Potency	Intravenous loading
Pethidine	0.1	0.5 to 1 mg/kg
Morphine	1	0.05 to 0.1 mg/kg
Methandone	1	0.05 to 0.1 mg/kg
Hydromorphine	5	0.01 to 0.02 mg/kg
Fentanyl	50-100	0.5 to 1 microg/kg
Sufentanyl	500-1000	0.025 to 0.05 microg/kg

Other opoid drugs used as analgesics

Tramadol

Opioid Activity
1. Tramadol produces antinociception via predominantly, a mu-opioid receptor mechanism.
2. No respiratory depression, sedation, or constipation, as observed with other opiates.
3. No analgesic tolerance.
4. No psychological dependence or euphoric effects in long-term clinical trials.

Monoaminergic Activity
1. Noradrenergic and serotonergic neurons originate in the brainstem and terminate in the dorsal horn of the spinalcord.
2. Monoaminergic pathway modulates the spinal processing of nociception through the section of nor epinephrine and serotonin
3. Tramadol's novel mechanism of analgesic action is partially due to its adrenergic action and
4. Enhanced secretion of serotonin and inhibits the reuptake of serotonin in the CNS by tramadol.

CPY2D6 Pathway
1. Tramadol is a racemic mixture of a (+)- and a (-)-enantiomer.
2. + enantiomer is selective agonist of mu-opiate receptors and preferentially inhibits serotonin reuptake.
3. -ve enantiomer mainly inhibits noradrenaline reuptake
4. Tramadol is a prodrug that requires transformation by the cytochrome P450 complex to the metabolically active 0- desmethyl-tramadol.
5. The parent molecule also produced analgesia via a monoaminergic action.

Efficacy
1. Effective and well-tolerated analgesic in all 3 forms of administration.(PO,IV,PR)
2. Onset of analgesia is within 30 minutes
3. Duration of action from 3 to 7 hours
4. Drowsiness is the most frequent side effect
5. No adverse effects were observed in the parturient after labor or in the newborn when given for labour pain relief.

Adverse Events

Dependence
1. Withdrawalsymptoms after abrupt discontinuation or reduction of dose.
2. hallucinations, paranoia, extreme anxiety, panic. Attack, confusion, and unusual sensory experiences can occurin rare cases.

Serotonin Syndrome
1. Minor possibility of this exists with both tramadol and tapentadol.
2. Avoid concurrent administration of SSRl's or selective-norepinephrine reuptake inhibitors, triptans, or tricyclic antidepressants.

Tapentadol
1. FDA approved tapentadol hydrochloride in 2008.
2. For oral treatment of moderate-to-severe acute pain in patients older than 18 years.

It is a centrally acting analgesic with 2 mechanisms of action in a single molecule: mu-opioid agonism and norepinephrine reuptake inhibition.

Table3. Major Difference between tramadol and tapentadol

Tramadol	Tapentadol
Racemic mixture of a (+) and A (-) enantiomer	Nonracemic compound
Has active metabolites	Has no active metabolites
Tramadol is a prodrug that requires transformation by the cytochrome P450 complex	No such thing is required
O-desmethyle-tramadol)the metabolite is actually the active form	Tapentadol itself is the active form
Poor metabolizer will not show adequate response to therapy	No such problem with Tapentadol

Tapentadol is as effective as oxycodone or morphine, with a lower incidence of gastrointestinal adverse side effects.

Pharmacokinetics
1. Oral absorption of tapentadolis rapid.
2. Is present in the serum in the form of conjugated metabolites
3. Its excretion was exclusively renal(99°/o: 69°/o conjugates;27o/o other metabolites; 3°/o in unchanged from}

REFERENCES

1. Inturrisi CE, Shultz M, Shin S, et al. Evidence from opiate binding studies that heroin acts through its metabolites. Life Sci1983; 33:773–776.
2. Traynor JR. The mu- opioid receptor. Pain Rev.1996; 3:221–248.
3. Gourlay GK.. Chronic pain: clinical pharmacology of the treatment of acute and chronic pain. In: Max M (Ed). Pain 1999-an updated review: refresher course syllabus. Seattle: IASP press, 1999, pp 433–442.
4. Bernard CM. Epidural and intrathecal drug movement. In: Yaksh TL (Ed). Spinal drug delivery, Amsterdam: Elsevier, 1999, pp 239–252.
5. Gourlay GK. Sustained relief of chronic pain: pharmacokinetics of SR morphine. Clin Pharmacokin 1998; 35:173–190.
6. Labroo RB, Paine MF, Tthummel KE, et al. Fentanyl metabolism by human hepatic and intestinal cytochrome P450 3A$: implications for inter individual variability in disposition, efficacy, and drug interactions. Drug Metab Dispos 1997; 25:1072–1080.
7. Gourlay GK. Treatment of cancer pain with transdermal fentanyl. Lancet 2001; 2:165–172.
8. Zeppetella G. An assessment of the safety, efficacy and acceptability of intranasal fentanyl citrate in the management of cancer related breakthrough pain: a pilot study. J Pain Symptom Manage 2000; 20: 253–258.
9. Takala A, Kaasalainen V, Seppala T, et al. Identification of human cytochrome P450 3A4 as the enzyme responsible for fentanyl and sufentanil N-dealkylation. Anesth Analg 1996; 82:167–172.
10. Vercauteren M, Boeckx E, Hangreefs G, Noorduin H, van den Bussche G. Intranasal sufentanil for perioperative sedation. Anaesthesia 1988; 43:270–273.

11. Mather LE, Woodhouse A, Ward ME, et al. Pulmonary administration of aerosolized fentanyl: pharmacokinetic analysis of systemic delivery. Br J clin Pharmacol 1998; 46:37–43.
12. Higgins MJ, Asbury AJ, Brodie MJ. Inhaled nebulised fentanyl for postoperative analgesia. Anaesthesia 1991; 46:973–976.
13. Plummer JL, Cherry DA, Cousins MJ. Estimation of methadone clearance: application in the management of cancer pain. Pain 1998; 33:313–322.
14. Eckhardt K, Li S, Ammon S, et al. Same incidence of adverse drug events after codeine administration irrespective of the genetically determined differences in morphine formation. Pain 1998; 76:27–33.
15. Intravenous and intranasal administration of oxycodone. Acta anaesthesiol Scand 1997; 41309–41312.
16. Desmeules J, Gascon MP, Dayer P. Magistris M. Impact of environmental and genetic factors on codeine analgesia. Eur J Clin pharmacol1991; 41:23–26.
17. Portenoy RK, Foley KM, Stulman J, et al. Plasma morphine and morphine-6-glucuronide during chronic morphine therapy for cancer pain: plasma profiles, steady state concentrations and the consequences of renal failure. Pain1998; 41:13–19.
18. Hewett K, Dickenson AH, Mcquay HJ. Lack of effect of morphine-3-glucuronide on the spinal antinociceptive actions of morphine in the rat: an electrophysiological study. Pain 1993; 53:59-63.
19. Gong Q1, Hedner J, Bjorkman R, Hedner T. Morphine-3-glucuronide may functionally antagonize morphine-6-glucuronide induced antinociception and ventilatory depression in the rat. Pain 1992; 48:249–255.
20. Goldman B. Diagnosing addiction and drug seeking behavior in chronic pain patients. In: max m (Ed). Pain 1999– an updated review: refresher course syllabus. Seattle: IASP Press, 1999, pp 1–20.
21. Doverty M, White JM, Somogyi AA, et al. Hyperalgesic responses in methadone maintenance patients. Pain 2001a; 90:91–96.
22. Fillingim RB (Ed). Sex, gender, and pain, progress in pain research and management. Vol 17. Seattle: IASP Press, 2000.
23. Gourlay GK, Kowalski SR, Plummer JL, Cousins MJ, Armstrong PJ. Fentanyl blood concentration-analgesic response relationship in the treatment of postoperative pain. Anesth Analg 1988; 67:329–337.
24. Miaskowski C, Gear RW, Levine RD. Sex-related differences in analgesic responses. In: Fillingim RB(Ed). Sex, gender, and pain, progress in pain research and management. Vol. 17. Seattle: IASP Press, 2000, pp 209–230.
25. Kieslowski CJ, Raffa RB, Porreca F. Tramadol and its enantiomers differentially suppress c-fos-like immunoreactivity in rat brain and spinal cord following acute noxious stimulus. EurJpain 1998; 2:211–219.
26. Lodge D, Jones M, Fletcher E. Non-competitive antagonists of N-methyl-D-aspartate. In: collingridge GL, Watkins JC, (Eds). The NMDA receptor, Oxford: Oxford University Press, 1994, pp 104–131.
27. Gorman AL, Elliott KJ, Inturrisi CE. The d- and l- isomers of methadone bind to the non-competitive site on the N-methyl-D-aspartate(NMDA)– receptor in rat forebrain and spinal cord. Neurosci lett 1997;223 :5–8.
28. Kumar Pramod. A text book of Pain. 1st Edn. New Delhi,CBS Publishers, 2005.
29. Kumar Pramod Drugs in Anaesthesia. 1st Edn.,Mumbai, NationalBooks,2018.

Chapter 7:

OPIOID DRUG DELIVERY

Current interest in improving the management of pain by the use of opioid analgesics has led to the search for newer methods of opioid drug delivery. Opioids can be given by (1) sublingual, (2) continuous subcutaneous infusion, (3) transdermal, (4) continuous spinal opioid infusion and (5) intraventricular injection. Each of these modes of administration shares the advantage that they can be used for continuous or repeated administration of an opioid analgesic when injections and oral dosing are to be avoided

Sublingual administration

Although the sublingual route is not a common route of administration for opioids, it offers a number of potential advantages over injections or the oral route (table 1) the total sublingual and buccal area is small compared to the gastrointestinal tract.

Table 1: Comparison of New Methods of Opioid Delivery[2, 3, 4]

Consideration	Continuous Spinal Infusion	Continuous Subcutaneous Infusion	Continuous Transdermal Delivery	Intra-ventricular Injection	Sublingual Application
Avoids im/sc injections	Yes	Yes	Yes	Yes	Yes
Avoids need for iv access	Yes	Yes	Yes	Yes	Yes
Circumvents oral absorption	Yes	Yes	Yes	Yes	Yes
Use by ambulatory	Yes	Yes	Yes	Yes	Yes
Ease of management	Responsible other	Responsible other	Self-administered	Responsible other	Self-administered
Complications	Infrequent but potentially serious	Infrequent, mild	Unknown	Potentially serious	Mild

The potential exists for a rapid absorption of drugs in this area is rich in blood and lymphatic vessels. In selecting the opioid that might be suitable for use by the sublingual route, consideration must be given to the principles governing absorption through the oral mucosa and to the physiochemical properties of the opioids (table 2). If the drug is administered in a solid dosage form, then the first step is the dissolution of the dosage form in the tissue fluids (figure 1).

Table 2: Physicochemical Properties of Opioids

Drug	Partition Coefficient	PKa
Morphine	0.00001	7.9
Hydromorphine	0.0001	
6-Acetylmorphine	0.0012	
Levorphanol	0.01	9.4
Heroin	0.043	

Meperidine	1.7	8.5
Fentanyl	19.68.4	8.4
Methadone	44.6	9.3
Buprenorphine	60.3	

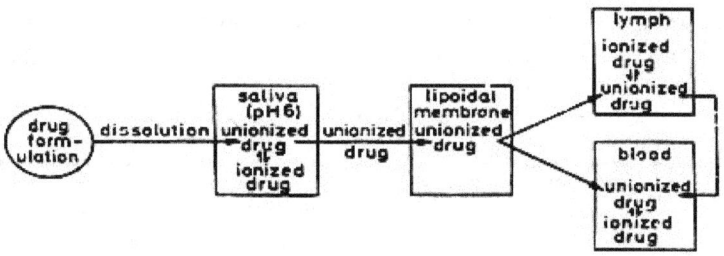

Figure 1: A schematic representation of the sublingual absorption of a drug that is ionized at physiological pH.[4]

Intranasal Administration

The absorption of opioid drugs from the nasal mucosa has been used to treat breakthrough or incident pain and also for preoperative sedation. Nasal spray bottles that deliver an accurate volume of solution (and therefore ,dose) as a spray per activation are used for this route of administration. Fentanyl, oxycodone and sufentanil have been effectively administered in this manner. The intranasal bioavailability for oxycodone and sufentanil was 45% and 78% respectively. Administration of intranasal sufentanil as either drops or a spray had essentially the same effect on the degree of postoperative sedation

Pulmonary Administration Using Aerosol or Nebulizated Solutions

Evidence suggests rapid, extensive but variable absorption of both morphine and fentanyl[10] after inhalation of drug solutions that have been aerosolized. In fact, the mean blood concentration-time profiles following pulmonary administration were similar to those seen with intravenous administration, which raises the possibility of a noninvasive option of the small droplets that constitute the aerosol, the absorption of opioid drugs from traditionally nebulized solutions is less efficient and results in lower bioavailability and more variable postoperative analgesia.

Rectal Administration

The rectal route is frequently used in patients who have difficulty in swallowing or have significant vomiting despite optimized antiemetic therapy. The absorption of drugs from the rectum is notoriously variable and depends greatly on the nature of the formulation used. Liquid rectal formulations (solutions or suspensions) frequently have reasonable, rapid and predictable absorption, but with low patient acceptance because the solution is difficult to hold in the rectum, particularly in ambulant patients. While rectal bioavailability of opioids from solid dosage forms can be extensive (greater than oral bioavailability of the same dose), it is highly variable and the precise anatomical location of the suppository in the rectum is a crucial factor governing the extent of avoidance of hepatic first-pass metabolism and hence rectal bioavailability [5].

While vaginal pessaries can also be used to administer opioid drugs, this route of administration is not greatly favoured by most female patients.

Continous subcutaneous infusion (CSCI)

Opioids injected subcutaneous in aqueous solution are generally rapidly absorbed with time to reach the maximum concentration in plasma from 10 to 30 min. faster or slower absorption is possible depending on the vascular of the site, the ionization and the lipid solubility of the opioid, the volume of the solution. Opioids, being relatively small molecules, are absorbed directly into the capillaries and the absorption process appears to be limited by blood flow. A prime determinant of the absorption rate from a subcutaneous site is the total surface area over which absorption can occur. Although the subcutaneous tissues are somewhat loose, and moderate amounts of fluid can be administered, the normal connective tissue matrix prevents indefinite lateral spread of the injected solution. The properties shown to be important for the absorption of opioids from the sublingual cavity will also influence subcutaneous absorption.

Coyle et al[5] have evaluated continous subcutaneous infusion of opioids using a portable infusion pump attached to a 27 gauge butterfly needle in the management of pain in cancer pts. Based on these observations, guidelines for the selection of the opioid and starting dose for CSCI are given in (table3).

Table 3: Guidelines for Continuous Subcutaneous Infusion (CSSI)

1. Most opioid analgesics available for parenteral use can be administered by CSCI (meperidine [pethidine] and pentazocine are irritating to tissues).
2. May initiate CSCI with the same opioid analgesic that patient have been receiving by the alternate route?
3. Starting dose is calculated using equianalgesic conversing tables (see table 5) with use of rescue doses and titration to effect.
4. Equipment: a portable infusion pump, drug delivery bas, and a 27-gauge pediatric butterfly needle.
5. Home management requires instruction of patient and family.

Table 4: Special Considerations with Continuous Subcutaneous Infusion (CSSI)

1. Local irritation at the site of administration (usually when volume exceeds 1 ml per hour)—more frequent rotation of site infusion
2. Pain breakthrough due to poor absorption from a particular site—change infusion site.
3. Rapidly escalating pain in terminal patients may necessitate the discontinuation of CSCI.
4. Availability of a clinical nurse specialist to assist in home management.
5.

The appropriate management of pts by the use of CSCI requires special considerations as outlined in table 4 and equianalgesic starting doses for some opioid administered by CSCI are given in table 5. these workers found that the steady state plasma morphine concentration varied from 13 to 24 ng/ml during CSCI with a dosage of 2 mg per hour for 12 days in a 22 yr old cancer pt[5].

CSCI has been demonstrated to be a relatively simple, safe and effective method for opioid administration to adults and children in pain. Additional studies are required to continue the development of guidelines of CSCI and determine whether any currently available opioids may possess pharmacokinetic or other properties that make them particularly useful for CSCI.

Continous transdermal delivery

The newest and perhaps most challenging method of opioid drug delivery involves the development of a transdermal drug delivery system (figure 2).

Table 5: Equianalgesic Conversion Ratios[6]

Opioid Analgesic	Equianalgesic Doses (mg)	
	PO	IM/SC
Morphine	30.0	10.0
Hydromorphone (Dilaudid	7.5	1.5

Levorphanol (Levo-Dromoran)	4.0	2.0
Methadone	20.0	10.0

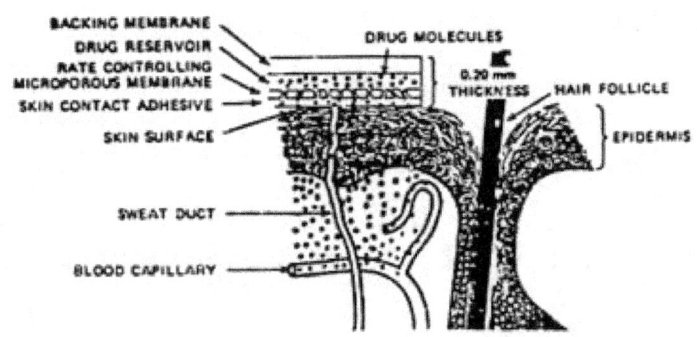

Figure 1: A schematic representation of the flow of drug from a transdermal delivery system through skin into the systemic circulation.

A continous transdermal delivery system for opioid administration offers a number of potential advantages including ease of self- administration (table 1). A critical consideration in the absorption of drugs applied to the skin surface is the properties of the epidermis. This is because despite its thinness the epidermis is a formidable barrier to the absorption of most drugs. Most of the resistance to drug diffusion encountered in the epidermis results from the ultra thin, outermost layer of dead cells called the stratum corneum, the intra cellular space of the corneum contains a unique protein called keratin. Together with a lipid rich medium comprising 15% to 20% of the total stratum corneum, the overall organization is designed to minimize water loss at the body surface. This organization also confers a high resistance to the diffusion of most chemicals. The physiochemical properties of a drug that make it suitable for transdermal delivery are

1. sufficient lipid solubility to penetrate tissue to the capillaries
2. adequate water solubility to allow fairly concentrated solutions (>1.0 mg/ml) to be incorporated into the drug reservoir
3. high relative analgesic potency since it reduces the bulk of the reservoir system.

These considerations have led to the use of the potent, highly lipid soluble opioid, fentanyl in a transdermal delivery system currently under development. Preliminary results indicate that after a lag period of 2-3 hrs, fentanyl appears in plasma and 12 hrs are required for steady state plasma fentanyl levels to be achieved. Additional pharmacokinetic and analgesic studies are required before this potentially useful drug delivery system can be adequately evaluated.

Continuous spinal opioid infusion (CSOI)

Spinal opioids offer potential advantages over systemic opioid administration including a substantially longer duration of analgesia at much loser dose. Furthermore, if the opioid remains localized to the site of administration then selective activation of spinal cord opioid receptors could provide segmental analgesia without supraspinally mediated adverse affects. Opioid analgesia is free of the sympathetic, motor and proprioceptive adverse effects produced by local anaesthetics. However, adverse effects occur with spinal opioids including sedation, nausea and vomiting, respiratory depression, urinary retention and pruritis[4]. The most feared adverse effect, respiratory depression, occurs as a consequence of rostral redistribution of opioid to supraspinal brainstem sites by movement in the CSF or systemic uptake into the circulation.

Opioid receptor densities are the highest in the marginal zone and in the substantia gelatinosa of the dorsal horn. These areas of spinal cord receive primary nociceptive afferent terminals of A delta and C fibers and microinjection of opioids suppresses noxious evoked activity of lamina V neurons. In addition the analgesic effects of intrathecal opioids are dose dependent, stereo specific, antagonized by naloxone and subject to the development of tolerance[7].

Table 6 lists some of the factors that determine the response to spinal opioids. It is well established that there are multiple opioid receptor types and that the μ, κ and δ receptor types are to be found in the spinal cord. There is a lack of opioids for use in humans that are highly selective for each of these receptors. However, animal studies have been encouraging[8] and the use of selective opioids and opioid peptides will no doubt improve the specificity of this mode of administration and may overcome the limitations imposed by tolerance.

Table 6: Factors Determining the Response to Spinal Opioids

1. Relative analgesic potency
2. Receptor selectivity
3. Pharmacokinetics in CSF and spinal cord
4. Tolerance to opioids

Table 7: Distribution of Opioids from CSF to Spinal Cord

Opioid	Brain: plasma Ratio	Cord's ratio	Initial Dose in Cord (%)
Morphine	0.046	0.06	3.8
Methadone	1.23	3.1	67.0
Fentanyl	10.58	34.7	95.8

Calculations by Bullingham et al[2] predict relatively little uptake of morphine from CSF into the spinal cord at equilibrium (table7). The persistent CSF morphine levels favor redistribution to supraspinal sites. Thus the low lipid solubility and limited uptake into spinal cord of morphine results in a slow onset of action while the slow egress from CSF and spinal cord results in a relatively long duration of action[4]. Furthermore, the supraspinal redistribution of morphine in CSF predisposes to effects mediated cephalad while respiratory movements may enhance the spread of morphine from spinal to supra spinal CSF with pharmacological consequences.

In contrast to morphine, methadone is very lipid soluble (table 2) and is rapidly taken up from the lumbar CSF into the spinal cord (table 7). Rapid egress occurs from CSF leaving a very little methadone available in CSF to move supraspinally. Thus lipid soluble opioids such as methadone are characterized by a more rapid onset but a shorter duration of action than morphine. The opioid fentanil presents a third pharmacokinetic profile. Its lipid solubility is similar to that of methadone resulting in rapid onset but it appears to possess high affinity at μ receptors, resulting in a longer duration of action. Respiratory depression is less common in pts who have developed some degree of opioid tolerance due to prior systemic administration of opioids. Yaksh et al[8] found that in morphine related tolerance rats very little cross tolerance occurs to the delta opioid receptor agonist, DADL, administered intrathecally. Moulin et al[10] found that intrathecal DADL produced safe and effective analgesia in cancer pts with some degree of tolerance to systemic opioids.

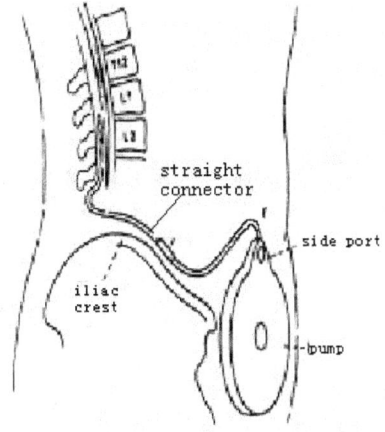

Fig 3. Infusaid pump with catheter in epidural space L1-L2

Cancer pain requires individualization of dose regardless of the route of administration. Cousins and Mather[4] have reviewed the use of long-term epidural catheters to administer opioids. Another innovation is a totally implanted system for continous spinal opioid infusion. In addition to the advantages indicated in table 1 CSOI avoids the use of neurolytic agents or neurosurgical procedures for pain control and allows pre operative assessment of the pts response to spinal opioids.

A schematic of the Infusaid model pump 400 is shown in figure 3. The pump includes a 47 ml drug chamber, which is under compression from a temp sensitive bellows. The pump delivers opioid at a constant low rate (2 to 4 ml/day) for 14 to 21 days into a silastic catheter, which is implanted under local, regional and general anaesthesia into the epidural or sub arachnoid space. The pump model also has and auxiliary side port (figure 4), completely by passing the pump mechanisms by implanting the pump in a subcutaneous pocket in the abdomen or chest (figure5).

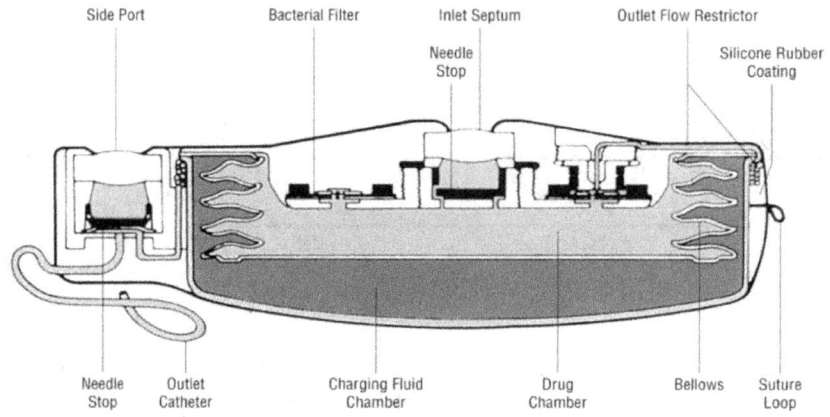

Fig 4. A cross section of infusaid implantable pump

However tolerance appears to develop rapidly in some pts and more slowly in others. Tolerance development with or without escalation in pain due to disease progression results in failures after 2-6 months of CSOI. To date, mechanical problems associated with the catheter system and CSF hyromas have been reported. No evidence of catheter induced spinal cord pathology or epidural abscess or meningitis was found in the series[3, 7].

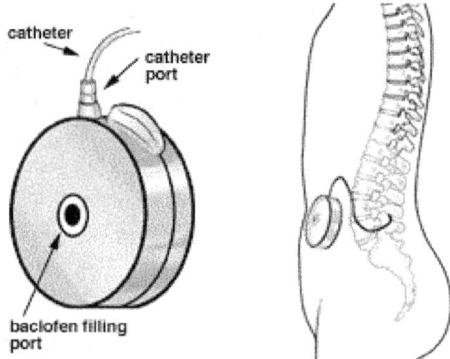

FIG.5. Spinal infusion pump

Parenteral Administration

The absorption of all opioids following either intravenous, intramuscular, or subcutaneous administration has been well characterized over a prolonged period .Patinnt controoed Analgesia has been in in use in postoperative and Intensive care wards.

Patient Controlled Analgesia (PCA) is a method of pain control that gives the patient the power to control their pain.
- Pain medication is administered through a computerized pump.
- The pump contains a syringe of pain medication as prescribed by a doctor that is connected directly to a patient's intravenous (IV) line.
  - The pump is set to deliver a small, constant flow of pain medication.
  - Additional doses can be self-administered as needed by the patient pressing a button.

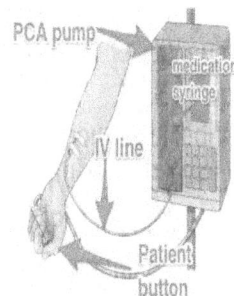

Fig 6. PCA pump

Table 8: Intravenous PCA opioids

Agent	Bolus	Lockout Interval	4 h Maximum Dose	Infusion Rate[a]
Fentanyl (10 μg/mL)	10-20 μg	5-10 min	300 μg	20-100 μg/h
Hydromorphone (Dilaudid) (0.2 mg/mL)	0.1-0.2 mg	5-10 min	3 mg	0.1-0.2 mg/h
Meperidine (10 mg/mL)[b]	5-25 mg	5-10 min	200 mg	5-15 mg/h
Morphine sulfate (1 mg/mL)	0.5-2.5 mg	5-10 min	30 mg	1-10 mg/h

Smart pumps: Highly sophisticated infusion technology used with both epidural & intravenous infusions. Incorporate multiple comprehensive libraries of drugs, usual concentrations, dosing units and dose limits, to avoid medication errors.

Fig 7: Smart pump

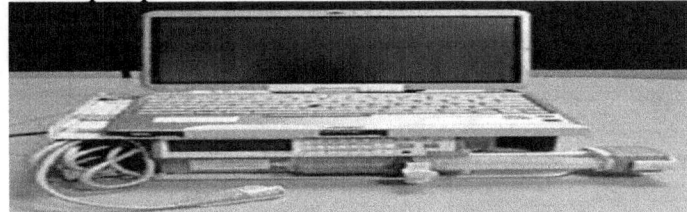

Intraventricular injection

Intraventricular injection of opioid has been reported to be of value in the management of chronic cancer pain. The procedure requires the implantation of an Ommata reservoir to allow IVT opioid administration. The selection of pts and guidelines for the use of IVT are discussed by Lobato et al[11]. table 1 compares IVT administration with the other methods we have discussed. The only opioid used in these reports was morphine in doses that ranged from a starting dose of 0.25 to 1 mg given 1 or 2 times a day[12]. to a maximum dose of 1 to 15 mg given 1 to 3 times per day. Nausea and vomiting occurred in 20% to 60# pts, and other opioid effects including drowsiness and disorientation were reported. The pts developed respiratory depression 4 to 9 hrs after the initial morphine dose. Complications included catheter obstruction and a meningitis, treated successfully with antibiotics. The development of tolerance required a progressive increase in dose. Pharmacokinetic studies confirm very high ventricular CSF levels of morphine, which decay with a t1/2 of 7 hrs[8]. IVT morphine is distributed to cisternal and lumbar CSF[8]. Since opioids can act at spinal and supraspinal sites to produce analgesia, the mechanisms of IVT analgesia may involve multiple sites. It can be assumed that IVT administration of opioids mediate adverse effects such as nausea and vomiting and sedation. It is unlikely that these limitations to the selectivity of IVT administration can be circumvented with available opioids.

References
1. Beckett A.H., Hossie R.D. Buccal absorption of drugs. In: Brodie B.B.,Gillette J.R, eds.,Handbook of experimental pharmacology, vol 28, Springer-verlag, New York, 1971, pp. 25-46.
2. Bullingham R.E.S, McQuay H.J., Moore R.A. Extradural and intrathecal narcotics. In: Atkinson R.S., Hewer C.L., eds., Recent advances in anaesthesia and analgesia, vol 14, Churchill Livingstone, New York, 1982, pp. 141-156.
3. Coombs, D.W., Maurer L.H., Saunders R.L., Gaylor M. Outcomes and complications of continuous intraspinal narcotic analgesia for cancer control pain, J. Clin. Oncol, 1984, 1414-1420.
4. Cousins M.J., Mather L.E. Intrathecal and epidural administration of opioids, Anaesthesiology, 1984, 276-310.
5. Coyle N., Mauskop A., Maggard J., Foley K.M. Continuous subcutaneous infusions of opiates in cancer pts with pain, Oncol. Nur. For., 1986 53-57.
6. Foley K.M. The treatment of cancer pain, N. Engl. J. Med., 1985, 213, 84-95.
7. Greenberg H.S. Continuous spinal opioid infusion for intractable cancer pain. In: Foley K.M., Inturrisi C.E., eds., Advances in pain research and therapy, vol 8, Paven press, New York, 1986 pp. 351-359.
8. Yaksh T L, Achison S R, Durant PAC, Characterisation of action and pharmacology of intrathecally administered DADL encephalin. In: Foley KM Intrurist CE eds. Advances in pain research and therapy, 8, Raven, New York, 1986, 303.
9. Payna R, Interrisi CE. CSF distribution of morphine, methadone and sucrose after intrathecal injection. Life Sci 1986, 37. 1139-1144.
10. Moulin D.E., Inturrisi C.E., Foley K.M. Cerebrospinal fluid Pharmacokinetics of intrathecal morphine sulfate and DADL encephalin Ann. Neurol., 1986, 20, 218-222.
11. Lobato R.D., Madrid J.L., Fatela L.V., Gozalo A., Rivas J.J., Saeabia R. Analgesia elicited by low dose intraventricular morphine in terminal cancer pts. In: Fields H.L., Dubner R., Cervero F., eds., Advances in pain and research and therapy , vol 9 , Raven press, New York, 1985, pp. 673-681

Chapter 8.

Psychotropic Drugs as Analgesics

Both the non-psychiatrist and the psychiatrist can find it hard to disentangle the way in which psychotropic drugs promote pain.

Fig 1: Cause responsible for pain.

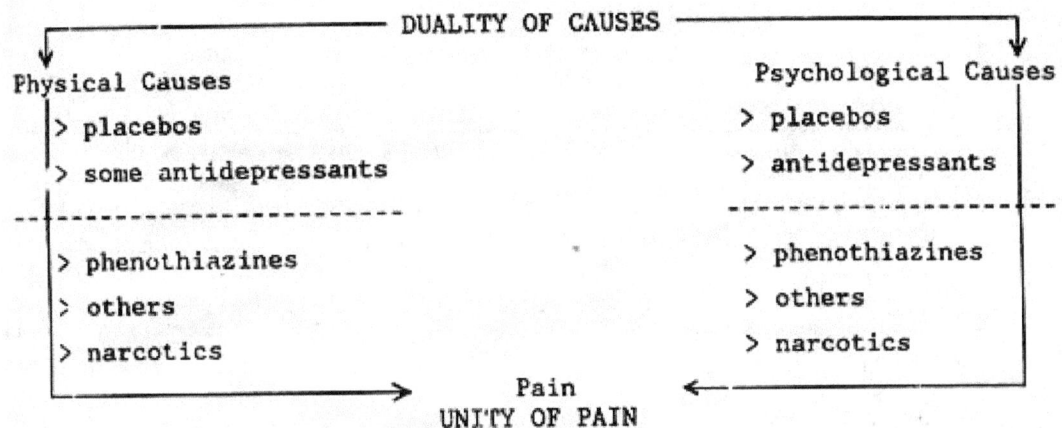

The above diagram indicates how to begin with the causes of pain and recognize that causes may be multiple whilst the final experience is unitary. Pain is not to be understood as a psychological experience at one time and a physical experience at another. It always is just one experience. However, it can have many different causes grouped either as physical or psychological. Thus there is duality of causes but monism of the final phenomenon. The final experience is always a psychological event.

Many different drugs may affect physical causes or psychological causes of pain[1,2]. for example, pain even when it is due to lesions, may be relieved by placebos, perhaps sometimes more than when it is due to hypochondrias is. Some anti depressants relieve pain, of course by relieving depression, which produces it. But other antidepressants may relieve pain because they have analgesic effects, even when there is no depression.

A few patients have no organic cause which can be recognizes for pain. At the same time they have pain and they are not depressed. That is to say they do not meet the criteria for a sad mood, low spirits, and associated phenomena. Magni et al[3] collected a group of patients who had such a pattern of pain and examined then systematically for other phenomena which are associated with depression like a family history of depressive spectrum disorders. They found that imipramine binding was reduced in patients with this pattern of illness in tha same direction as pts with depression but not to the same extent. In an additional study these authors demonstrated that there was a response of the pain to antidepressants, particularly in those pts who had a reduced number of imipramine binding sites and who had a family history of depressive disorders[4]. This suggests that there are sometimes patients whose cerebral pathophysiology is such that they will respond to antidepressants, in the same way as pts with depression, but who lack the evidence of a depressed mood.

1. De afferentation pain e.g. Causalgia, phantom pain, and thalamic pain.
2. Pain from carcinoma.
3. Pain from major lesions e.g. rheumatoid arthritis or osteoarthritis.
4. Pain from minor lesions with concomitant psychological change.
5. Pain from musculoskeletal disturbances e.g. Fibrositis syndrome or mechanical back pain.

Several drugs overlap in their functions. Carbamazepine is an anticonvulsant and was first used in neurology. It is now well and widely established for the relief of trigeminal neuralgia. It has been suggested that it will ameliorate the mood, especially of epileptic pts but more recently of others. It is now used to relieve manic-depressive illness and depression. It prevents manic-depressive illness in some patients and perhaps depression as well and my even are antidepressant.

It is a drug, which overlaps, in its neurological and psychiatric effects. It is commonly used for other pains besides trigeminal neuralgia. It should be considered particularly

1. Recognizable nerve damage.
2. Sharp or stabbing or jabbing pains.

By contrast, lithium carbonate is used primarily in psychiatry and has been spread to neurology. Its first use is for manic-depressive illness. It is known that in relatively small doses it is helpful for a number of cases of chronic cluster headache. The latter is an organic disease probably related to sympathetic dysfunction.

Table 1: Drugs used inPsychiatry.

Drug	First Use	Second Use
Carbamazepine	Epilepsy, trigeminal Neuralgia	Manic-depressive illness
Lithium	Manic-depressive Illness	Chronic cluster headache
Diazepam	Anxiety	Muscle relaxant

Another drug used first in psychiatry and then on physical grounds is diazepam, which is used for anxiety and also for muscle relaxation. At present, clonazepam appears to be coming to the fore as a potential drug for the relief of pain. Formerly, it was mostly considered to be a Benzodiazepine, which happened to be useful for epilepsy, myoclonic jerks and perhaps rare dystonic disorders.

Phenothiazines

Phenothiazines are widely used for pain[6]. The rationale for their use is that they have numerous central and peripheral effects including a local anaesthetic action in the laboratory[7,8]. There is also laboratory evidence of analgesia being induced by them in mice.

Possible uses

They have been put forward or recommended for use with thalamic or central pain and other de afferentation pain e.g. causalgia, neuralgias, neuropathy, and phantom pain, disc lesions. They are also potentially helpful with carcinoma. Sometimes they are used for pain, which causes insomnia, or for persistent troublesome pain for which no other control is available e.g. Cluster headache.

Intravenous methotrimeprazine has been shown to be comparable with morphine[2]. Two single dose trials of phenothiazines compared with narcotics have shown them to be comparable with each other[1,7]. However the longer trials do not support case reports which have suggested the benefit of phenothiazines.

Disadvantages

These include the production of depression. This is perhaps a controversial statement, but anyone who has seen a patient control pain by raising the dose of methotrimeprazine, develop depression which was removed by an increased dose of anti depressant and then reduce both phenothiazines and anti depressant simultaneously without a recurrence of the depression, until the next time the phenothiazines was raised, is unlikely to feel that there is nothing in the statement. Further, a number of patients regularly complain of dysphoria or unpleasant subjective feelings when they are given phenothiazines. Thus many will not take them and it is unwise to persuade a patient to feel wretched one way in order to cure the wretchedness of pain with a given drug. If patients reject phenothiazines for pain because of dysphoria, never urge them further.

Sedation is both an advantage and a disadvantage of phenothiazines. Anticholinergic effects are common and well recognized and include hypotension, constipation and retention of urine. Tardive dyskinesia and Parkinsonism are important side effects for which care must be taken. They lead to a simple precaution. If phenothiazines are used, monitor the patients regularly for tardive dyskinesia. Warn the relatives of the patients. Undertake liver function tests and blood dyscrasias occasionally.

Favored phenothiazines are methotrimeprazine, fluphenazine, pericyazine and chlorprpmazine.

Antidepressants

Antidepressants are probably the most widely used psyhotropic medication for pain.

Rationale
1. Serotoninergic drugs promote antinociceptive effects via the peri acqueductal gray matter. They promote stimulation-produced analgesia. Many antidepressants are serotoninergic. Hence it is often thought that serotoninergic antidepressants will be the most effective analgesics.
2. Tricyclic antidepressants and monoamine oxidase inhibitors potentiate opiate analgesia.
3. The mouse writhing test is positive for amytriptyline at least.

Objections
1. The rat hot plate tail flick test is negative for most or all antidepressants.
2. Non depressed patients did not respond in at least one trial to the use of amitriptyline.
3. Zimelidine is more serotoninergic than amitriptyline but less analgesic[10].
4. Maprotiline is reportedly effective in tension headache and is highly catecholinergic. But tension headache depends upon a psychological mechanism as well as a physical one.

Evidence -There are a number of adequate positive control trials of anti depressants compared with placebo in the treatment of organic conditions causing pain e.g.

Table 2: Anti depressants

Condition	Drug (NO. Of Trials) [1,2]
Arthritis	Imipramine
Arthritis	Dibenzepin
Diabetic neuropathy	Amitriptyline
Diabetic neuropathy	Imipramine
Low back pain	Clomipramine
Migraine	Amitriptyline
Neoplasm	Imipramine
Post-herpetic neuralgia	Amitriptyline

The key test of antidepressants as an analgesic without depression being present was undertaken by Watson et al[11]. In this study using amitryptyline double blind vs. placebo, 24 pts with post herpetic neuralgia were studied of whom only one showed a worthwhile response to placebo whilst 16 showed a good or excellent response to amitryptyline. The Beck depression inventory scores indicated that 14 out of the 23 pts were not depressed. 11 of these 14 had good to excellent pain relief. In the whole study, using amytryptiline and placebo, only 1 pt responded to placebo. The response to amitryptyline in the non depressed pts compared with the placebo is significant at the level< 0.01

Perhaps other antidepressants besides amitryptyline are analgesic, but the evidence has not been brought forward. Likely candidates include imipramine and perhaps doxepin. As already mentioned, zimelidine is not particularly analgesic. One controlled trial does support it but did not distinguish well between depressed and non-depressed pts. Another trial, open and comparative between amitriptyline and zimelidine showed amitriptyline to be much better[10].

It is unlikely that the serotoninergic effects of amitriptyline account for its special antidepressant benefits, in relation to migraine it is said that it may have some calcium channel blocking effects which might account for its analgesia but this does not appear to be the favored explanation in relation to other types of pain such as post herpetic neuralgia. Salter and Henry[9] have produced evidence that adenosine may be related to the modulation of pain. Their evidence is based on the fact that adenosine mediates the depression of spinal dorsal horn neurons, which is induced by the peripheral vibration in the cat. In other words, adenosine mediates the depression of spinal. It might be the case that the analgesic effect of antidepressants is related to some other feature than their serotoninergic characteristic, perhaps their adenosinergic than zimelidine. Dipyridamole is adenosinergic and some initial open observations suggest that it has analgesic qualities.

Disadvantages

They have numerous Anticholinergic effects particularly in the case of the most effective one, amitryptyline. Weight gain is a problem as well as dry mouth, constipation and some times retention of urine, hypotension, cardiac arrhythmias and very rarely glaucoma. If antidepressants are combined with phenothiazines as is sometimes advantageous for the control of pain, these effects are increased.

Other psychotropic drugs

Benzodiazepines are sometimes used for pain. They relieve anxiety and may act upon the muscle contraction effect. An increasing role has been suggested for clonazepam. Narcotics of course also have psychotropic effects but are mainly considered to be analgesics.

Nonsteroidal anti-inflammatory drugs may work psychologically but presumably only through a placebo action. The following table summarizes the relative strength of some of these efts.

Table 3: Other psychotropic drugs

Drug	Physical causes	Psychological causes
	Effects	
Placebo	+/-	+/-
Some or all anti depressants	+++	
Phenothiazines	+	+/-
Benzodiazepines	+	+
Lithium carbonate	+/-	+/-
Carbamazepine	++	+/-
Narcotics	++++	+
NSAIDs	++	+/-

Some or all antidepressants are highly effective as analgesics in certain circumstances. Narcotics are the most effective analgesics in physical circumstances but less so in psychiatric illness. Phenothiazines are of less use as a rule for pain from psychological causes than they are for pain from physical causes. For Carbamazepine the same is true. Lithium carbonate is useful for very specific cases of either physical or psychological illness and the same may be true for Benzodiazepines.

References:
1. Bloomfield S., Simard-Savoie S., Bernier J., Tetreault L. Comparative analgesic activity of lovomepromazine and morphine in pts with chronic pain, Can. Med. Assoc. J., 90, 1964, 1156-1159.
2. Lasagna R.G., DeKornfeldt T.J. Methotrimeprazine: a new phenothiazine derivative with analgesic properties, . Am. Med. Assoc., 178, 1961, 887-890.
3. Magni G., Andreoli F., Arduino C., et al. 3-H Imipramine binding sites are decreased in platelets of chronic pain pts, Acta Psychiat. Scand., 1987.
4. Magni G., Andreoli F., Arduino C., et al. 3-H Imipramine binding sites in chronic pain pts treated with mianserin. Acta Psychiat. Scand, 1987.
5. Melzack R., Wall P.D. Pain mechanisms: a new theory, Science, 150, 1965, 971-979.
6. Monks R., Merskey H. Psychotropic drugs. In: Wall P.D. Melzack R., eds., Textbook of pain, Churchill Livingstone, Edinburgh, 1984, 526-637.
7. Montilla E., Fredrik W.S., Cass L.J. Analgesic effect of methotrimeprazine and morphine, Arch. Intern. Med ., 111, 1963, 91-94.
8. Ncordenbos W. Pain, Elseiver, Amsterdam, 1959,
9. Salter M.W., Henry J.L. Evidence that adenosine mediates the depression of spinal dorsal horn neurons induced by peripheral vibration in the cat, Neuroscience, in press, 1987.
10. Watson C.P.N., Evans R.J. A comparative trial of amitryptyline and zimelidine in post herpetic neuralgia, Pain, 23, 1985, 387-394.
11. Watson C.P.N., Evans R.J., Reed K., Merskey H., Golsmith L., Warsh J. Amitryptyline versus placebo in post herpetic neuralgia, Neurology, 32, 1982, 671-673.

Chapter 9.

Anti Epileptic and Membrane Stabilizing Drugs as Analgesics

Drugs that have the capacity to interfere with impulse generation have the potentially therefore to switch off excitable cells. If the drugs affected some neurons more than other neurons, then the possibility arises that certain specific circuits could be silenced. The excitability of the neuron resides in its sodium channels. These are discrete aqueous pores that span the membrane and exist in an open and closed state. At resting membrane potentials the sodium channel has a closed molecular configuration. When the membrane is progressively depolarized, an increasing number of sodium channels change from the closed resting form to an open active form. This voltage dependent increase in sodium conductance results in an in rush of sodium ions generating the depolarizing phase of the action potential. The action potential is terminated because the sodium channel can exist in the open state only for a short self limited period; it rapidly decays to a closed state i.e. however different from the closed resting state. The difference is that this closed form of the channel cannot be opened by depolarization of the membrane, it is effectively inactivated (figure 1). The inactivated form of the channel can be converted to the resting closed form. It is the proportion of sodium channels at the resting membrane potential that are in the inactivated or resting state that determines the excitability of the neuron[1].

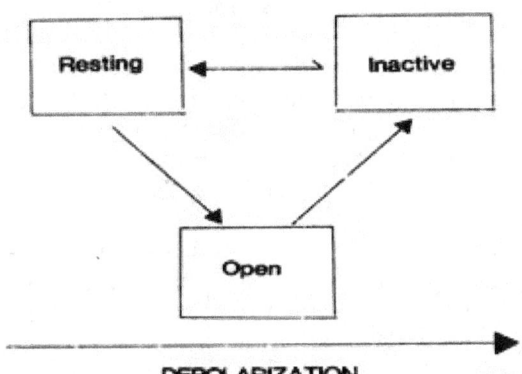

Figure 1: The sodium channel is a voltage-dependent protein that spans the neuronal membrane. At resting membrane potentials the channel is closed, but can be activated by depolarisation to the open form. The active form rapidly decays to a closed inactive form.

Three classes of drugs have the capacity to interact with the sodium channel (figure 2). The first is that class of which tetrodotoxin TTX is the best example. This toxin, produced by the puffer fish, binds to sodium channels in a non-voltage dependent way and prevents the channel from opening. The second class is exemplified by the aromatic linked tertiary amines[2] and the anti epileptics diphenylhydantoin and carbamazepine[3]. these drugs, when they are in the cationic form appear to bind specifically in a classic manner to a voltage dependent receptor on the inner surface of the molecule that is only exposed when the membrane is depolarized. Having bound to the receptor, these drugs alter the distribution of the sodium channel so that most of the channels are maintained in the inactive form. The third class of drugs are the uncharged or lipophillic form of the local anaesthetics and the general anaesthetics which interact with the sodium channel in a non receptor mediated way to alter macroscopic permeability i.e. membrane in inactive state.

Two factors could be involved in the antinociceptive or analgesic actions of membrane stabilizing drugs. The first relates to the concept of conduction safety and the second to use or frequency dependent block.

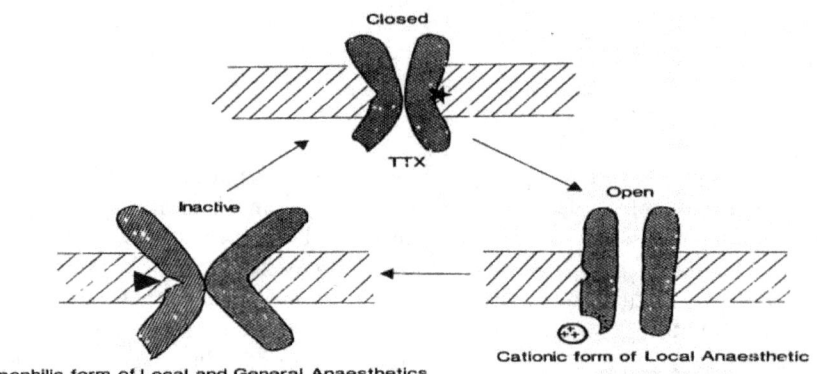

Figure 2: A representation of the three different ways that drugs can interact with the sodium channel. Only membrane stabilising drugs such as lidocaine or procaine and anti-epileptics such as carbamazepine or diphenyl-hydantoin interact with the receptor in a voltage-dependent way.

Conduction safety

Under normal circumstances, depolarization activates sufficient sodium channels to generate more inward current than is required to produce a full overshooting action potential. The margin of safety is of the order of seven. Conduction will fail if either the threshold rises high enough or the amplitude of the spike decreases reducing the safety factor below 1. the conduction safety of the neuron is not distributed homogenously along its surface (figure 3). Branch points, where impedance mismatches can occur, area of lower density of sodium channels, variations in transition kinetics, Schwann or glial cell influences, ionic concentration gradients, all can influence conduction safety. It is possible that certain neurons have a lower conduction safety than others and therefore would be more sensitive to membrane stabilizing drugs. If C primary afferent neurons were particularly sensitive, because for e.g. of the small size of their terminal branches, then systemic administration of sodium channel blockers could produce a greater effect on these than on other neurons.

Frequency or use dependence

The major effect of membrane stabilizing drugs or the anti epileptic drugs diphenylhydantoin and Carbamazepine is to bind to the sodium channel once it has been activated.

The interaction of these drugs with the channel is therefore voltage dependent. Consequently cells which fire at high frequencies with repetitive bursts or show sustained depolarization will be more susceptible to the actions of the drugs than those cells which fire infrequently. If certain particular types of afferent input produce a prolonged depolarization or elicit high frequency discharges, then this input would be more susceptible to blockade by the membrane stabilizing drugs than inputs that did not have these effects. C afferent fibers do have the capacity to produce prolonged depolarization of dorsal horn neurons. This may partly explain the more selective action of lidocaine or tocainide on C than on A afferent fiber evoked activity[4].

In clinical conditions, the membrane stabilizing drugs could be effective either on those sensory conditions resulting from C inputs or those conditions associated with abnormal paroxysmal activity in primary afferent or second order neurons, such as trigeminal neuralgia. Development of safe, effective sodium channel blocking drugs that can be administered orally would appear to be a priority for the future treatment of many intractable pain conditions.

References:

1. Strichartz G.R., ed. Local anaesthetics. Handbook of experimental pharmacology, vol. 81, Springer-Verlag, Berlin, 1987.
2. Wiesenfeld-Hallin Z., Lindblom U. The effect of systemic tocainide lidocaine and bupivacaine on nociception in the rat, Pain, 23, 1985, 357-360.
3. Wilbur M. Pharmacology of diphenylhydantoin and Carbamazepine action and voltage sensitive sodium channels, Trends Neurosci. April 1986, 147-151.
4. Woolf C.J., Wiesenfeld-Hallin Z. The systemic administration of local anaesthetics produces a selective depression of C afferent fiber evoked activity in the spinal cord, Pain, 23, 1985, 361-374.

Chapter 10.

Evaluation of Pain and Pain Imaging

Five pearls of Evaluatiuon
    EVALUATE
    USE A SCALE TO DOCUMENT   PAIN LEVEL & RESPONSE
    USE APPROPRIATE DRUG & MODALITY
    FOLLOW RECOMMENDATIONS
    MULTISPECIALITY APPROACH

Dimensions of Pain measurement

    Intensity -what we usually measure
    Affective -effect on mood, attitude etc.
    Context – implications of pain, expectations, consequences
    Comparisons with usual / worst pain
    Treatment thresholds – when to treat?

Clinical assessment

a) Presenting complaint
 – immediate problem
b) History of present illness –
- Onset – abrupt or slow
- severity of pain and possible aetiology.
- Duration - acute or chronic.
- Character - burning, cramping, aching, deep, superficial, boring, shooting
C) Site - clue for source
 Referred pain possibility should always be considered.
- Radiating pain
- Severity
- Timing - pattern and degree of fluctuation and frequency of remissions
- Exacerbating and relieving factors

RATING SCALES

Self reporting pain severity scoring systems for adults – GOLD STANDARD
- Record at rest and with movement
- Correlate well, generally reliable
- Ensure patient understands the method well & its purpose to avoid confusion.

    1. Categorical Rating Scales (CRS)
    widely applicable verbal method employing different descriptors of pain
     - no, mild, moderate, severe pain
    2. Visual Analog Scale (VAS) 7.5/10
    10 cm line requires pt to mark their current pain severity on the continuum. VAS scale is measured from the no pain point to the pain estimate.

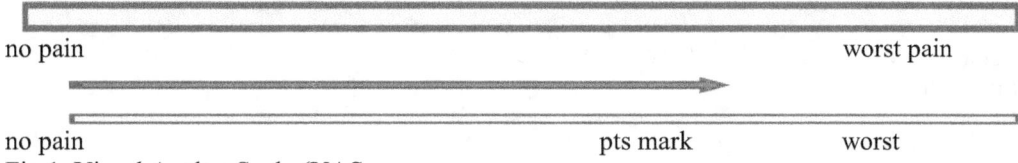

no pain   pts mark   worst

Fig 1. Visual Analog Scale (VAS

3. Verbal Numerical Rating Scale (VNRS)
asks pt to estimate their severity as a number
0 = no pain and 10 = worst possible pain
4. McGill Pain Questionnaire
measures sensory, affective and other miscellaneous aspects of pain

Past history
- Any systemic illness

- Exposure to surgery
- Treatment taken for pain

Personal history
- Occupation
- Habits
- Marital life
- Family disputes

Physical examination
- General
- Vitals
- Systemic- affected system
- Neurological Ex- higher functions, cranial nerves, sensory & motor ex, reflexes, gait & specific tests : trigger point detection etc

Non organic signs:
1. Tenderness
2. Simulation
3. Distraction
4. Regional disturbances
5. Over reaction

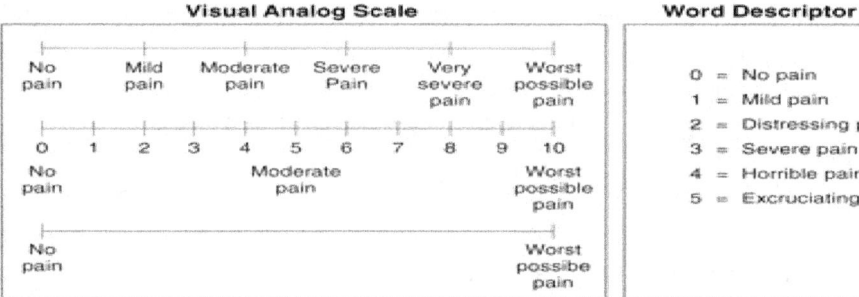

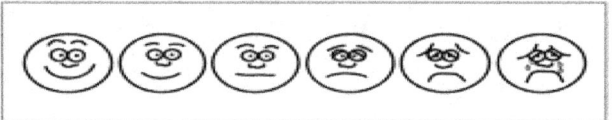

Fig 2: Pain scales

Assess
- Temperature,
- Pulse rate,
- Blood pressure,
- Respiratory rate
- Sedation along with pain.

Paediatric Pain Scales
- Oucher Scale
- CHEOPS: Children Hospital of Eastern Ontario Pain Scale
- CRIES: Crying, Requires O2, Increased vital signs Expression, Sleepless
- COMFORT Behaviour Scale: Neonate < 3 years
- DSVNI : Distress Scale for Ventilated Newborn Infant
- Revised Comfort: Ambuci et al 1982; measures other constructs than pain; upto 9 years; ICU ventilation, Surgical setting

- N-PASS: Neonatal Pain Agitation and Sedation Scale
- DEGR: Douleor Enfant Gustave Roussy

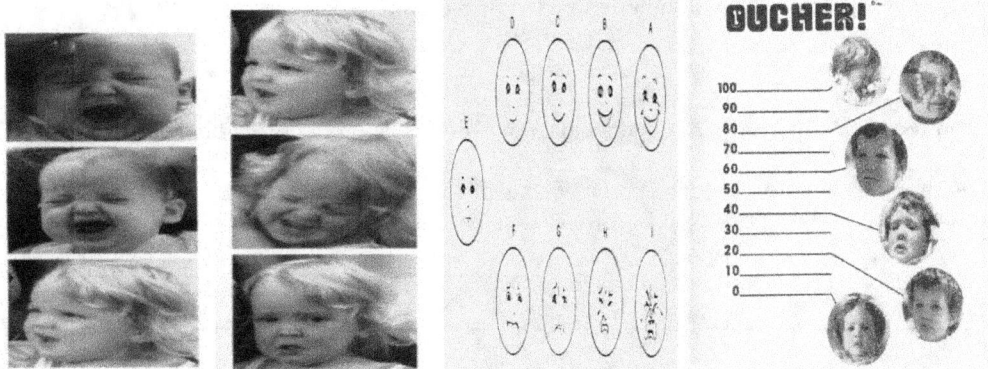

Fig 3: Pain assessment by face of the child.　　Fig 4: A. Faces Pain Scale B. Oucher Scale

Non-complaining, still child
? an ideal patient
- still because of pain
- no complains to avoid injections

Table 1: **CRIES** Scale

CRIES (Krechel et al. Ped Anaesth 1995)			
	0	1	2
Crying	No	High Pitched	Inconsolable
Requires O_2 for Sat > 95	No	< 30%	< 30%
Increased vital signs	HR and BP= or < Preop	HR or BP< 20% of Preop	HR or BP > 20%of Preop
Expression	None	Grimace	Grimace/grunt
Sleepless	No	Wakes at Frequent Intervals	Constantly awake

OBJECTIVE PAIN SCALE (Hannallah, 1987)

BLOOD PRESSURE
< /= 10% preop……………...　0
> 10-20% preop……………..　1
> 20% preop………………….　2

CRYING
Not crying……………………　0
Crying responds to TLC…....　1
Crying does not respond
  to TLC……………………..
localize……　1

MOVEMENT
None………………………...　0
Restless…………………….　1
Thrashing…………………..　2

AGITATION
Asleep or calm………………　0
Mild…………………………...　1
Hysterical……………………　2

VERBAL EVALUATION OR BODY LANGUATE
Asleep or states no pain…...　0
(Preverbal child-No special posture)
　　　　　　　　　　Mild pain/cannot
(Preverbal child-Flexing extremities)
Moderate pain/can localize…　2
(Preverbal child-Holding location of pain)

Back pain
  Acute: lasting ≤3 months
o Chronic: lasting >3 months
These are of 5 basic types
　　Local pain - Caused by activation of pain-sensitive nerve endings near affected part of the spine.
　　　Site - near the affected part

Table 2: Assessing Children's' Distress in the PICU

Alertness	Blood Pressure
Deeply asleep 1	Blood pressure below baseline 1
Lightly asleep 2	Blood pressure consistently at baseline 2
Drowsy 3	Infrequent elevations of 15% or more during observation period 3
Fully awake and alert 4	Frequent elevations of 15% or more above baseline (more than 3 during observation period 4
Hyper alert 5	Sustained elevation of 15% or more 5

Referred to the back - ƒ Abdominal or pelvic in origin. Unaffected by posture.
Pain of spinal origin - Restricted to the back or referred to lower limbs

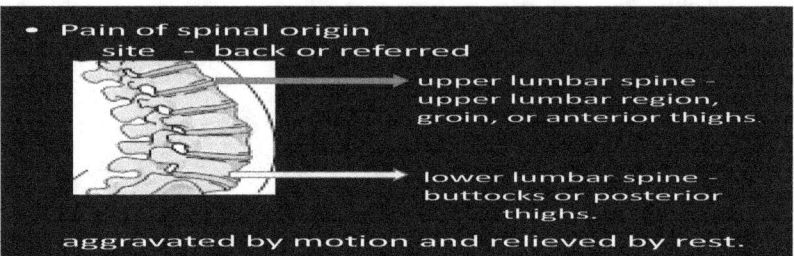

Fig 5: Pain of spinal origin

Radicular pain - Radiates from spine to leg in specific nerve root territory.
- ✓ Typically sharp
- ✓ Elicited by - Coughing, sneezing, or voluntary contraction of abdominal muscles
- ✓ Increase in postures that stretch the nerves and nerve roots.

Pain associated with muscle spasm   Accompanied by taut paraspinal muscles and abnormal posture, dull pain.

History
- Understanding the type of pain
- Risk factors for underlying cause of back pain
    - Age > 50 years
    - Prior diagnosis of cancer / medical illness
    - Intravenous drug use
    - Glucocorticoid use
    - No relief with bed rest
    - Urinary incontinence or recent nocturia
    - Focal leg weakness or numbness
    - Pain radiating into the leg(s) from the back
    - Chronic infection (pulmonary or urinary)
    - Pain increasing with standing and relieved by sitting
    - History of spine trauma

Physical examination
Significant signs-
- Unexplained fever, weight loss
- Positive SLR sign, crossed SLR sign, or reverse SLR sign
- Percussion tenderness over the spine or costovertebral angle
- An abdominal mass (pulsatile or nonpulsatile)
- A rectal mass

Focal sensory loss (saddle anesthesia or focal limb sensory loss)
Leg weakness
Spasticity or reflex asymmetry

Inspection
- ✓ Lateral curvature of the spine (scoliosis)
- ✓ Asymmetry in the paraspinal muscles suggests muscle spasm.

Palpation
- ✓ May elicit pain over a diseased spine segment

Hip pain
- ✓ May be confused with spine pain
- ✓ Can be reproduced by internal and external rotation at the hip with the knee and hip in flexion (Patrick sign) and by tapping the heel with the examiner's palm while the leg is extended

SLR sign
Elicited by passive flexion of extended leg at the hip with patient in supine position
The maneuver stretches L5/S1 nerve roots and sciatic nerve passing posterior to the hip.
SLR is positive if the maneuver reproduces the pain.

Reverse SLR sign
Passive extension of leg backwards with patient standing
The manoeuvre stretches L2–L4 nerve roots and femoral nerve passing anterior to the hip.

Crossed SLR sign
Positive when SLR on 1 leg reproduces symptoms in the opposite leg or buttocks
Nerve/nerve root lesion is on the painful side.

Pain referred from visceral organs may be reproduced during:
Palpation of the abdomen (pancreatitis, abdominal aortic aneurysm)
Percussion over the costovertebral angles (pyelonephritis, adrenal disease)

Neurologic examination
Includes a search for
  Weakness,
  Muscle atrophy,
  Focal reflex changes,
  Diminished sensation in the legs, and
  Signs of spinal cord injury

Table 3: Lumbar radiculopathy

Lumbosacral Nerve Roots	Reflex	Sensory	Motor	Pain Distribution
L2[a]	—	Upper anterior thigh	Psoas (hip flexion)	Anterior thigh
L3[a]	—	Lower anterior thigh, Anterior knee	Psoas (hip flexion), Quadriceps (knee extension), Thigh adduction	Anterior thigh, knee
L4[a]	Quadriceps (knee)	Medial calf	Quadriceps (knee extension)[b], Thigh adduction, Tibialis anterior (foot dorsiflexion)	Knee, medial calf, Anterolateral thigh
L5[c]	—	Dorsal surface—foot, Lateral calf	Peroneii (foot eversion)[b], Tibialis anterior (foot dorsiflexion), Gluteus medius (hip abduction), Toe dorsiflexors	Lateral calf, dorsal foot, posterolateral thigh, buttocks
S1[c]	Gastrocnemius/soleus (ankle)	Plantar surface—foot, Lateral aspect—foot	Gastrocnemius/soleus (foot plantar flexion)[b], Abductor hallucis (toe flexors)[b], Gluteus maximus (hip extension)	Bottom foot, posterior calf, posterior thigh, buttocks

a – reverse SLR +
b – majority innervation by this root
c – SLR

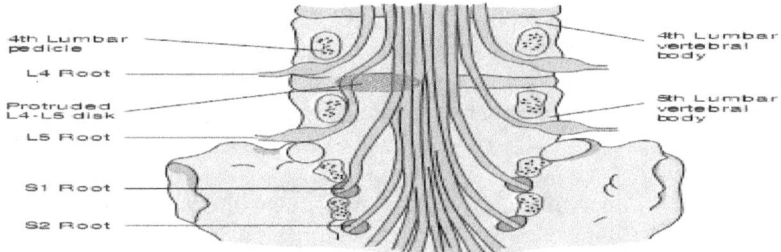

Fig 6: Compression of L5 – S1 nerve root by herniated disc

Pain Imaging
• MRI and CT myelography
  ✓ Tests of choice for evaluation of spine
  ✓ MRI is superior for the definition of soft-tissue structures.
  ✓ CT myelography provides optimal imaging of bony lesions and is tolerated by claustrophobic patients.
• **Plain film radiography**
  ✓ Spine fracture especially when risk factors are present.

Tumour

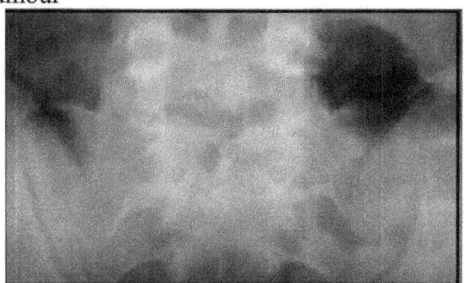 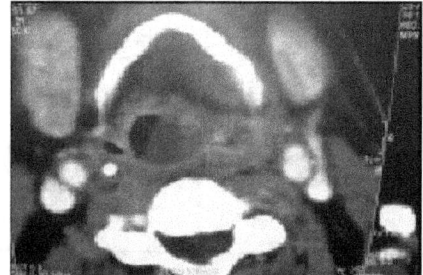

Fig 7 a : X-ray Lumbosacral spine in Spina bifida   Fig 7 b: CT Neck glossopharyngeal neuralgia
laryngeal

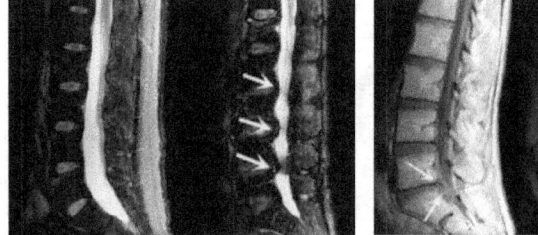 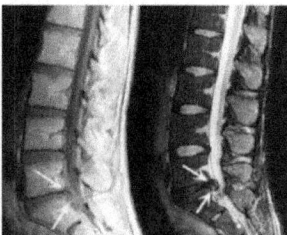 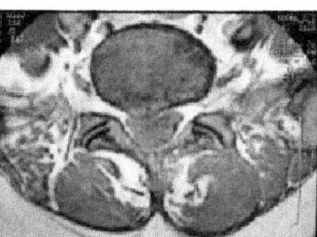

Fig 8. : MRI of lumbar herniated disk; left S1 radiculopathy-arrows outlining disk margins   Sagittal T2 reveals a protruding disk at L5-S1 level displaces the central thecal sac

Diagnostic Procedures
Neuro imaging and electrophysiologic studies.
EMG: For radiculopathy- Pattern of muscle involvement indicates the nerve root(s) responsible

CANCER PAIN
Causes of pain in cancer
  ➢ Cancer itself – pressure on any organ, bone, nerves or blood vessels
  ➢ Cancer treatment –
  ➢ Chemotherapy & radiotherapy – pain due to mucositis, peripheral neuropathy
  ➢ Surgery – acute post operative pain, phantom limb pain, stump pain, etc.

Assessment of pain in cancer

Initial evaluation
Identify cause of pain
Detailed history –
pain intensity , character
Physical examination –
 neurological
Psychological assessment

Pain evaluation
A Ask about pain regularly
B Believe the patient and family in their reports of pain and what relieves it
C Choose pain control options appropriate for the patient, family and setting
D Deliver interventions in a timely, logical and coordinated manner
E Empower patients and their families to choose the modality

Table 4: **Elements of cancer pain assessment**

Elements of cancer pain assessment	
Factor	Question
Intensity	How sever is your pain?
Character	How would you describe your pain?
location	Where is your pain?
Radiation	Does your pain go anywhere?
Timing	When does your pain occur?
Correlated factors	What makes your pain better or worse?
Implications of pain	How does this pain affect your daily living?
Meaning of pain	What does the pain mean to you?

Headache
 - Quality, location, duration, and time course of the headache and
- Conditions that produce, exacerbate, or relieve it
- Pain intensity –
rarely diagnostic value, important from the patient's perspective
Quality is helpful for diagnosis. - Tension-type- tight "band like" or dull, deeply located, and aching pain.
- Jabbing, brief, sharp cephalic pain, often multifocal (ice pick–like),
- Throbbing quality and tight muscles about the head, neck, and shoulder girdle - migraine.

Table 5: **Headache Symptoms That Suggest a Serious Underlying Disorder**

"Worst" headache ever
First severe headache
Subacute worsening over days or weeks
Abnormal neurologic examination
Fever or unexplained systemic signs
Vomiting precedes headache
Induced by bending, lifting, cough
Disturbs sleep or presents immediately upon awakening
Known systemic illness
Onset after age 55

Table 6: CHRONIC PELVIC PAIN

	History	Relevance
1.	Age	Reproductive age group
2.	Parity	Infertility, Nulliparity – endometriosis, PID Multiparity – pelvic relaxation, osteopenia
3.	Occupation	Long standing, heavy weight lifting – pelvic congestion syndrome
4.	Pain History (pneumonic – ODD PAINS)	Onset: usually gradual or insidious Duration: more than 3 to 6 months Distribution: pain mapping Precipitating event: surgery, accident, death of loved one Aggravating or relieving factors: defecation, coitus Intensity: visual analog scale Nature: sharp shooting, dull aching Symptoms associated: bowel-bladder symptoms
5.	Treatment History	medical, surgical, physiotherapy, psychiatric
6.	Personal History	addiction, drug abuse, bladder-bowel habits, sleep pattern, contraceptive use, sexual relations, social life, physical or sexual assault
7.	Menstrual History	dysmenorrhea, menorrhagia or other menstrual abnormalities, premenstrual symptoms
8.	Family History	endometriosis, cancers, depression or other psychiatric problems
9.	Obstetric History	number of pregnancies and their outcome; abortions (how, why, when); antenatal problems like excessive weight gain, proper calcium intake; mode of delivery (vaginal or cesarean), details of delivery (duration, instrumentation, episiotomy); postnatal period, breast feeding, interval between successive pregnancies

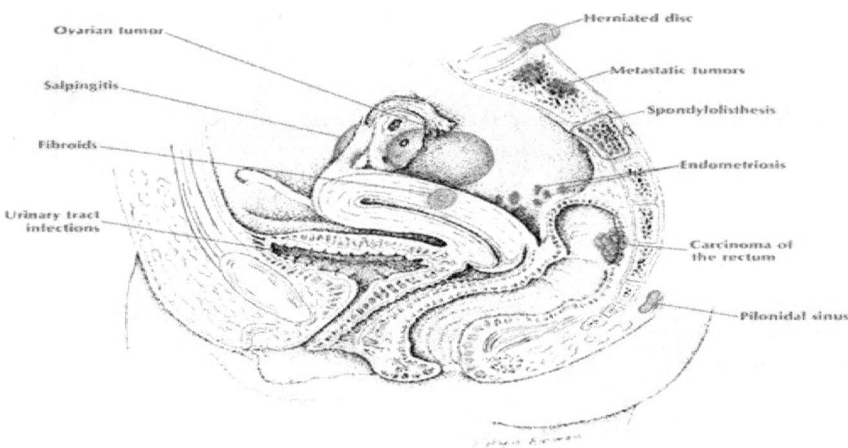

Fig 9: CAUSES OF PELVIC PAIN

Diabetic neuropathy
Types:
-Early – intermittent tingling / numbness, mainly in feet
-Later – intense, constant pain
- Painless neuropathy – ulcer painless, surrounded by callous, at toe or bottom of feet

Classification of diabetic neuropathy-

Symmetric
1. Distal primarily sensory polyneuropathy
2. Autonomic neuropathy
3. Chronic proximal motor neuropathy

Asymmetric
1. Acute or subacute proximal motor neuropathy
2. Cranial mononeuropathy

3. Truncal neuropathy
4. Entrapment neuropathy in the limbs
Foot examination
Physical examination
Neurological examination
Mechanical/thermal sensitivity
Sympathetic activity
EMG – rule out other myalgia
Nerve conduction velocity study
Quantitative sensory testing
Nerve or skin biopsy
Blood studies – for diabetes

Activity recorded during EMG.
A. Spontaneous fibrillation potentials and positive sharp waves.
B. Complex repetitive discharges recorded in partially denervated muscle at rest.
C. Normal triphasic motor unit action potential. D. Small, short-duration, action potential seen in myopathic disorders. E. Long-duration polyphasic motor unit action potential seen in neuropathies

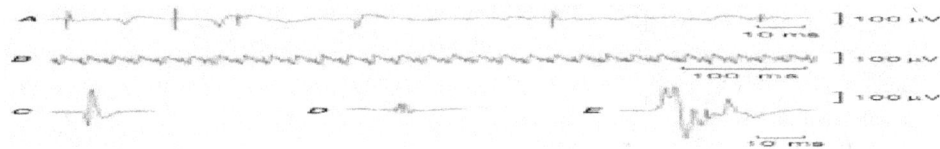

Fig 10: Activity recorded during EMG.

Causes of Neuropathic pain

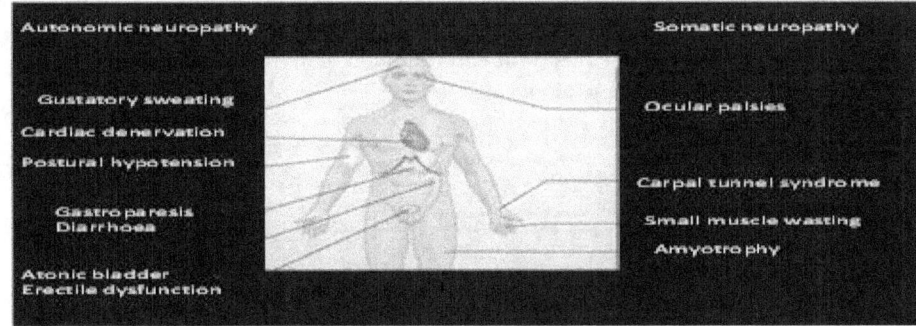

Fig 11: Causes of Neuropathic pain

Post herpetic neuralgia
Sequelae of acute herpes zoster infection
Starts: within 3 – 4 weeks
Seen more commonly in elderly & immuno compromised patient

Assessment
History: herpes zoster infection before 4 – 6 weeks
- unilateral pain in a dermatomal distribution.
Thoracic > facial > cervical
Nature of pain –
- Bursts of vibrating pain to stigmatized area
- Reflex sympathetic dystrophy – burning pain in the segment
- Hypersensitivity in scarred area
finally the area may become numb
Dormant during sleep
Physical examination-
- Areas of hyperpigmentation & scarring in areas of prior vesicular eruption

- Allodynia, dysesthesia, hyperesthesia
- Pain induced disruption of social activities, mood, depressed effect, poor sleep

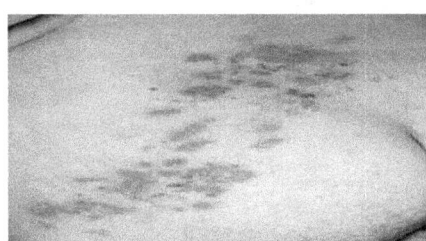 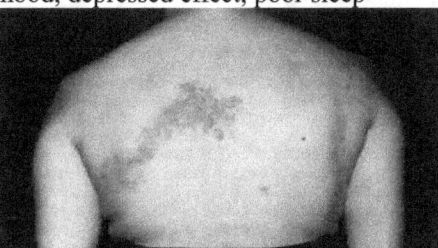

Fig12: Herpes zoster - A. Hemorrhagic vesicles and pustules. B. VZV affecting a dermatome

Pain Assessment in critically Ill & Cognitively Impaired Patients

Pain Assessment in Critically Ill Patient
    Inadequate & Incomplete assessment
    Inadequate Pain Management

Issues in Critically Ill Patients:
Moribund, altered consciousness
Less cooperation, altered sensorium
Patient too sick, mentally incompetent
Heavily medicated, on ventilator
Altered pain assessment
Assessment & resuscitation simultaneous
Cognitively impaired, aging, child, dementia

Methodologies for Pain Assessment
A. Subjective – Patient rated (cognitive patient)
B. Objective – Care giver rated (Patterns of particular behavior – hand on forehead in headache)
C. Review medical records for pain inducing pathology (painful neuropathy in DM)
D. Diagnosis – Physical exam, Lab studies (problems inducing pain eg. fracture, UTI)

Observational Items in Pain Rating Systems
- Facial expression
- Body posture
- Vocalizations
- Appetite
- Interactivity

INTUBATED – Guiding Principles for Assessment of Pain
1. SELF-REPORT: Attempted Hampered by
 - Delirium, Cognitive & communication limitations, level of consciousness, presence of end tracheal tube, sedatives and neuromuscular blocking agents.
Delirium – wax and wane and impact ability to self report.
Serial assessment for the ability to self report should be conducted

2. Potential causes of Pain/Discomfort:
Existing medical conditions, trauma, surgical/medical procedures- invasive instrumentation, drawing blood, suctioning, turning, positioning, drain and catheter removal and wound care Immobility, hidden infection, early decubiti.

Observation of Patient Behaviour:
1. Facial expression – grimace, frown, wincing.
2. Physical movement ,immobility, increased muscle tone increases pain
3. Tearing, diaphoresis in sedated, paralysed patients autonomic responses to discomfort
4. Behaviour pain scales not appropriate in paralysed flaccid patients.Analgesic trial –Distress versus pain behaviour .Further assessment- Changes in physiology, vital signs.

Table7: ABCD Bundle

ABCDE Bundle	Tools
Awaken	**Wake Up and Breath Protocol**, performed jointly every 24 hours by a Nurse and Respiratory Therapist: • Safety Check → Spontaneous Awakening Trial (SAT) • Safety Check → Spontaneous Breathing Trial (SBT)
Breathe	
Choose Medication & Coordinate Care	**Daily, interprofessional rounds** assess each patient daily, in which the team adjusts treatment and medications, as necessary, and sets goals for the day: • Ventilation • Medications • Mobility If the patient is delirious, the team figures out possible causes, aided by questions such as those embodied in "Stop, THINK, and (perhaps) Medicate"
Delirium Assessment	**Monitor pain, agitation, and delirium**, using the following tools: • Critical Care Pain Observation Tool (CPOT) • Richmond Agitation and Sedation Scale (RASS) • Confusion Assessment Method for the ICU (CAM-ICU) or Intensive Care Delirium Screening Checklist (ICDSC)
Early Mobility	**Early Mobility Protocol** provides a safety check and series of progressive goals to increase patient mobility: • Safety Check → Progressive Mobility

4. Care giver Ratings of Pain & Pain relief-Physicians, nurses, family members.Simple category scale – No pain to slight, moderate or severe pain/ pain relief**.**

Limitations – 1: Care giver judgments are not true, only inferred.2. Pain is a subjective experience, cannot be observed truly.3. Rater's expectations, past experience, belief about patient's conditions distorts judgment. 4. Rater's bias – knowledge of patients conditions, stereotyping (racial, gender, age, social groups) multiple, well trained raters, well defined criteria.5. Attempt an analgesic trial appropriate to the intensity of pain based on patient pathology and analgesic history. Explore other causes if used. causing pain if behavior continues. 6. Establish a procedure for pain assessment: Attempt self report/ why it cannot be Identify pathologic conditions/ procedure.

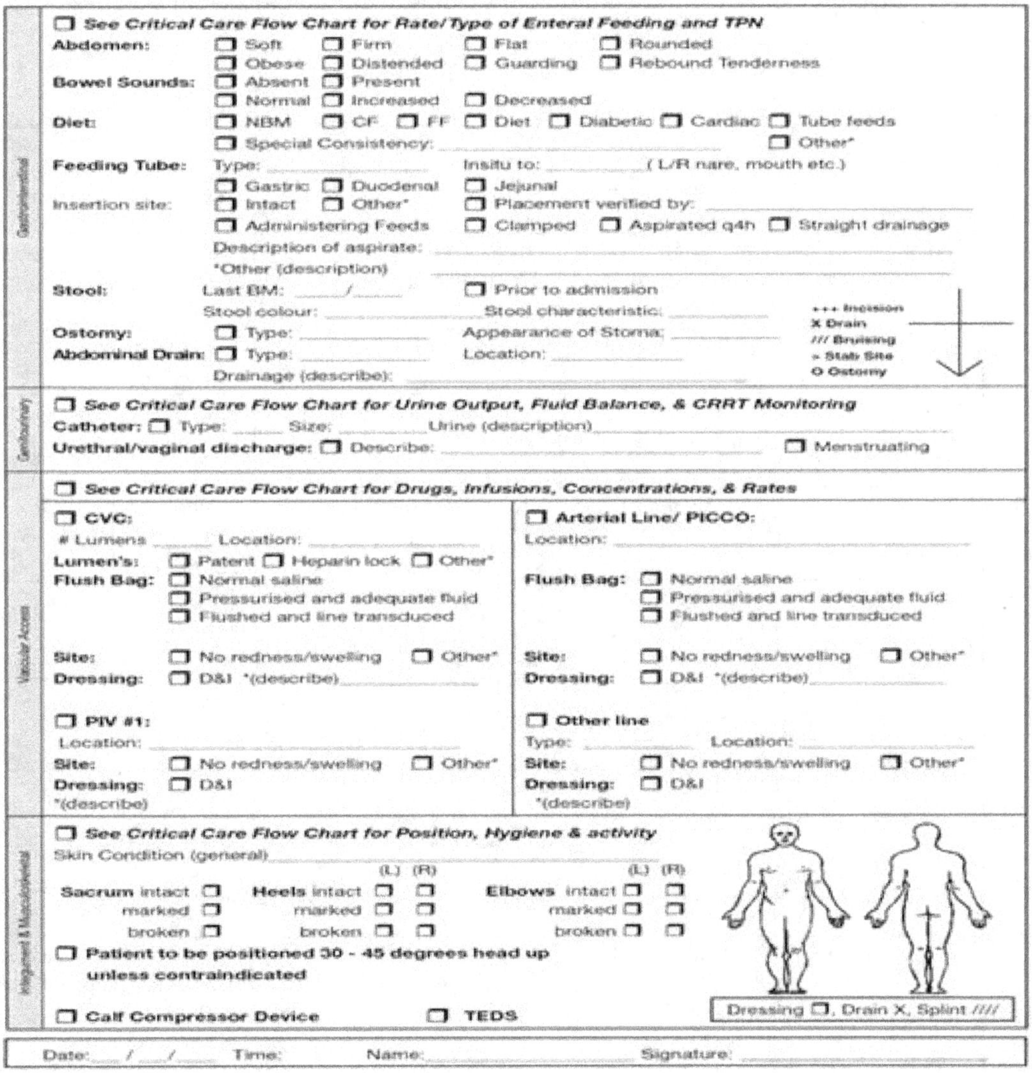
Gastrointestinal

❐ See Critical Care Flow Chart for Rate/Type of Enteral Feeding and TPN

Abdomen: ❐ Soft ❐ Firm ❐ Flat ❐ Rounded ❐ Obese ❐ Distended ❐ Guarding ❐ Rebound Tenderness

Bowel Sounds: ❐ Absent ❐ Present ❐ Normal ❐ Increased ❐ Decreased

Diet: ❐ NBM ❐ CF ❐ FF ❐ Diet ❐ Diabetic ❐ Cardiac ❐ Tube feeds ❐ Special Consistency: ❐ Other*

Feeding Tube: Type: Insitu to: (L/R nare, mouth etc.) ❐ Gastric ❐ Duodenal ❐ Jejunal

Insertion site: ❐ Intact ❐ Other* ❐ Placement verified by: ❐ Administering Feeds ❐ Clamped ❐ Aspirated q4h ❐ Straight drainage

Description of aspirate:

*Other (description)

Stool: Last BM: / ❐ Prior to admission

Stool colour: Stool characteristic:

Ostomy: ❐ Type: Appearance of Stoma:

Abdominal Drain: ❐ Type: Location:

Drainage (describe):

+++ Incision
X Drain
/// Bruising
» Stab Site
O Ostomy

Genitourinary

❐ See Critical Care Flow Chart for Urine Output, Fluid Balance, & CRRT Monitoring

Catheter: ❐ Type: Size: Urine (description)

Urethral/vaginal discharge: ❐ Describe: ❐ Menstruating

Vascular Access

❐ See Critical Care Flow Chart for Drugs, Infusions, Concentrations, & Rates

❐ CVC:
Lumens Location:
Lumen's: ❐ Patent ❐ Heparin lock ❐ Other*
Flush Bag: ❐ Normal saline ❐ Pressurised and adequate fluid ❐ Flushed and line transduced
Site: ❐ No redness/swelling ❐ Other*
Dressing: ❐ D&I *(describe)

❐ Arterial Line/ PICCO:
Location:
Flush Bag: ❐ Normal saline ❐ Pressurised and adequate fluid ❐ Flushed and line transduced
Site: ❐ No redness/swelling ❐ Other*
Dressing: ❐ D&I *(describe)

❐ PIV #1:
Location:
Site: ❐ No redness/swelling ❐ Other*
Dressing: ❐ D&I
*(describe)

❐ Other line
Type: Location:
Site: ❐ No redness/swelling ❐ Other*
Dressing: ❐ D&I
*(describe)

Integument & Musculoskeletal

❐ See Critical Care Flow Chart for Position, Hygiene & activity

Skin Condition (general)

Sacrum intact ❐ marked ❐ broken ❐
Heels (L) (R) intact ❐ ❐ marked ❐ ❐ broken ❐ ❐
Elbows (L) (R) intact ❐ ❐ marked ❐ ❐ broken ❐ ❐

❐ Patient to be positioned 30 - 45 degrees head up unless contraindicated

❐ Calf Compressor Device ❐ TEDS

Dressing ❐, Drain X, Splint ////

Date: / / Time: Name: Signature:

Fig 13: Pain Assessment Chart

Pain Assessment Scales:
1. Numerical Analogue Scale
   "0" – No pain, "10" – worst pain
   How would you rate your pain
2. Visual Analogue Scale

   0 |————|————|————|————|————|————|————|————|
   No Pain   **Worst Pain**

3. **Verbal Descriptive Scales**:
0-no pain; 1-3 mild pain; 4-6 moderate pain; 7-10 worst pain
4. Face Scales (Pediatric/Adult)

Table 8: Non verbal painaid scale.

Items*	0	1	2
Breathing independent of vocalization	Normal	Occasional labored breathing. Short period of hyperventilation.	Noisy labored breathing. Long period of hyperventilation. Cheyne-Stokes respirations.
Negative vocalization	None	Occasional moan or groan. Low-level speech with a negative or disapproving quality.	Repeated troubled calling out. Loud moaning or groaning. Crying.
Facial expression	Smiling or inexpressive	Sad. Frightened. Frown.	Facial grimacing.
Body language	Relaxed	Tense. Distressed pacing. Fidgeting.	Rigid. Fists clenched. Knees pulled up. Pulling or pushing away. Striking out.
Consolability	No need to console	Distracted or reassured by voice or touch.	Unable to console, distract or reassure.
			Total**

Table 9: FLACC SCALE (0 to 10)

Categories	0	1	2
Face	No particular expression/ smile	Occasional grimace or frown, withdrawn, disoriented	Quivering chin, clenched jaw
Legs	Normal position or relaxed	Uneasy, restless, tense	Kicking or legs drawn up
Activity	Lying quietly, normal position. Moves easily	Squirming, shifting, tense	Arched, rigid or jerking
Cry	No cry (awake or asleep)	Moans/ whimpers, occasional complaining	Crying, screams, sobs, frequent complaints
Consolability	Content, relaxed	Reassured occasional touching, or being talked to	Difficult to console/ comfort

Table 10: Modified FLACC, Non verbal Pain Assessment Tool (FRAAC)

Score	0	1	2
Face (F)	1. Unwrinkled brow 2. Unclenched jaw 3. Blank/content expression	1. Distressed appearance 2. Worried expression 3. Wrinkled brow 4. Turned down mouth corners	1. Alarmed/ fearful expression 2. Open eyes/ Pleading expression 3. Clenched jaw 4. Scowling/ stern face
Respiration (R)	1. Normal unlabored 2. Barely audible	1. Respiration difficult breathing, increased sound 2. Look more strained 3. Increased	1. Gas exchange not good 2. Episodic rapid breaths 3. Gasping 4. Very loud, strained.

Activity(A)	1.Lying quietly 2.Open position 3.Moves easily/flaccid 4.Nontense muscles 5.Appears restful	1.Squirming/uneasy 2.Fidgeting 3.Clenched fists 4.Not content 5.Slightly restless	1.Arched/rigid 2.Jerking 3.Forceful touching 4.Tugging/rubbing body parts 5.Legs drawn up/arms flailing, writhing
Audible(A)	No sound/quiet	1.Moans/Whispers 2.Expressed pain 3.Hushed low sound 4.Crying	1.Loud guttural moans 2.Unpleasant sound/noise 3.Scream./yell
Consol ability (C)	Contentment	Reassured by sound of loved one/soft touching/caressing distractible	Inconsolable, Unable to comfort through distraction

Behavioral pain scale (BPS)

BPS Intubated patient   BPS Non Intubated patient
1   2   3   4   1   2   3   4

Fig 14: BPS scale (1+2+3 = Total BPS Value)

Table 12: ICU PAD care Bundle

PAIN	AGITATION	DELIRIUM	
• % of time patients are monitored for pain ≥4x/shift • Demonstrate local compliance and implementation integrity over time in the use of ICU pain scoring systems	• % of time sedation assessments are performed ≥4x/shift • Demonstrate local compliance and implementation integrity over time in the use of ICU sedation scoring systems	• % of time delirium assessments are performed Q shift • Demonstrate local compliance and implementation integrity over time in the use of ICU delirium assessment tools	Assess
• % of time ICU patients are in significant pain (i.e., NRS ≥ 4, BPS ≥ 6, or CPOT ≥ 2) • % of time pain treatment is initiated within 30" of detecting significant pain	• % of time patients are either optimally sedated or successfully achieve target sedation during DSI trials (i.e., RASS = -2 – 0, SAS = 3 – 4) • % of time ICU patients are under sedated (RASS >0, SAS >4) • % of time ICU patients are either over sedated (non-therapeutic coma, RASS <-2, SAS <3) or fail to undergo DSI trials	• % of time delirium is present in ICU patients (CAM-ICU is positive or ICDSC ≥ 4) • % of time benzodiazepines are administered to patients with documented delirium (not due to ETOH or benzodiazepine withdrawal)	Treat
• % of time patients receive pre-procedural analgesia therapy and/or non-pharmacologic interventions • % compliance with institutional-specific ICU pain management protocols	• % failed attempts at SBTs due to either over or under sedation • % of patients undergoing EEG monitoring if: – at risk for seizures – burst suppression therapy is indicated for ↑ ICP • % compliance with institutional-specific ICU sedation/agitation management protocols	• % of patients receiving daily physical therapy and early mobility • % compliance with ICU sleep promotion strategies • % compliance with institutional-specific ICU delirium prevention and treatment protocols	Prevent

Table 13: CAM-ICU care

Feature 1: Acute Onset or Fluctuating Course	Score
Is the pt different than his/her baseline mental status? OR Has the patient had any fluctuation in mental status in the past 24 hours as evidenced by fluctuation on a sedation scale (i.e., RASS), GCS, or previous delirium assessment?	Either question Yes →
Feature 2: Inattention	
Letters Attention Test (See training manual for alternate Pictures) Directions: Say to the patient, "I am going to read you a series of 10 letters. Whenever you hear the letter 'A,' indicate by squeezing my hand." Read letters from the following letter list in a normal tone 3 seconds apart. S A V E A H A A R T Errors are counted when patient fails to squeeze on the letter "A" and when the patient squeezes on any letter other than "A."	Number of Errors >2 →
Feature 3: Altered Level of Consciousness	
Present if the Actual RASS score is anything other than alert and calm (zero)	RASS anything other than zero →

Table 14: Medscape Score

Indicator	Description	Score	
Facial expression	No muscular tension observed	Relaxed, neutral	0
	Presence of frowning, brow lowering, orbit tightening, and levator contraction	Tense	1
	All of the above facial movements plus eyelid tightly closed	Grimacing	2
Body movements	Does not move at all (does not necessarily mean absence of pain)	Absence of movements	0
	Slow, cautious movements, touching or rubbing the pain site, seeking attention through movements	Protection	1
	Pulling tube, attempting to sit up, moving limbs/ thrashing, not following commands, striking at staff, trying to climb out of bed	Restlessness	2
Muscle tension Evaluation by passive flexion and extension of upper extremities	No resistance to passive movements	Relaxed	0
	Resistance to passive movements	Tense, rigid	1
	Strong resistance to passive movements, inability to complete them	Very tense or rigid	2
Compliance with the ventilator (intubated patients)	Alarms not activated, easy ventilation	Tolerating ventilator or movement	0
	Alarms stop spontaneously	Coughing but tolerating	1
OR	Asynchrony: blocking ventilation, alarms frequently activated	Fighting ventilator	2
Vocalization (extubated patients)	Talking in normal tone or no sound	Talking in normal tone or no sound	0
	Sighing, moaning	Sighing, moaning	1
	Crying out, sobbing	Crying out, sobbing	2
Total, range			0-8

Other Behavior Scores: Adult, ICU, Dementia
1. BPS: Behavioral Pain Scale (Payen,2001)
2. CPOT: Critical Care Pain Observation Tool (Gelinas)
3. ADD: Assessment of Discomfort in Dementia Protocol (Kovach 1999)
4. CNPE: Nonverbal Pain Indicator Long Term Acute Care Setting (Feldt 1998)
5. Doloplus 2: Lefebre – Chapiro 2001
6. NO PAIN – Nursing Assisstant Administered Instrument to   Assess Pain (Snow et al 2003)
7. PACSLAC: Pain Assessment Scale for seniors with Severe Dementia (Puchs-Lacelle 2004)
8. PAINAD: Pain Assessment in Advanced Dementia Scale (Lane 2005)

Paediatric Pain Scales: Pain assessment by face of the child.
- DSVNI : Distress Scale for Ventilated Newborn Infant (tested in ventilated new borns ICU,procedural pain – Sparshott 1966)
- COMFORT Behaviour Scale: Neonate < 3 years

- Revised Comfort: Ambuci et al 1982; measures other constucts than pain; upto 9 years; ICU ventilation, Surgical setting
- N-PASS: Neonatal Pain Agitation and Sedation Scale
- DEGR: Douleor Enfant Gustave Roussy
- CHEOPS: Children Hospital of Eastern Ontario Pain Scale
- CRIES: Crying, Requires O2, Increased vital signs, Expression, Sleepless

Assessment and Management of Pain

Patient Education
1. Explain the pt's right to have pain assessed and managed
2. Discuss potential post operative/ procedural pain
3. Explain that effective pain relief is part of Pt Tt plan
4. Explain the pt's report of unrelieved pain is essential & instruct in how to report pain
5. Discuss that staff will respond quickly to reports of pain
6. Provide information about potential treatments including risks/ benefits/ side effects/ limitations

SCREENING
1. Confirm presence/absence of pain & intensity of pain
2. Ask "Do you have pain that you would like us to address? And have you had pain in the recent past that concerns you?"
3. Perform at- inpatient – outpatient visit – post procedures – with the routine nursing assessment unsolicited patient report of pain – time of discharge

ASSESSMENT
1. Choose a pain assessment scale appropriate for patients age/condition
2. Complete documentation including pain, intensity/quality, location, characteristics, and aggravating/relieving factors.
3. Set a real time patient comfort goal, with patient input- goal may relate to other factors – functional status, quality of life.

Pharmacology -Systemic Analgesics –
   1. Opioids(Fentanyl)
   2. Tranquilizers (Midazolam)
   3. NSAIDS-No sedation, Cardioresp Depr
   4. Dissociative (Ketamine)
   5. Adjuvants (Clonidine)

Table 15: Opoids- doses, routes.

Drug	Dose iv/id/PCA	Duration (mts)
1. Sufentanil	10 to 20 µg	20 – 45
2. Morphine	5/10 – 15 mg	30-60 / 120-180
3. Fentanyl	25-50/ 100 µg 10-25 µg PCA	20-40/ 30-60
4. Nalbuphine	10-20/1-3µg PCA	120-240
5. Butorphanol	1-2 µg/kg	120-240
6. Remifentanyl	0.1-0.5µg/kg PCA	2 - 3
7. Tramadol	100 µg/ kg	180

Post assessment Implementation of Treatment Plan
1. Initiate within one hour of pain identification and assessment
2. Include patient's comfort goal in plan
3. Use population- specific guidelines where applicable
4. Use pharmacology and/or non pharmacologic modalities as indicated
5. Continue treatment until patient comfort goal is reached

REASSESSMENT:
Performed within one hour of any pain intervention.2. Include intensity, quality, location, characteristics, aggravating & alleviating factors.3. Use same pain rating scale for all assessments, if scale is changed, note in medical record.4. Reassess comfort goal as appropriate.

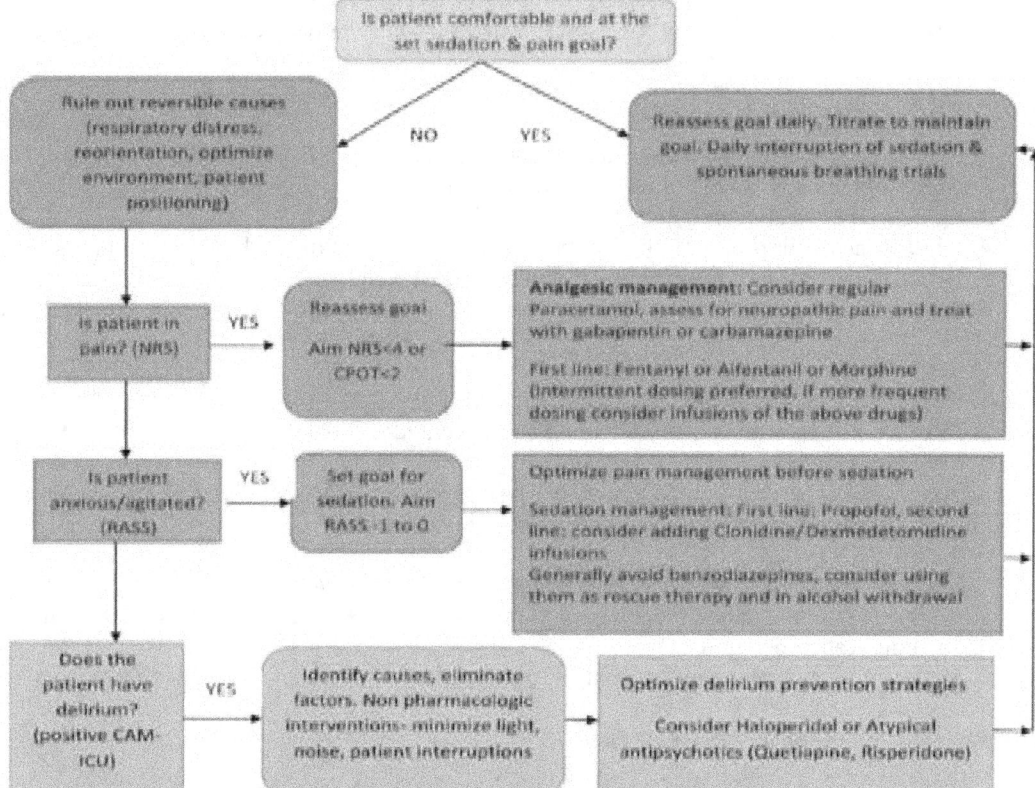

Fig 15: Medscape Reassessment flow chart

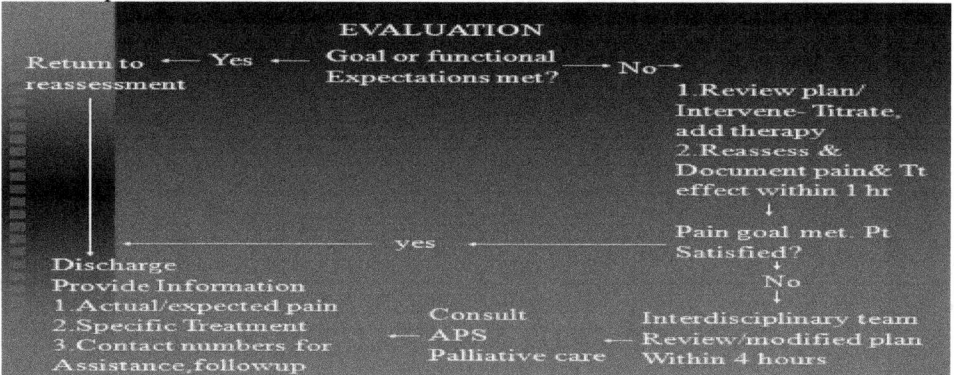

Fig 16. ICU Evaluation flow chart

Pain imaging

Spinal cord central pain:-
64-94% of patients with spinal cord injury have central pain. Etiology includes trauma (65%), iatrogenic (12%) inflammatory neoplasm, skeletal or vascular and congenital lesions.

Brain central pain:-
98.6% incidence caused by brain lesions are more intractable than those arising from spinal cord. It is caused by vascular causes, iatrogenic trauma, infra temporal infection, syringo bulbia and degenerative diseases. Right side lesions are involved in stroke induced pain having thalamus involvement.[1]

Treatment:-
=>Surgical: - The pain can disappear after removal of the tumor. Trauma pain can be relieved by exploring and excising the patient's atrophic cortex. Thalamic pain syndrome relieved by resection of post central gyrus. Cordotomy, trigeminal dorsal root entry zone, PVG stimulation relieves pain.

Features of central brain pain: - Central pain is of burning, cold, numb, tingle, sting, or itchy or aching bruise, sore, throbbing, cramping, tight or tearing.
Patho physiology is similar to peripheral neuropathic pain. The pain delays from a few weeks to months.[1]
Pattern of sensory loss:- Hemi body sensory loss- 46.5%, associated sensory-20.5%, hyperpathy, allodynia or both-6.8%, touch, position, vibration, sensory loss-5.5%

FUNCTIONAL IMAGING IN BRAIN:-

Functional imaging is a promising tool for investigating the mechanism of central pain. Cesaro et al found that stimulating the affected half of body, so as to produce hyperpathia in patients with stroke induced hyperpathic pain, produced thalamic hyperactivity in the SPECT scans, but this was not seen after stimulation of the unaffected side.[2] Patients without hyperpathia did not show this hypersensitivity to stimulation. It was hypothesized that loss of function of inhibitory thalamic neurons after a stroke result in disinhibition of medial thalamic nucleus and possibly pain. There was a reduced perfusion in parietal lobe further reduced by induced allodynia attributed to cortical inhibition. The injection of Propofol reduced brain central pain for 5 min during which cerebral hypoperfusion improved.[3]
Flirato et al[4]- in stroke patients studied with SPECT scans, found that patients with thalamic lesions tend to have superficial pain, while those without it tend to have deep pain. In the former there was reduced back ground neural activity and reduced O_2 consumption in thalamus. The central pain resulted from a chemical imbalance between glutaminergic and GABAergic mechanisms in transmission between sensory thalamus and cortex, which opposing glutaminergic and potentiating GABAergic transmission, by administering Ketamine or Propofol respectively.
Spinal cord pain functional imaging: An associated spinal cord injury, peripheral neuropathic or cancer pain, diminished perfusion of the human contra lateral thalamus in SPECT and PET. These changes could be normalized by relief of the pain by resection of syrinx in case of spinal cord or by cordotomy in cancer pain.[2]

Imaging the Brain during Pain
The large volume of the human forebrain in relation to the spinal cord suggests that descending modulatory influences are more important in humans than in other species. In humans the forebrain occupies 85% and the spinal cord 2% of the volume of the central nervous system,[1] but in rats the corresponding percentages are 44% and 35%, respectively. The human corticospinal tract contains almost a million fibers, but the spinothalamic tract contains only a few thousand. Consequently, descending forebrain influences are likely to play a uniquely important role in humans. Brain imaging depicts the activity of multiple supraspinal structures ranging from the brainstem to the forebrain. Supraspinal processing of nociceptive information activates somatic and autonomic reflexes, neuroendocrine responses, attention, arousal, evaluation of the spatiotemporal and physical features of the stimulus, hedonic experience, mnemonic functions, cognitive processes, and the ascending and descending control systems that mediate and modulate these activities and their interactions. To understand how multiple neuronal populations contribute to distinct nociceptive responses, and how they unite to produce integrated responses, requires conjoint analysis of conscious behavior and the activity of multiple synaptic populations.

Imaging Pathological Pain Most acute pain subsides with wound healing, but unfortunately, sometimes pain from injuries may persist, as in chronic complex regional pain syndromes (CRPS).[2] In animal models, continuing afferent activity originates spontaneously from damaged nerve fibers and from their cell bodies in the dorsal root ganglion. Evidence also suggests long-term changes in the physiology of spinal and supraspinal neurons, perhaps exaggerated by abnormal inputs from damaged peripheral nerves. Functional reorganization of sensory neurons in the spinal cord, thalamus, and cerebral cortex of animals occurs after peripheral injury with or without nerve damage. It was demonstrated that the intensity of phantom limb pain experienced by amputees correlates with the extent of functional reorganization of the somatosensory cortex. Patients with central pain provide evidence that central lesions alone may produce chronic pain in the absence of any nociceptive input.[3] These examples emphasize the need for information about supraspinal systems, including the forebrain, to better understand pathological pain of peripheral or central origin.

Types of Functional Imaging Functional imaging includes single photon emission computerized tomography (SPECT), positron emission tomographic (PET) studies of glucose metabolism or receptor binding, and electrophysiological methods such as magnetoencephalography (MEG) and high-density electroencephalography (EEG) with equivalent current dipole analysis (ECD). This brief review will concentrate on PET and functional magnetic resonance imaging (fMRI) methods to detect changes in regional cerebral blood flow (rCBF).

Physiological Basis for SPECT, PET, and MRI Imaged brain events correspond to activity in populations of synapses. The energy demand of synaptic activity requires rapid increases in local blood flow to deliver glucose and oxygen. Several experiments have demonstrated the close coupling of synaptic neurotransmitter release, recycling, and glucose utilization,[4] the global cerebral blood flow increased during brain activity. The, speciall optical sensors can monitor the reflectance of different wavelengths of light by synaptic populations as they respond to specific stimuli. Signals detected by this optical imaging originate within a few hundred microns of evoked synaptic activity and are thus capable of defining anatomical boundaries within the synaptic neuropil.. In PET activation, radiolabeled water or CO_2 is used, and the accumulated count of radioactivity provides an estimate of the regional cerebral perfusion during the scan (about 1 minute). This value is compared across conditions (e.g., pain or no pain) to obtain estimates of task-related or stimulus-specific changes in rCBF. When a population of active synapses uses oxygen, oxyhemoglobin is changed locally to deoxyhemoglobin. The different magnetic resonance signals of these two forms of hemoglobin make fMRI possible. The amplitude of the signal is proportional to the rCBF, which (as in PET) correlates with functional measures of neuronal activity. Among the advantages of fMRI is the lack of radiation, which offers the opportunity to repeat individual studies frequently. fMRI provides better spatial resolution than PET or SPECT. A disadvantage of fMRI is that ferromagnetic materials, present in most electronic devices and recording instruments, cannot be brought near the scanner magnet. Subjects with implanted ferromagnetic metal prostheses or other devices thus cannot be studied with fMRI. Another disadvantage of fMRI is that the imaging of resting (unstimulated) activity and the statistical analysis of the responses of the whole brain are less well established than for PET.

What PET and fMRI Reveal about Pain

Many discrete brain structures are active during pain. Although for many years multiple brain structures and pathways were known to participate in the processing of nociceptive information activity with the perception of pain which correlates specifically with synaptic activity in the primary and secondary somatosensory cortex (S1 and S2) and the anterior cingulate cortex. PET and fMRI studies have confirmed that activation of a network of interactive subsystems consistently occurs during perception of pain. Pain-related activity is found most frequently within the medial midbrain, thalamus, lentiform nucleus, cerebellum, and the insular, prefrontal, parietal (including S1 and S2), and anterior cingulate cortices. Thus, sensory, motor, association, and limbic systems combine to mediate the multiple components of the pain experience and response.

Normal group differences in pain perception are associated with differences in brain activation. There are differences in the spatial pattern and intensity of synaptically induced rCBF during different forms and intensities of innocuous and noxious thermal stimuli, the perceived differences between acute skin and acute muscle pain reflect differences in the intensity and spatiotemporal pattern of neuronal activity within overlapping sets of forebrain structures.

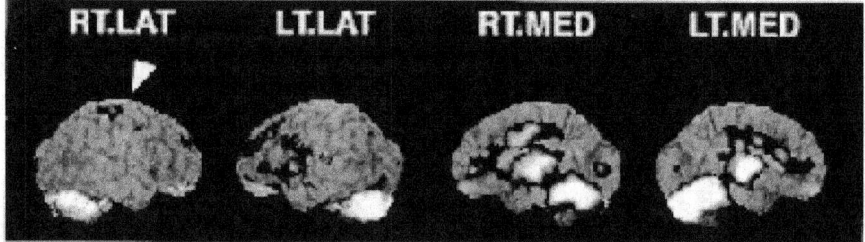

Figure 1: - Significant pooled rCBF increases (averaged across 11 normal subjects) during immersion of the left hand in painfully cold (1°C), compared to mildly cool (29°C) water. Responses significantly ($P < 0.05$) above global blood flow are shown in gray scale (white corresponds to $P < 0.0001$). Arrow indicates a response in the right (contralateral) sensorimotor cortex. Note the strong responses in the cerebellum, bilateral thalamus, and anterior cingulate gyrus (mid-anterior and perigenual regions).[7] Both male and female subjects rated 40° C contact heat stimuli as warm and 50°C stimuli as painful, and activation of the contralateral prefrontal cortex, insula, and thalamus overlapped completely in males and

females. However, females rated the 50° C stimuli as more intense than did males, and showed significantly more intense activation of the responding areas, [7] perception and brain activation were similar

The functional specificity of pain-activated brain regions can be identified in imaging experiments intensity in normal subjects, pain unpleasantness correlated with the intensity of rCBF response in a far anterior (dorsal perigenual) region of the anterior cingulate cortex, but not in the S1 cortex. The information about pain intensity was widely distributed among many, but not all, pain-activated regions, including the cerebellum, these brain structures are highly heterogeneous in function. In fMRI experiments designed to separate the perception of pain from the anticipation of pain, the activation of certain regions is better correlated with anticipation of pain than with pain perception. Unique patterns of forebrain activation occur in neuropathic pain. Imaging studies of pain caused by damage to the peripheral or central nervous system reveal that there is a thalamic hypoactivity at rest in patients with central neuropathic pain. [8]Painful dysesthesiae of the left hemibody and face following a lacunar infarction at the lateral edge of the right ventral posterior lateral thalamus on sensory examination revealed deep pressure allodynia on the left and symmetrical cutaneous heat pain thresholds. At rest, rCBF was less in the right thalamus than the left. The noxious heat stimulation (55°C) is equally painful on either side. During noxious heat stimulation of the right (normal) side, there was a slight reduction in rCBF in the left thalamus compared to its value at rest. When noxious heat was applied to the patient's left (abnormal) side, there was a strong rCBF increase in the right (contralateral) thalamus compared to the left. These results suggest that pathological hypoactivity in the resting hemithalamus masks an underlying hyper-responsiveness to noxious stimulation. This pathological hyper-responsiveness may be due to a loss of resting inhibitory activity within the thalamus

Therapeutic Implications of Pain Imaging: Understanding the pathophysiology of chronic, severely painful conditions could suggest preventive measures and physical or pharmacological methods targeted specifically against maladaptive central adaptations. Researchers must first distinguish between adaptive, neutral, and maladaptive reorganization. Anatomical and physiological differences among patients may require new, genetically based technology. Therapy may include local delivery of growth factors or specific suppressors, neurosurgical stimulation, or ablative procedures. Ultimately, defining each patient's pathophysiology will allow effective interventions to target specific sites and pathways based on information obtained through imaging that patient's pain.

References
1. Kumar P. Textbook of Pain.2nd edition. New Delhi CBS publishers.
2. Merskey H, Bogduk N. Classification of Chronic Pain: Descriptions of Chronic Pain Syndromes and Definitions of Pain Terms. Seattle: IASP Press, 1994.
3. Casey KLE. Pain and Central Nervous System Disease: The Central Pain Syndromes. New York: Raven Press, 1991.
4. Sokoloff L. In: Lassen NA., et al. (Eds). Brain Work and Mental Activity. Copenhagen: Munksgaard, 1991 52-64.
5. Casey KL, et al. In: Bromm B (Ed). From Nociception to Pain. New York: Raven Press, 1994.
6. Casey KL, Minoshima S. In: Jensen TS, et al. (Eds). Proceedings of the 8th World Congress on Pain. Seattle: IASP Press, 1997, pp 855-866.
7. Paulson PE. Pain perception and brain stimulation. Pain. 1998;76:223-229
8. Casey KL, et al. Abstracts: 9th World Congress on Pain. Seattle: IASP Press, 1999, pp 435-436.

Chapter 11.

Peripheral Nerve Blocks

Basis for use of peripheral nerve blocks:- To interrupt the nociceptive input at its very source or blocking the nociceptive impulses coursing in the peripheral nerves. This also interrupts abnormal reflex mechanisms contributing towards path physiology of some pain syndromes and blocking sympathetic hyperactivity. Low concentrations of local analgesics block unmyelinated C and B fibers and small unmyelinated delta C fibers with only a minor interruption of somatic motor functions. The neurolytics also acts in the same way on unmyelinated fibers sparing the other sensations e.g. touch, temperature and motor functions for a prolonged period.

Indications for nerve blocks

(1) Diagnostic Blocks (a) Ascertain specific nociceptive pathways.
    (b) Help determine mechanism of chronic pain syndromes.
    (c) Aid differential diagnosis of the site and cause of pain.
    (d) Determine patients' reaction to the pain relief.

(2) Prognostic Block (a) Predict the effects of neurolytic block/ surgery
    (b) Afford the patient to experience the numbness and other side effects and help patient to decide whether or not to have it done.

(3) Therapeutic Blocks (a) Control acute post operative and traumatic pain.
    (b) Breaking of vicious circle involved in the pain syndrome.
    (c) Provide temporary relief to permit other therapies or development of accessory muscle functions mobility.

Causes of Failures

(1) Inadequate knowledge of pain syndromes.
(2) Inadequate evaluation of patients.
(3) Inadequate management of patients before and after the block.
(4) Lack of appreciation of specific indications, limitations and possible complications of these procedures.
(5)

Basic principles of application of nerve block

(1) Ample knowledge of pain syndromes and therapeutic measures.
(2) Devoting adequate time and effort to evaluate the patient through history, examination and assessment of pain syndromes.
(3) High skill with the knowledge of anatomy, pharmacology and side effects.
(4) Patients must be fully informed about the procedure.

Diagnostic / Prognostic blocks require:

(a) Precise localization of nerves to be blocked with x-ray image intensifier.
(b) Injection of small volumes (2-4 ml) of local analgesics, avoiding spillage to adjacent nerves.
(c) No decisions made till 2-3 blocks produce consistent results.

Careful assessment of patients by physician for results

(a) Reaction of patient to needle insertion to evaluate pain threshold.
(b) Ascertain if intended nerve has been blocked.
(c) Evaluate efficacy of block in relieving pain, patho physiology and duration of pain relief.
(d) Record results in detail in patient's chart.

Equipments for peripheral nerve blocks

(1) Needles: - 22SG- 15cm, 12cm, 8cm. 25SG- 4cm, 3cm, disposable needles.
(2) Ring forceps
(3) Syringes – 1ml, 2ml, 5ml, & 10ml (preferably leur lock)
(4) Bowls for antiseptic and spirit.
(5) Gauge pieces 5-10 pieces.
(6) Local anaesthetic vial

(7) Neurolytic solution vial or ampoule (phenol, alcohol)

Table 1: Clinical characters and doses of local analgesics [1]

Character	Lignocaine	Bupivacaine	Prilocaine	Etidocaine
Latency(speed of onset)	Fast	Fast	Moderate	Very fast
Penetration	Marked	Moderate	Moderate	Moderate
Duration	45 min	90-120 min	1 hr	> 90 min
Optimal concentration- infiltration spinal nerve & plexuses	0.25 0.5-1.0	0.05 0.25-0.5	0.25 0.5-1.0	0.1 0.5-1.0
Maximum concentration(mg/kg)	3-5	2	6	2

Side effects and complications of regional analgesia
(1) Systemic Toxic reactions – excessive close infection, intravenous infections.
(2) A very high or total spinal anaesthesia due to dural puncture accidentally.
(3) Pneumothorax- brachial, caeliac, intercostal and Para vertebral blocks.
(4) Neurological complications – neuropathy, dysfunction.
(5) Other systemic reactions – psychogenic responses to local analgesics, anxiety, allergic reactions, idiosyncratic reactions. Prevented by aspiration, treatment by oxygenation and artificial ventilation, vasopressors, i/v fluids.

Neurolytic Agents[2]
(1) Absolute alcohol – 95% hypobaric, causes burning sensation for 2-5 mins. Side effects – neuritis.
(2) Aqueous phenol - 5% Hyperbaric, no initial burning sensation. Selective analgesic action (?), ease of injection. Less neuritis.
(3) Phenol in Glycerol – 5-8% solution. Not used now a days. Difficult to inject.
(4) Chlorocresol – 4-6% solution, hyperbaric, selective analgesia.

Premedication: - A barbiturate or anxiolytic drug is must for successful regional & peripheral nerve block.

Monitoring and resuscitation equipments:[3]
A careful monitoring of pulse, BP, twitching of eye muscles is needed for early local analgesic toxicity or sympathetic block. In the patients having cardiac diseases an ECG monitor is applied. Watch of respiration & Spo2 (pulse Oxymeter) may be needed. The x-ray or image intensifier is useful guide for nerve block.
The cardiac respiratory resuscitation instruments must be at hand. ECG defibrillator monitor, and i/v line with a pint of 5% dextrose / saline running, a tilting table, ambu-bag or anaesthesia machine with facilities for endotracheal intubation. The oxygen can be supplied by ventimask, nasal mask or by anaesthetic machine.

Drugs: - for emergency cardiac support. Atropine, Adrenaline, Antiemetics, Midazolam, Vasopressors, and Antierrythmics etc. must be available in nearby tray.

Oral analgesics used alongwith peripheral nerve blocks are aspirin, non steroidal anti-inflammatory drugs, opioids, tricyclic antidepressants and antiemetics.

The peripheral nerve blocks are used in combination with oral analgesics. Sometimes, catheters are placed for continuous/bolus injections of local analgesics. In cancer patients continuous infusion of 50% alcohol has been reported in some regional cancer centers with success. The catheters must be taken care well by preventing infection, breakage, blockade and kinking especially during their removal. A simple artery forceps clamped over the epidural catheter, if left for a few hours will remove it on its own due to its weight. The catheters are put in the in-patients as continuous watch is needed for any complication. Some times epidural catheters are left for many weeks in cancer patients for relief of pain. Currently many implantable devices are available which deliver analgesics in graded concentration for chronic pain relief.

The peripheral nerve blocks are used as one of the tools of the pain relief and not as a pan ace for it. The knowledge of anatomy and physiology of various nerves comes in handy for anesthesiologist who is using peripheral nerve blocks in the surgical operations for anesthesia. However, some enthusiastic surgeons manage local infiltration blocks for small procedures e.g. skin grafting, hydrocele, inguinal and femoral hernia, and caudal blocks. The ophthalmologist has been using local anesthetic drugs as surface analgesia and retro bulbar block , but complications like over dosage are quite frequent due to less appreciation and lack of knowledge about pharmacology and side effects of the drugs and technique. A better training for eye and general surgeon will help them performing many operative procedures in the field areas or now a days fashionable medical campus. However there is no replacement of the adequate knowledge and the treatment. Anesthesiologist also can not be absolved of the under use of regional epidural and peripheral nerve blocks even in major centers. However for a pain clinician a proper training of peripheral nerve blocks is a must.

Peripheral nerve blocks

Indications of somatic nerve blocks fall in to two categories (1) Diagnostic and treatment of cancer pain.
(2) Management of Neuralgias.

Dermatomes (fig.-1) is the area of skin predominantly innervated by a single spinal segment e.g. the C5 dermatome overlies the deltoid region. The dermatomes are not constant in all individuals. There is a particular confusion of cervico thoracic and lumbo sacral junctions. Foerster (1933) provided a chart of dermatomes by sectioning adjacent dorsal roots leaving a zone of remaining skin sensation. He also used electrical stimulation of the distal end of divided dorsal roots to produce cutaneous vaso dilatation approximating its dermatome. His dermatomal map is still in clinical use. When a patient describes pain radiating down an extremity or trunk, it is important to recognize and record the exact distribution of pain and the dorsal nerve involved. This helps in treating the pain by a peripheral nerve blockade as well.[5]

Fig. Dermatomes[4]

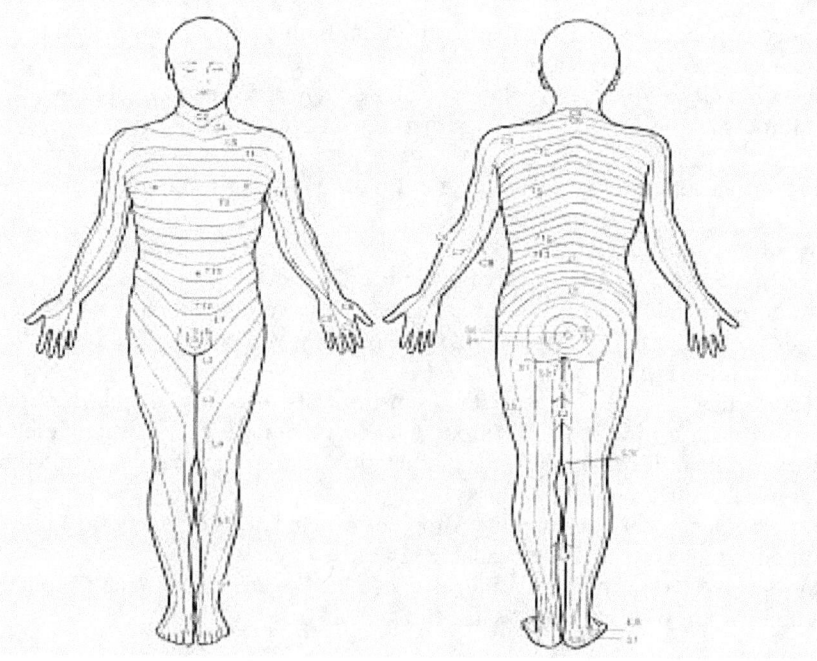

References
1. Textbook of Pain, 2nd Ed, CBS Pub New Delhi 2008.
2. Kumar Pramod - Terminal cancer care 2nd Edition, CBS Medical Pubs, New Delhi 2005.
3. Kumar Pramod - Guide to Peripheral Nerve Blocks 1st Edition CBS Medical Pubs, New Delhi 2008.
4. Kumar Pramod - A Handbook of pain management & related symptoms in cancer, Samvedana, Indraprastha Apollo Hospital New Delhi, 2003.
5. Kumar Pramod - Illustrated Atlas on peripheral nerve blocks Anaesthesia Dept. Jamnagar 2002.

Chapter 12.

Peripheral Nerve Blocks of Head & Neck Pain Relief

Gasserian Ganglion Block
- The needle inserted through a skin wheal skin overlying the second upper molar tooth directed to the midpoint of zygomatic arch, viewed from the front, directed to the pupil, depth marker set 1.5 cm.
- Eliciting paresthesia, a CSF drop over the hub of needle confirms successful block.
- 1-1.5 ml of aqueous phenol 5% or absolute alcohol, CT guided

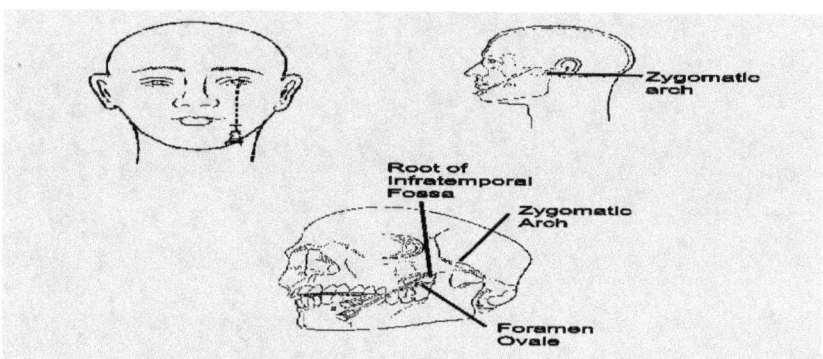

Fig 1: **Gasserian Ganglion Block**

Maxillary Nerve Block
- Mark skin just below the midpoint of the zygomatic arch.
- Needle is inserted straight on the lateral pterygoid plate. needle is withdrawn, redirected 1 cm anterior, superior, reaches till pterygopalatine fossa, maxillary nerve parasthesia

Fig:2:   Maxillary Nerve Block.   Fig 3:: Mandibular Nerve Block

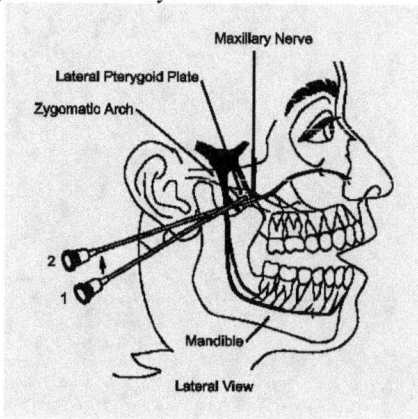 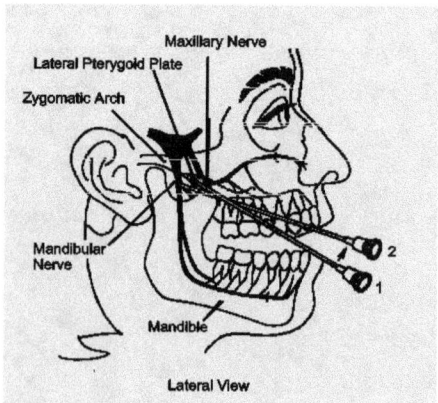

Mandibular Nerve Block
- Needle 1 is withdrawn reinserted 1 cm posterior and superior.
- Its point contacts the mandibular nerve just below foramen ovale.
- 2-3ml local analgesic/ neurolytic is injected

Terminal Branches of Trigeminal Nerve Blockade
- Supraorbital, infraorbital and mental nerves their exits from respective foraminae same plane as the pupil.

- 1-2 drops of neurolytic solution is injected

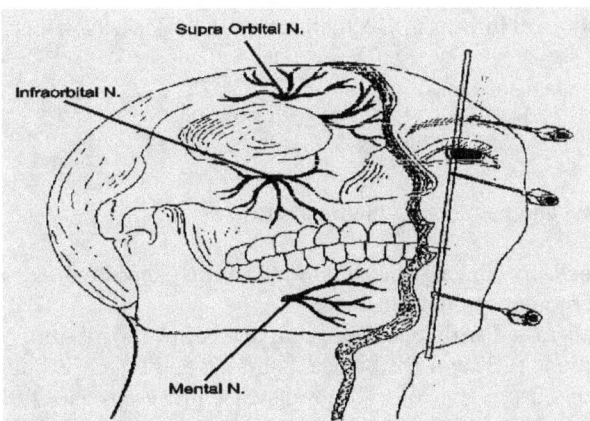

Fig 4: **Terminal Branches of Trigeminal Nerve Blockade**

Spenopalatine ganglion block
- Small cotton wick 4 to 5 cm long is winded down as in an oil lamp inserted into the nares involved.
- Local analgesic instillation breaks the cycle of pain which disappears after 3 to 4 days.

Surgical procedures
- Cryotherapy-cooling probe
- Damage the nerve/ganglion
- Relief >1year
- Anaesthesia dolorosa ,parasthesia, keratitis

Gangliolysis
- Lowest rate of complication –parasthesia
- Better control over extent of sensory loss
- Long term relief, low cost.
- **Procedure-** fluoroscopic control, G A
- Needle 2.5 cm to corner of the mouth in occlusal plane into foramen ovale.
- 60 Hz current – elicit paresthesia
- Radiofrequency lesion in ganglion
- Fogarty balloon catheter (#4) into Meckel's cave and inflate for 1-10 min (80%) success

Microvascular decompression
- 85% success – 5year
- Suboccipi8tal craniotomy under GA
- Visualize Trigeminal nerve under microscope near pons
- Repositioning of offending artery
- Coagulating a vein
- no sensory loss

Trigeminal Retrogasserian Neurectomy-Sectioning of trigeminal nerve root between ganglion and pons
- Approach posterior fossae
- Partial rhizotomy – reduces anesthesia dolorosa

Trigeminal Tractom- Section of trigeminal tract in medulla
- Loss of pain and temperature sensations
- No sensory loss

Stereotactic radiosurgery-Lesion made in trigeminal nerve root near pons
- Linear accelerator
- Gamma knife – cobalt 60

- Intersection of 210 beams used
- CT, MRI, contrast cisternography
- Pain relief – 77%, No risk of surgical infection, GA, hematoma, CSF leak, facial weakness, brain stem injury or hearing loss.
- Side effects – facial parasthesia, sensory loss.

Cervical Plexus Block:

Indications:- Thyroid surgery analgesia and pain due to malignancies.

Block 1. Superficial cervical plexus block- local analgesic solution (2 -5 mL) deposited along the line drawn on the posterior border of the sternomastoid muscle.
Deep cervical plexus block- three wheals raised with local analgesic just below the mastoid process (C2), second one finger breadth below wheal one (C3) and third wheal is drawn one finger breadth below the second wheal (C4) vertebrae, tubercle of Chassaignac of C6 on transverse process is a useful landmark. A 5 cm needle is inserted transversely about 2 - 4 cm deep till it reaches transverse process. After a negative aspiration test local analgesic or neurolytic is deposited. A single needle prick can also be used at C3 transverse process mastoid muscle and than redirecting it cephalad & caudad blocking all points.
Fig 5: Cervical Plexus BlocK

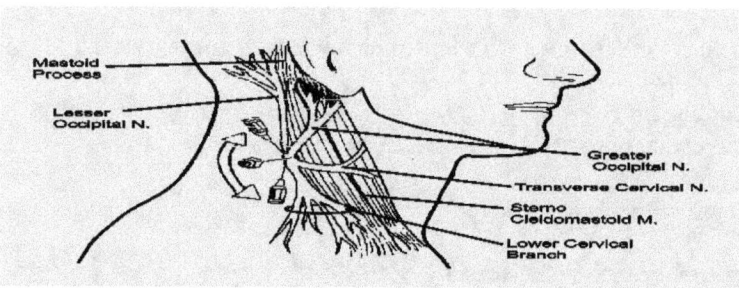

Stellate Ganglion Block

- Patient lying supine neck extended without a pillow. Wheal raised two fingers breadth lateral to jugular notch similar distance above clavicle, on the medial border of sternomastoid, palpating tubercle of Chassaignac transverse process. A needle directed backwards till it reaches bone. Withdrawn 0.5 cm & 10 mL of local analgesic/neurolytic injected. Horner's syndrome, lacrimation and red eye.

Fig 6:- Stellate Ganglion Block.   Fig 7:- Glossopharyngeal Nerve

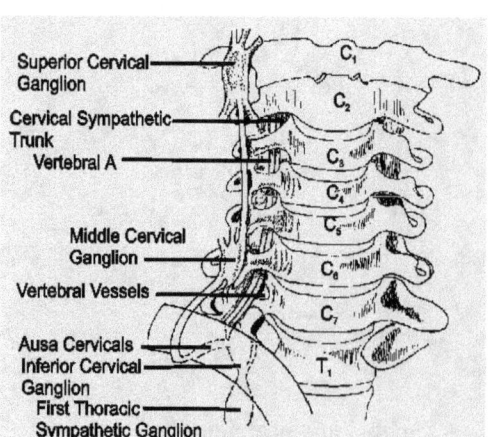 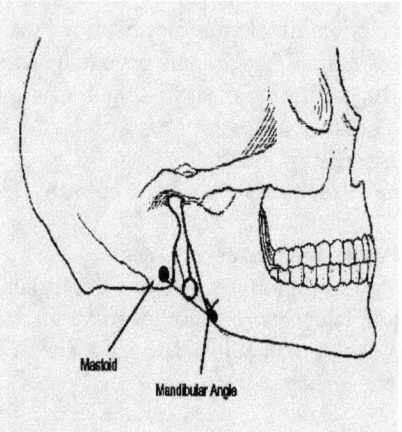

Glossopharyngeal Nerve

- Glossopharyngeal nerve, arises from jugular foramen, supplies posterior part of tongue and oropharynx.
- Patient in supine position, head lying rotated to opposite side, line drawn, joining tip of mastoid process and the angle of jaw. A wheal at midpoint, needle inserted perpendicular, it strikes the mastoid process 2-4cm, needle is withdrawn, reinserted anterior to the styloid process 0.5cm deeper, reaches glossopharyngeal nerve The vagus nerve is posterior to the styloid process

References

1. Textbook of Pain, 2nd Ed, CBS Pub New Delhi 2008.
2. Kumar Pramod - Terminal cancer care 2nd Edition, CBS Medical Pubs, New Delhi 2005.
3. Kumar Pramod - Guide to Peripheral Nerve Blocks 1st Edition CBS Medical Pubs, New Delhi 2008.
4. Kumar Pramod - A Handbook of pain management & related symptoms in cancer, Samvedana, Indraprastha Apollo Hospital New Delhi, 2003.
5. Kumar Pramod - Illustrated Atlas on peripheral nerve blocks Anaesthesia Dept. Jamnagar 2002.

Chapter 13

Peripheral Nerve blocks of trunk

The intercostal nerve block is done either at the angle of the rib or in the posterior axillary line with patient in lateral or supine position respectively. A needle is introduced near the lower border of the rib hitting it and slided past it, 3mm internally. 2-3 ml of 1.5-2 % lignocaine or even neurolytic solution can be used in trauma, fracture rib, cancer, herpes and other painful condition of the chest and rib resection. The midaxillary block misses the lateral cutaneous nerve.

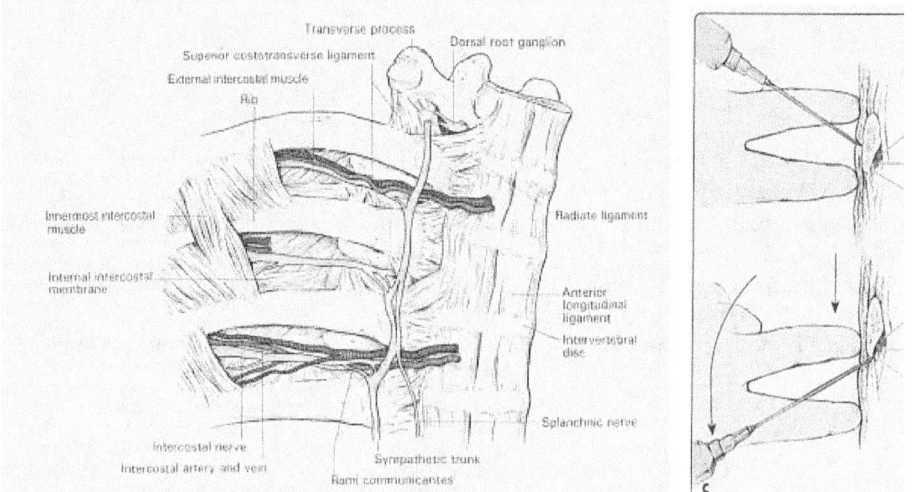

Fig 1: Anatomy and technique of intercostal nerve block.
    Side effects:- Pleural irritation or puncture.
    Geriatric patients: - The spines are fused so lateral approach is easier.

Techniques of spinal anesthesia:-

Intrathecal injection:- The patient in sitting or lateral position is painted and draped. A 25-27 SG lumbar puncture needle is introduced through an already formed wheal near the midpoint of lumbar vertebral spinous space. The needle punctures skin, subcutaneous tissue, supraspinous- interspinous ligaments and ligamentum flavum. There is loss of resistance to the needle which marks crossing the ligamentum flavum. In the lateral approach only ligamentum flavum is pierced. There is a click feeling as soon as the dura is punctured which is confirmed by a free flow of cerebro spinal fluid. Local analgesic 3-4 ml of Bupivacaine 0.25%, opiods is being injected through the needle and patient is made to lie supine with slight head up tilt to prevent reduction in blood pressure. After five minutes neurolytic drug Phenol can be injected.

    Side effects: - Hypotension, tachycardia, Bradycardia, nausea, regurgitation, headache, respiratory depression, neurological problems, backache at the site of puncture. Later is due to trauma to the tissues and multiple punctures.

Epidural block is given using an 18 SG touhy's needle which allows an epidural catheterization for prolonged analgesia and anesthesia. The procedure is same except dura is not punctured as in spinal intrathecal injection. This block has the advantage of no headache and more controlled segmental analgesia. Its use in trained hand is better and safer.

    Side effects: - Same as intrathecal injections except headache. An occasional total/ high spinal due to accidental puncture which is treated by endotracheal intubation, IPPV with vasopressor if needed. Surgery should be continued as planned as the patient regains consciousness and respiration as the local anesthetic effect wears off.

Spinal anesthesia in children: - Children vary in size and anatomy. Dura and spinal cord are at lower levels in infants and epidural space is shallow. The epidural fat is loose , more areolar so easy catheterization . The nerves are thin and incompletely myelinated, so onset of analgesia is faster with decreased concentration of local anesthetic drug.

Anatomical Difference: - Lower end of spinal cord is at L3 level in neonate, which moves upto L1 after 1 yr of age. Dura is at the lower level S4 and moves upto S2 level after 1 yr. The amount of CSF is 4ml /kg in neonate which reduces to 3ml/kg in small child and 2ml/kg in an adult. Skin to subarachnoid depth is 1.5cm. Psychological fear is to be taken care in children.

Low plasma protein binding enables more of the drug to remain in the active form upto 2 yrs of age, so danger of LA drug toxicity which can be masked by general anesthesia.

A 22SG Quincke needle (3.75cm) is used in children with 3mg/kg of lignocaine. Spinal opioids can lead to respiratory depression, nausea and vomiting.

Caudal epidural block:-
Technique of block:- With patient in supine or lateral position a wheal is raised over the sacral hiatus and entering the sacro coccygeal membrane at angle of 45 degree to the skin . Once the membrane is punctured the needle is depressed at angel of 30 degree entering the sacral canal for 2-3 cm. After aspiration and feeling of crepitus, after air injection in the canal, after a test dose of 8ml, upto 30ml local analgesic solution is injected.

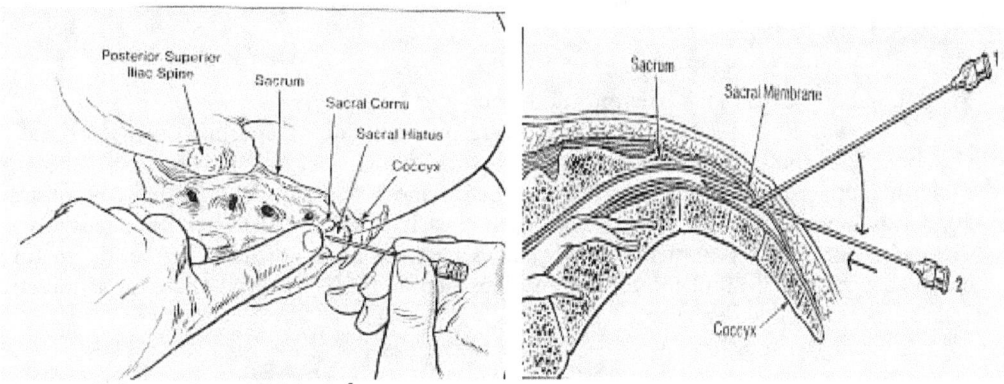

Fig 2. Technique of caudal block [3]

Indications: - Surgery in lower pelvis, Gynecology, forceps delivery, orthopedic operations, low back pain, pelvic pain.

Disadvantages: - (1) Anatomical variations (40%) (2) lack of control of height of analgesia (3) intrathecal injection (4) hypotension (5) infection.

Lumbar plexus block [4]:- Patient is in prone position with pillows flexing the lumbar spine or in lateral position with affected side up. Skin wheals are raised 5cm lateral to the upper borders of the spinous processes of L2, L3, L4 vertebrae just anterior to transverse process. A 15 cm needle is introduced through each wheal at right angle to the skin for 4-5 cm till it reaches transverse process. The needle is slightly withdrawn and directed upwards and inwards to pass in between transverse processes for 3-4 cm deep, to strike antero lateral aspect of the body of vertebrae. After careful aspiration, 10ml of 1% lignocaine is injected at each side. In the lateral approach wheal is raised at the apex of lumbar triangle formed by lower border of 12th rib, superior border of iliac crest and lateral border of para vertebral muscle (8cm lateral to mid point). The needle is inserted at an angle of 15* until it strikes body of vertebrae.

Indications: - Raynaud's disease, Burger's disease, traumatic vasospasm, thrombophlebitis, delayed healing of fractures, causalgias, Labour pain, renal colic.

Side effects: Intra dural puncture, intra vascular injection, shock, hemorrhage.

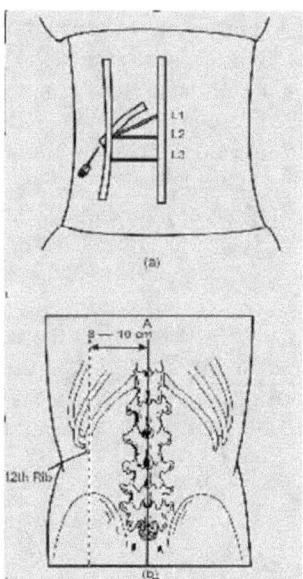

Fig 3. Lumbar plexus block Anatomy and technique [4]

Caeliac plexus block: - Two in number lying on each side of midline, on the aorta at the level of L1 vertebra. With the patient in prone position, spine of L1 vertebra is identified. Wheals are raised four finger breadth from the spine on each side below the 12th rib. A 20 cm needle is inserted at 45* to the median plane, facing inwards and upwards. It strikes body of L1 vertebra, partially withdrawn and directed more laterally until its bevel glances past the L1 body for a further 1 cm for 7 cm. After a careful aspiration 10-20ml solution of absolute alcohol (50%) or local analgesic is injected on each side. This block is given under sedation.

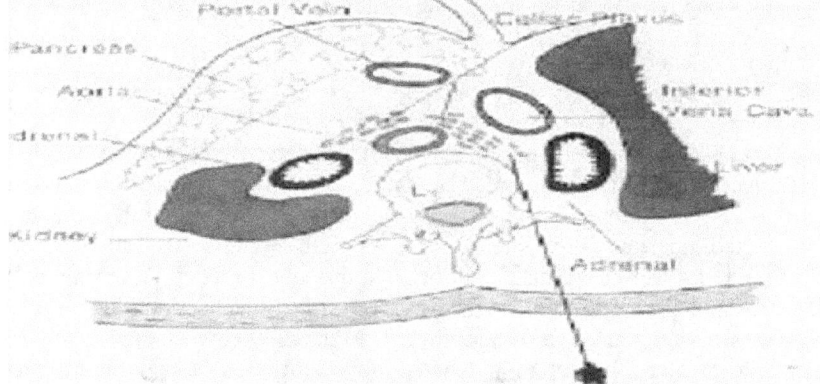

Fig 4: Posterior approach Caeliac Plexus block
Indications:- Acute pancreatitis, abdominal cancer.
Side effects: - Hypotension, puncture of aorta, renal vessels.

Superior Hypogastric plexus block:-
This plexus is formed by joining of lumbar sympathetic chain, branches of aortic plexus, Nervi erigentis (S2-S4). It divides in to left and right branches supplying inferior Hypogastric, ureter, testicular plexus, and sigmoid colon. It is situated on L5-S1 body near bifurcation of common iliac vessels. With patient in lateral position a skin wheal is raised in the midline at superior inter gluteal crease just above the anus. Stylet is removed from a 22SG 10cm needle which is bent 2.5 cm from its hub at 30* angle. Needle is inserted under fluoroscopy anterior to coccyx till its tip reaches sacro-coccygeal junction and position continued by injecting 2 cc of contrast medium. 4ml of 1% lignocaine or 10% phenol injected.

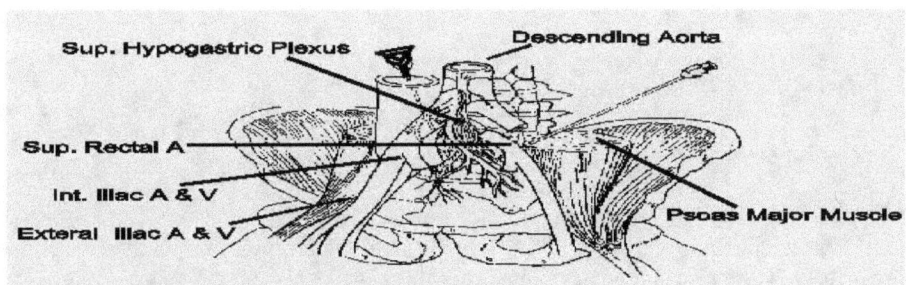

Fig 5. Technique of superior Hypogastric block [4]

Indications: - Cancer of pelvis, endometritis, inflammation and adhesions.

Technique of superior Hypogastric plexus block:- Skin wheal is raised 5-7 cm lateral to midline at L4-L5 interspace. A 20cm 22SG needle is directed midline at 30* cauded and 45* mesiad till it reaches L5 body, redirected again less mesiad till it walks off the body 1 cm further. After contrast medium confirmation, neurolytic agent is injected.

Femoral nerve block:- A wheal is raised one finger breadth in the outer ring of femoral artery, just below the inguinal ligament. A needle is inserted for 3-4 cm till the pulsations of the artery is transferred to the needle and 20 ml of 2% lignocaine is injected. The nerve lies beneath the deep fascia.

Indications:- Operations 5 cm below the patella & on lower femur when femoral nerve block is combined with sciatic nerve block.(2) for operation above the knee , lateral femoral cutaneous or obturator block.

REFERENCES
1. Raj PP .Practical management of pain , 3rd ed,St louis,Mosby year books,1998
2. Loeser JA, Bonica's management of pain, 3rd ed, Philadelphia, Iippincott-William & Wilkins,2001.
3. Wall PD & Melzack R. Textbook of pain(3rd) ed Edinburg z Churchill, Livingstone, 1994.
4. Kumar Pramod, Atlas on peripheral nerve blocks, Jamnagar ISSP Con 2002.

Chapter 14:

Lower Extremity Peripheral Nerve Blocks

Familiarity with anatomy and block technique
- Knowledge about the extent and limitation of each block
- Review the relevant anatomy prior to block
- Know the potential complications: phrenic nerve palsy in interscalene nerve block.
- Appropriate patient selection
- Amenable surgeon who can wait
- Failed block: GA/Sedation

Methods to Decrease the Risk of Nerve Injury from PNB
1. Aseptic technique
2. Blunt b**evel & insulated needles**
3. Use needles of appropriate length
4. Slow needle advancement
5. Slow **incremental injections** (15-20 ml/min)
6. Properly functioning nerve stimulator
7. **Avoid paresthesia** during injection
8. Choose appropriate local anesthetic drug
9. **Avoid blocks in anaesthetized patients**
10. **Avoid repeating block after failed block**

Nerves of Lower Limb

Lumbar plexus-
1. Lateral cutaneous N -L2-3.
2. Femoral nerve (L2-4)
3. Obturator nerve - L2--4
4. Genitofemoral N (L1-2)
5. Ilioinguinal, Iliohypogastric

Sacral plexus (S1-3) –
1. Sciatic nerve-L4,5,S1,3
2. Posterior cutaneous nerve of thigh S1,

3. Blocks Involving Lumbar Plexus
- Psoas Compartment Block-Posterior
- Femoral Nerve Block-Anterior
- Lateral Femoral Cutaneous N Block
- Fascia Iliaca Compartment Block
- Obturator Nerve Block

Psoas Compartment Block L4-L5 –
- Draw a line 5 cm parallel to spinous processes till it crosses PSIS. Mark where it crosses intercristal line.
- Advance needle perpendicular to skin until contact with L4 transverse process
- Withdraw needle & redirect 5° to 10° cranially to slide off the transverse process
- Incrementally inject 25-35 ml local anesthetic.

Psoas Comparment Block: Risks and Complications
- Epidural diffusion <1 to 16%
- Spinal anesthesia
- Intravascular injection:
  Seizures, Cardiac Arrest, Death
- Unilateral sympathectomy
- Renal subcapsular hematoma

- Psoas muscle hematoma
- Nerve Injury

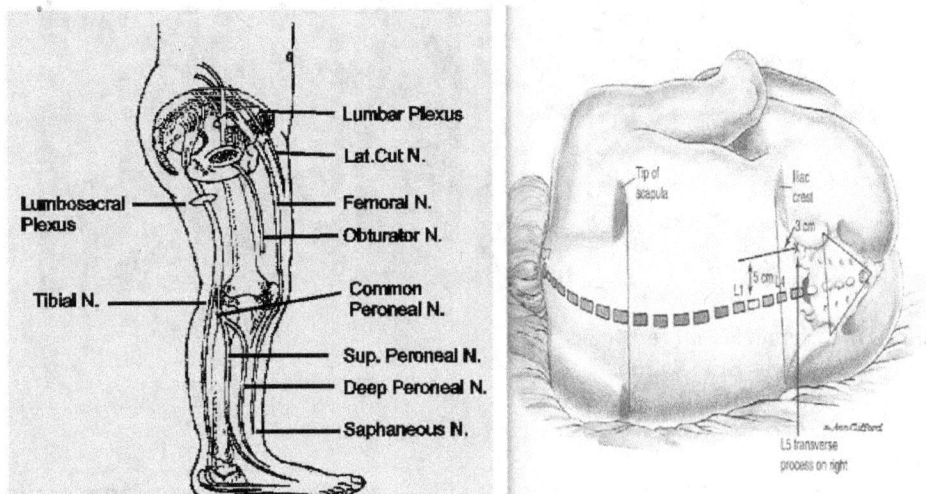

Fig1a: Nerves of lower limb. compartment block

Fig 1b: Surface landmarks of Psoas

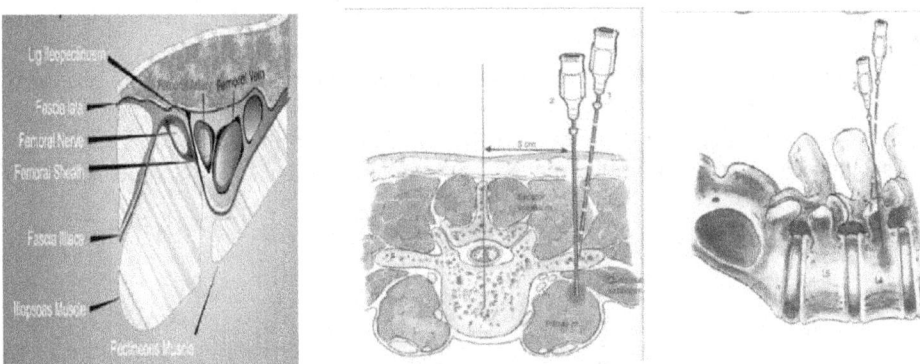

Fig 2 a: Psoas Comparment – Anatomy   Fig 2b: Spread of local anaesthetic in lumbar plexus block

Psoas compartment block – Clinical tips
- Avoid medial angulation as epidural/ intrathecal injection may occur.
- Useful for intra/ post operative analgesia in surgery for a fractured femoral neck.
- Of little value for total hip replacement because the hip joint is also innervated by the sciatic nerve and the cutaneous innervation will include the sub costal nerve.

Subcostal nerve: Clinical Tips
- A branch of T12 intercostal N. Blocked in conjunction with the lumbar plexus for hip surgery
- Landmarks: Anterior superior iliac spine, Iliac crest
- Technique: Using 22 G 80 mm needle make SC infiltration backwards from the anterior superior iliac spine along the iliac crest using 8 – 10 ml of solution

Femoral Nerve Block
- Position – Supine.
- Landmark: Inguinal crease, Femoral artery
- Continuously palpate femoral artery
- Shallow infiltration of local anesthetic
- Insert 4 cm insulated needle, Saggitaly, Slightly Cephalad, lateral to Femoral A.
  Fig: Anatomy of Psoas Comparment

Fig 3. STEPS OF FEMORAL NERVE BLOCK

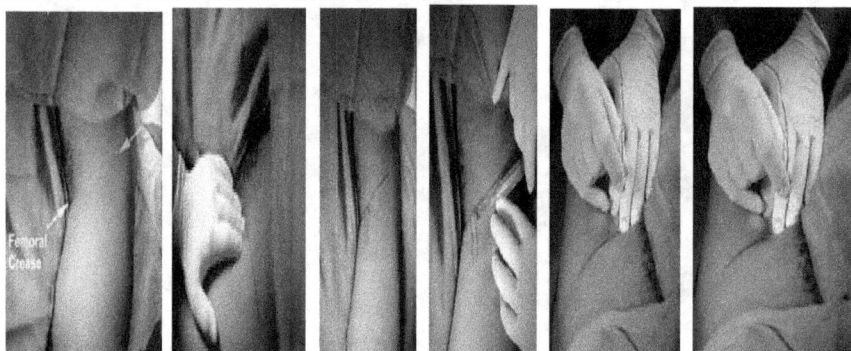

Clinicl Tips: Femoral Nerve Block
- Quadriceps Stimulation
- Patellar Twitch (0.2 – 0.5 mA)
- Failure to obtain quadriceps twitch on first needle pass

1. Redirect 10° to 15° laterally
2. Withdraw and reinsert 1 cm laterally Inject 15 – 25 ml of local anesthetic Sartorius stimulation is often achieved Medial/ anterior thigh contraction. Redirect laterally and deeper – elicit patellar ascension as quadriceps contract

Uses: Surgery for anterior thigh, knee or femur.

Winnie's 3 in 1 block
- As in femoral nerve block, placement of LA in femoral canal will result in proximal spread in to the psoas compartment
- Block 3 nerves: Femoral Nv, Obturator Nv, LFC Nv (3 in 1)
- Fascial sheath surrounding the lumbar roots extends into the femoral canal & acts as a closed conduit for the spread.

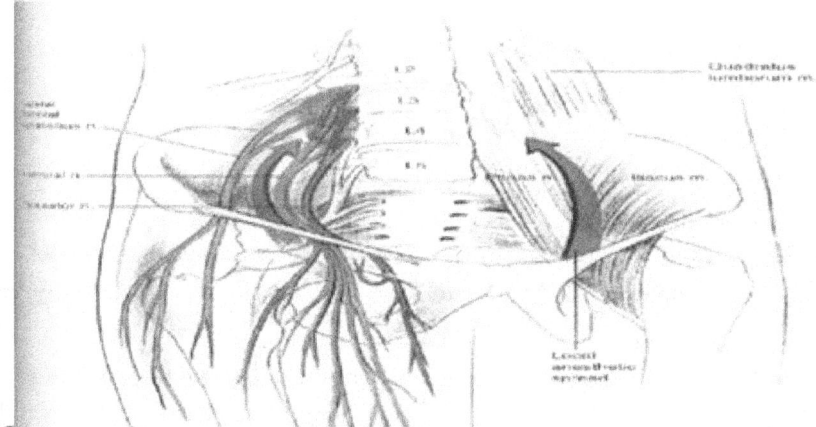

Fig 4: Nerves of Lower limb.

Lateral cutaneous nerve block:
- A wheal raised 1 finger breadth below & medial to the anterior superior iliac spine below inguinal ligament.
- A needle is inserted perpendicular to the skin & 10m LA deposited between skin & iliac bone, & below fascia lata.
- Indications: - Skin grafts of thigh when used with femoral nerve block

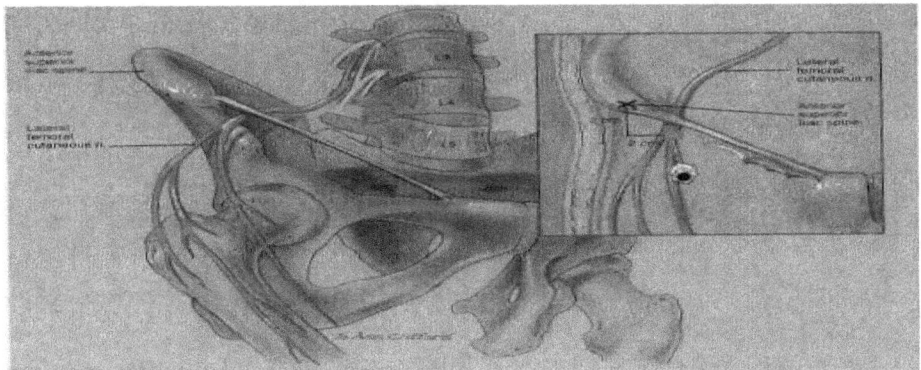

Fig 5: Lateral cutaneous Nerve block

Fascia Iliaca Compartment Block
- Insertion point :1 cm caudad to lateral and medial two thirds of inguinal ligament
- Insert perpendicular to skin.
- Advance needle to first loss of resistance (Fascia Lata).
- Advance needle to second loss of resistance (Fascia Iliaca).
- Inject 30 ml LA.
- AnalgesiaAnterior / Lateral thigh,Femoral shaft,Knee surgery

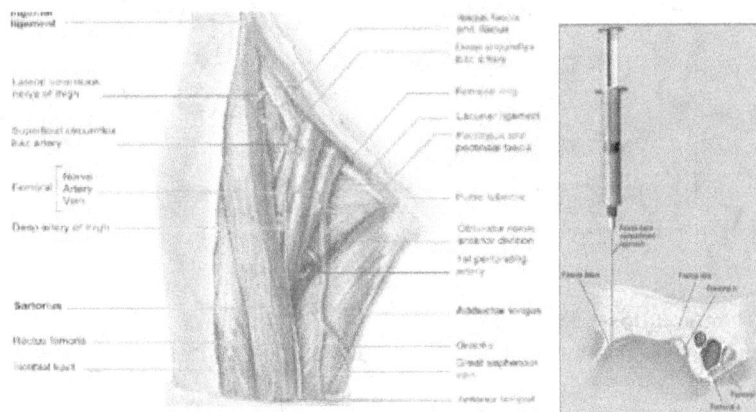

Fig 6: Fascia Iliaca Compartment Block

Obturator N block
- A wheal raised 1 cm below & lateral to pubic tubercle & a 5 cm needle introduced till it strikes bone.
- An 8 cm needle inserted in the track of first one & moved laterally aiming ASIS, a resistance of obturator membrane & adductor motor stimulation seen (2), Inject 10 ml LA.
- Clinical Tip Adductor spasm
- Knee surgery. Analgesia below pubic symphysis (with sciatic N block) for fracture of femur, skin graft.

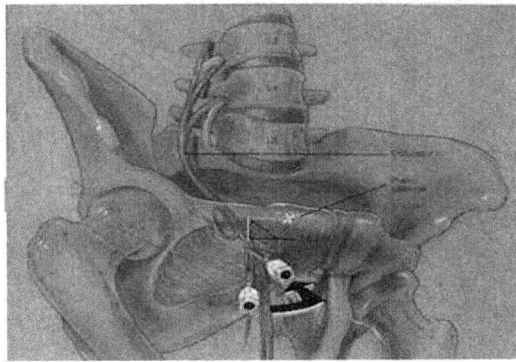
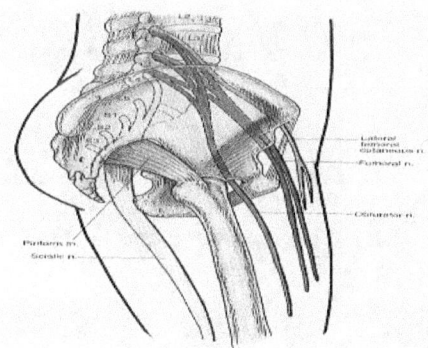

Figure 7a: Obturator block.   Fig 7b: Sciatric Nerve

Sciatic Nerve

- Leaves pelvis through greater sciatic foramen under the pyriform muscle and lying between the ischial tuberosity and the greater trochanter.
- Divide into lateral and medial popliteal nerves.
- Supplies the skin of the back of leg and the sole of the foot.

Indications- fractures around ankle, foot, knee, lower leg, ligation of varicose vein (with femoral block).

Sciatic N Block

- Posterior Approach: Patient in Sim's recovery position and arrange the knee, greater trochanter and posterior superior iliac spine in a line.
- Draw a line connecting PSIS & greater trochanter. At its midpoint drop a perpendicular line to intersect another line joining the greater trochanter & the sacral hiatus
- Insert a 22 G 10 cm needle perpendicular to skin at 8-10cm depth & elicit foot eversion (peroneal) & plantar flexion (tibial). Inject 15 – 20 ml of LA solution.

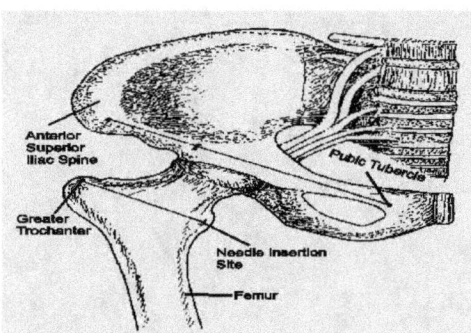 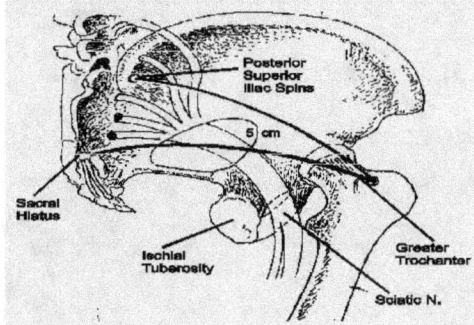

Fig 8: Sciatic Nerve Block

Sciatic Nerve– Clinical tips

- Only the classical posterior approach guarantees block of the posterior cutaneous nerve of the thigh
- If the nerve cannot be identified immediately, walk along the perpendicular line
- The onset of the block is slow –up to 60 min.
- The tibial & peroneal components may divide anywhere from the sciatic notch to the popliteal fossa. Aim for foot inversion & plantar flexion.
- Avoid adrenaline containing solutions as the nerve has a poor blood supply

Sciatic nerve block

- Ant. Inferior & lateral approaches
- Anterior approach: Supine position, Line of inguinal ligament trisected in 3 equal parts. A line is drawn parallel to above from greater trochanter. From the junction of inner & middle third of inguinal ligament, a perpendicular is drawn to the lower line & a wheal is raised at this point. A 10-15 cm needle inserted backwards and outwards till it meets the femur.
- A marker placed 5cm from the skin, needle partly withdrawn, redirected slightly medially just beyond the point where needle touched the femur,Inject 20-30 ml of LA .

Popliteal fossa

- A diamond shaped structure with sciatic nerve at the lateral border of the apex.
- The common peroneal nerve runs along the lateral border of the lower apex and blocked there- dorsiflexion
- The tibial nerve runs lateral to Popliteal vein and artery and blocked at the crease of knee joint –planter flexion

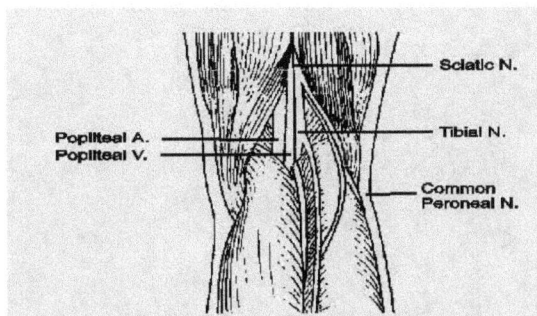

Fig 9: Popliteal Fossae Anatomy & Nerve Block

Popliteal Block: Lateral Approach
- Position – supine.
- Leg extended with foot at 90 degree angle to table Site of insertion :Intersection
- of vertical line drawn from upper edge of patella & groove between lateral border of biceps femoris and vastus lateralis
- 10 cm needle inserted at a 30 degree angle posterior to horizontal plane
- Tips:Elicit inversion response, If eversion direct needle posteriorly

Popliteal N B – Clinical tips
- The sciatic nerve is two nerves loosely bound together; commonly dividing into the tibial & peroneal nerves, 5 – 12 cm above the popliteal crease. In a small proportion of people it is separated for its entire course.
- High volume popliteal techniques – often block both the nerves, but individual localization of each nerve may improve the success rate.

Intra articular block
- This block is indicated for knee arthroscopy.
- Landmarks: Medial border of patella.
- Technique: Fully extend the knee.
- Identify the gap between the medial border of the patella & femur.
- Insert a 22G 50mm needle into the knee joint.
- Inject 30ml of 0.5% L -bupivacaine with adrenaline. Onset 40 min & duration 3 – 5 hrs.
- Inject portal sites with 1% lidocaine by surgeon.

Intraarticular – Clinical tips
- Sterile technique is of the utmost importance when injecting into a major joint
- Addition of morphine 2 – 5mg may improve postoperative analgesia
- Adrenaline containing solutions have the advantage of minimizing bleeding into the joint.

Saphenous nerve block at the knee

Indication: Ankle,foot surgery. Patient in sitting position, leg externally rotated.

A terminal branch of femoral which is subcutaneous below sartorius muscle at the medial side of the knee joint A line is drawn from the anterior border of medial epicondyle along the crease of knee joint till posterior border of medial epicondyle. A wheal is raised at midpoint in the subcutaneous tissue avoiding vein.

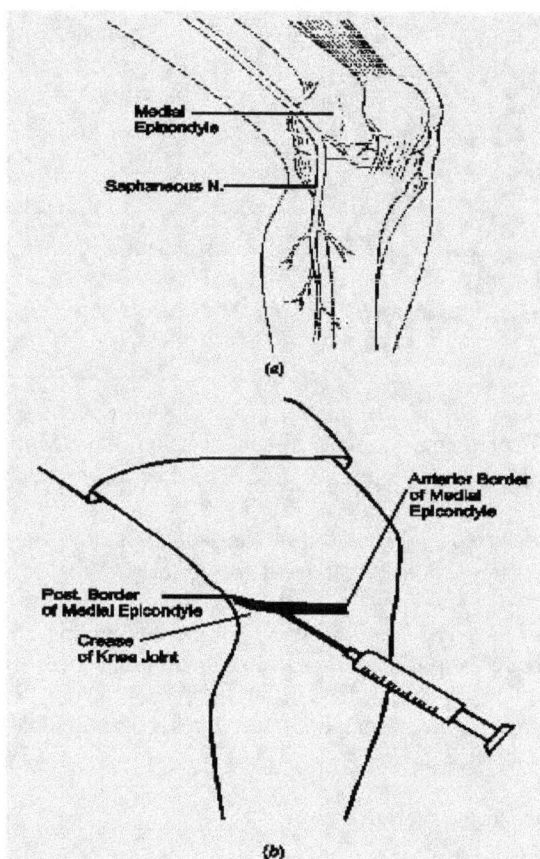
Fig 10:.Saphenous nerve block at the knee

Cutaneous nerve distribution of ankle
- Front of the ankle joint nerve supply: deep peroneal & superficial peroneal nerve.
- Back of ankle joint up to heel and anterior & posterior sole of foot is supplied by sural nerve.

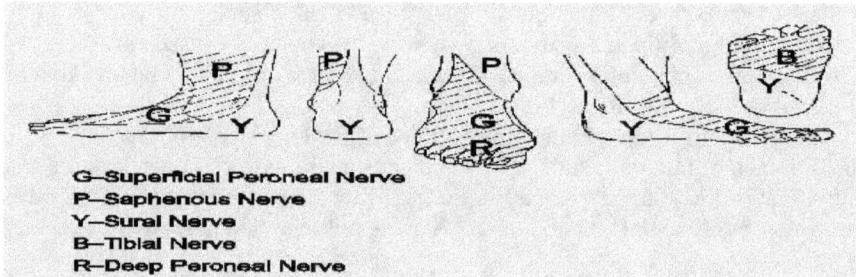
Fig 11.Cutaneous nerve distribution of ankle

Ankle block
- A s/c & intradermal wheal is raised circumferentially around ankle above medial malleolus.
- Sural nerve Blocked on line joining medial and lateral malleolus, below and posterior to the lateral malleolus.
- Posterior tibial nerve Prone Pt Blocked through a point on circular wheal just internal to tendo Achilles', deep to flexor retinaculum near the palpable posterior tibial artery. The nerve blocked behind medial malleolus using 10 ml LA.

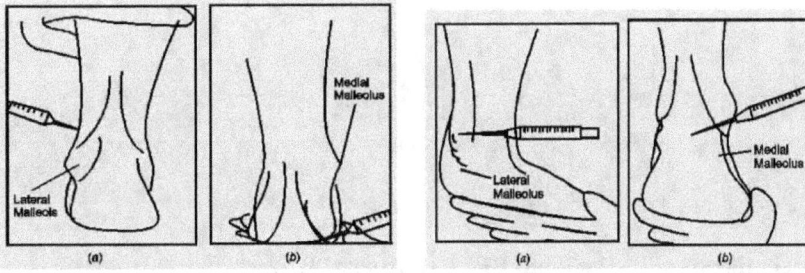

Fig 12: Ankle Blocks   Fig 13: Superficial Peroneal Saphenous & anterior Tibial N

Superficial peroneal nerve

It is blocked above the ankle joint by a subcutaneous wheal extending from the front of the tibia to lateral malleolus. It supplies front of the foot.

Saphenous nerve

It is blocked anterior to the medial malleolus using 10 ml of LA. It blocks the skin just below and above the internal malleolus.

Anterior tibial nerve

It is blocked midway between most prominent points of medial & lateral malleoli on circular line of infiltration in front of ankle joint. Needle pointed medially towards anterior border of medial malleolus and LA injected between the skin & bone

Digital Nerve Blocks
- Metatarsal Approach: 22 G 50mm needle at mid metatarsal level, 6ml .
- Digital Approach: A 22 G 50mm needle distal to metatarso-phalangeal joint, 3-6 ml
- Web Space: A 23 G 25mm needle into the web space, 6 ml
- Avoid adrenaline containing solutions.

References

1. Textbook of Pain, 2nd Ed, CBS Pub New Delhi 2008.
2. Kumar Pramod - Terminal cancer care 2nd Edition, CBS Medical Pubs, New Delhi 2005
3. Kumar Pramod - Guide to Peripheral Nerve Blocks 1st Edition CBS Medical Pubs, New Delhi 2008
4. Kumar Pramod - A Handbook of pain management & related symptoms in cancer, Samvedana, Indraprastha Apollo Hospital New Delhi, 2003
5. Kumar Pramod - Illustrated Atlas on peripheral nerve blocks Anaesthesia Dept. Jamnagar 2002

Chapter 15:

PERIPHERAL NERVE BLOCKS IN CHILDREN

Bier (1899) used spinal Anesthesia in 11 yr. old.

Reasons for underutilization of Regional Block (Eather, 1975)
Lack of experience.
Fear of adverse effects and
Lack of patient co-operation.
By 1990 there was an increased awareness about post operative analgesia due to –
Better ambulation of patient
Use of general anesthesia before regional block takes care of patient's cooperation
Fewer side effects.

General considerations
Children vary in size and Anatomy (Table 1)
Dura and spinal cord reach lower levels in infants.
Epidural space shallow
Epidural fat is looser, more areolar. Easy catheterisation.
Thin ligaments & fasciae – less resistance to needle tip.
Thin and incompletely myelinated nerves - ↑ onset, conc. of L.A.,
High parenteral acceptance (90%) but restless child (40%).

PERCEPTION OF PAIN IN CHILDREN
Motivational pain
Slow or True pain
C fibers – fully functional
Cognitive pain (Evaluative component)
A delta fiber
Not fully developed
Influenced by environment, socio cultural and past experiences
Difficulty
Communications
Assessment

PHYSIOLOGICAL CONSIERATIONS
Frightened by new environment
Cannot distinguish between adjacent parts e.g.. Forearm with arm.
No concept of parasthesia, differential block (localization of nerve by peripheral nerve stimulator)

PSYCHOLOGICAL CONSIDERATIONS
Pain free postoperative period which helps the patient as well as the relatives and the medical team
Persistence of motor/ sensory block – frightening (needs careful explanation)

CONTRAINDICATIONS
Infection
Bleeding disorders
Allergy
Uncorrected hypovolemia
Vertebral anomalies
Degenerative compressive neuronal disorders
Parent's refusal

Indication of Sole regional Anaesthetic
Premature infants requiring surgery below umbilicus
Risk of post-operative apnoea – NM diseases.
Chronic airway or pulmonary diseases eg. Tracheomalacia, asthma
Malignant hyperthermia
Post-operative, malignant and vascular spastic pain.

Anatomic differences in Children & Adults:

Anatomy Variable	Neonate	Small child 1 Yr.	Adult
Lower end of spinal cord	L3	L1	L1
DURA	S4	S2	S2
CSF/Kg	4 ml	3 ml	2 ml
Epidural Fat	Loose	Loose	Firmly Packed

Dosage of Local Anaesthetics (in mg/kg):

	Topical	plain soln.	Injection Epinephrine
Bupivacaine	-	2.5	2.5 – 3
Lignocaine	3	5	7 – 10
Mepivacaine	5	5	7
Etidocaine	-	3	3 – 4

Toxicity of L.A. in Children
Low Plasma protein concentrations.
Enabling more of drugs to remain active (till 1yr. age.)
Leads to Neurological toxicity at lower conc.
Reduced metabolism due to decreased plasma pseudo-cholinesterase & decreased hepatic microsomal activity.
Larger cardiac output leads to ↑ conc. and shorter duration.
General Anaesthesia may mask the signs of L.A. toxicity.

Specific blocks in children – Caudal Analgesia
Better cardiovascular stability.
Easy to perform & reliable up to/> 10K.g. B.W.
Rare but serious complication as with any regional block
In awake patient., psychological trauma and restlessness present.

Anatomy: Sacrum formed by fusion of five sacral vertebrae.
Sacral hiatus is the non-fusion of 5th vertebral arch.
Large bony processes on either side are sacral cornua.
Variable anatomy of sacral hiatus.
Sacral hiatus more cephalad and dural sac nearer.
Less resistance to cephalad spread of L.A.

Technique:
In lateral position identify hiatus by finger between cornua.
Taking antiseptic care using 23 G, 2.5 cm long needle over syringe filled with L.A.
Needle is placed midline at 60° to coronal plane.
Needle advanced ventrally till sacrococcygeal membrane is punctured.
Then lower the needle to 20° angle and advance 2-3 mm.
After negative aspiration L.A. injected in increments.
Analgesics used – Buprenorphine, clonidine.

Volumes of L.A. for caudal block (Armitage, E.N., 1986)

Volume (ml/kg)	Dermatomal level
0.5	Sacral
0.75	Inguinal
1.0	Lower thoracic
1.25	Mid thoracic

Continuous caudal in children:
    Easier cephalad access than lumbar epidural
    Less traumatic to spinal cord
    20 S.G. Touhy or Crawford needles (3.75-5 cm long) with 24G catheter or 2 2 gauge I.V. catheter over needle.
    Two occlusive dressing at gluteal crease and cephalad to catheter
    Used for high risk infants for GA or P.O. Analgesia.

Lumbar Epidural block:
    Used as an adjunct to GA for P.O. analgesia.
    Less chances of feco-urinary contamination as in caudal.
    Depth of epidural space from skin increases with age (10-18mm)
    Loss of resistance technique can lead to air embolism.
    Intravenons micro drip infusion with air bubble technique.
    Short (2.5 to 4 cm); Tuohy needle with short bevel, 20 SG with 24 Catheter.
    Bupivacaine infusion: loading 2 mg/kg, infusion 0.2 to 0.4 mg/kg/bw.
    Analgesic – morphine, fentanyl, sufentanil, butorphanol.
    Respiratory depression, nausea and vomiting.

Spinal Anaesthesia:
    Used in infants for high risk of P.O. apnoea following G.A.
    L.P. performed at L4/L5 interspace
    Skin to S.A. space depth is 1 to 1.5 cm.
    A 22 gauge, 3.75 cm Quincke needle used.
    Less distinct pop of ligenants & dural puncture.
    Less cardiovascular changes (<5 yr.age) - ↓ vagal activity, No venodilatation.
    Shorter duration of L.A. in younger age.
    Respiratory depression negates sedation in infants
    Lignocaine dose – 3mg/kg of 5% sol. (7.5% with Adrenaline)
    Incidence of post spinal headache is smaller than adults.
    Spinal opioids lead to resp. depression, nausea & vomiting.

Pediatric extremity blocks:
    Bony land marks easily palpable.
    Less co-operative to needle placement.
    No concept of parasthesia – P.N.S. is helpful.
    Propofol: 1 to 1.5 mg/kg bolus than 100-150 µg/kg/min.
    Bupivacaine: (0.25%) 0.25 mg/kg. Lignocaine: (0.25 to 0.50%) 5mg/kg.
    Radial, median and ulnar nerves blocked at wrist.

Axilliary Block:
    Safe and easy to perform.
    Nerves are superficial. Deep injection leads to failure.
    Technique is same as in adults.
    Musculocutaneous nerve block is more frequent.
    Catheters can be employed for continuous infusion.

Interscalene / parascalene block:
    Best for shoulder and upper arm involvement.
    Peripheral nerve stimular is used in lieu of parasthesia.
    Interscalene groove is easily palpable.
    Parascalene block is safer than supraclavicular block.

Intravenous Regional Anaesthesia:
A butterfly canula inserted into the hand.
Extremity is exsanguinated by gravity.
Tourniquet pressures: 180-240 mmHg. (Upper hand), 350 mmHg for lower limb.
Dose: 3 mg/kg (0.5%) lignocaine.
Keep tourniquet minimum for 20 minutes.

Lower Extremity Blocks:
Sciatic Nerve Block
Given under GA using anterior approach and using loss of resistance.
Employed in combination with femoral or lumbar plexus blocks.
Anterior approach (Mc Nicol & Salens) (supine)
A lineis drawn from anterior superior iliac spine to pubic tubercle.
A second line is drawn parallely medially from greater trochanter.
A perpendicular line is drawn from medial and middle parts of 1st to 2nd line.
Needle walks past the femur, enters thigh muscles.
Loss of resistance after sciatic neurovascular comp. is reached.
Peripheral nerve stimulator elicits dorsiflexion (tibial) or planter flexion (common peroneal n.) of foot.

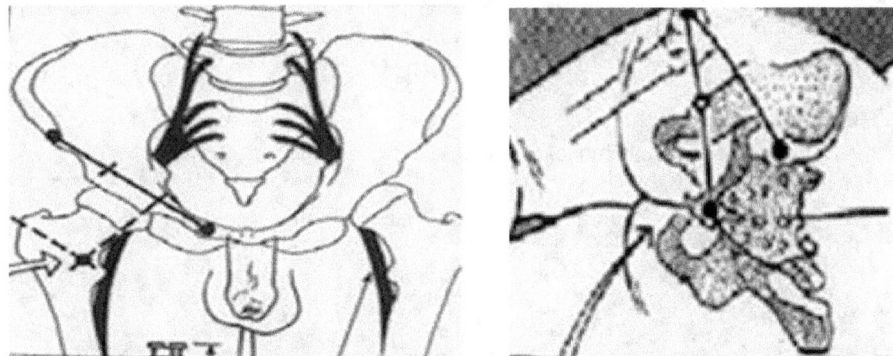

Fig :. Sciatic Nerve Block (Anterior & Classical Labat's approach)

Posterior approach: (Lateral Position)

Labats line – perpendicular line from midpoint of line drawn between superior border of greater trochanter and post.sup.iliac spine.
Winnie Modification for Ht,-Line between greater trochanter & sacral Hiatus.
Sciatic nerves are entered at the intersection of these lines.

Femoral Nerve Block:
Located lateral to femoral artery, deeper to faciae lata & Iliaca.
Used for analgesia, femoral shaft fractures.
After Quadriceps muscle contraction – L.A. is injected.

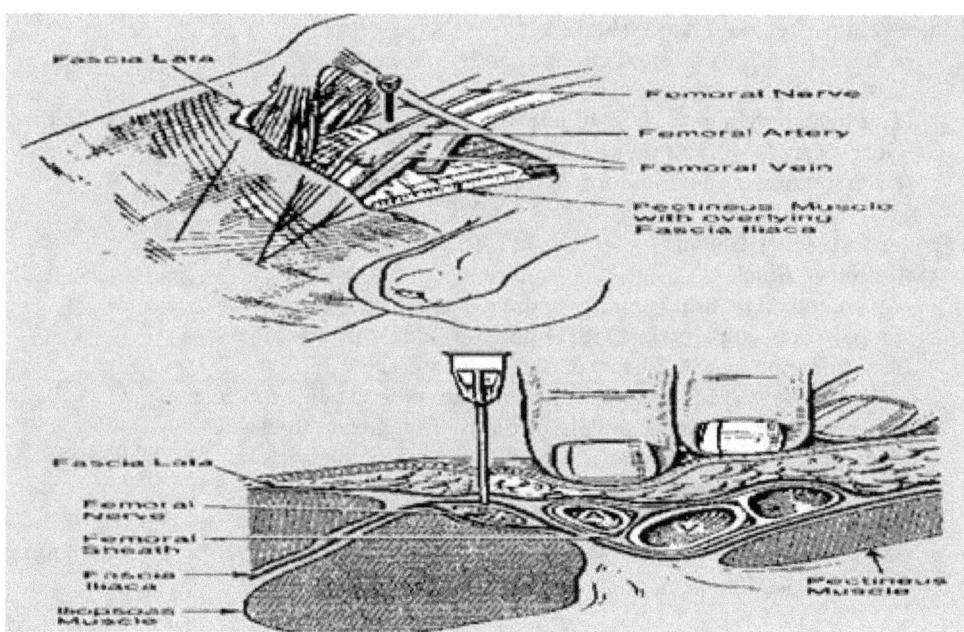

Fig 2. Femoral Nerve Block:

Lateral Cutaneous N. of thigh:
- Used for skin grafts and muscle biopsies.
- Injection medial to Ant. Sup. Iliac spine.
- First loss of resistance felt at External oblique aponeurosis and second after needle crosses ext. Oblique muscle & enters fascial canal.

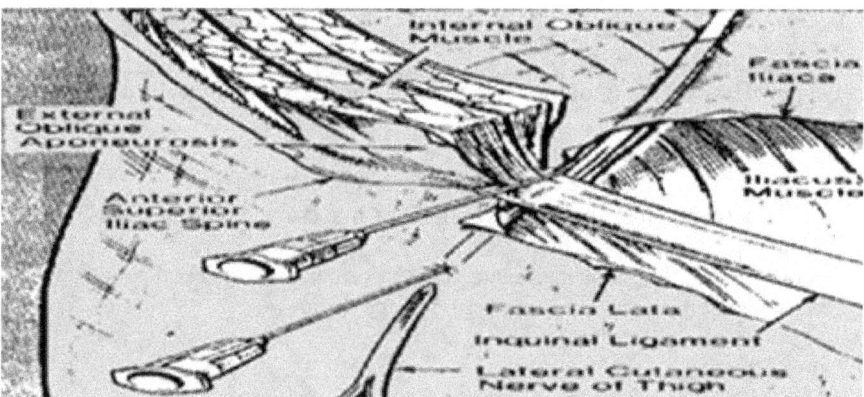

Fig 3: Lateral Cutaneous N. of thigh

Nerve blocks at the knee: For P.O. analgesia, severe muscle spasm.
- Tibial nerve blocked in prone position, placing a needle lateral to middle point of a line drawn from the apex of popliteal fossa and the midpoint of a line between femoral condyles.
- Nerve stimulator locates nerve 0.5 cm deeper to popliteal fascia.

Common Peroneal N. leaves tibial nerve at the apex of popliteal fossa.
- Runs laterally just medial to biceps femoris muscle, below popliteal fascia.

Saphenous nerve: Infiltration just posterior to medial border of tibia near long saphenous vein just below the knee.

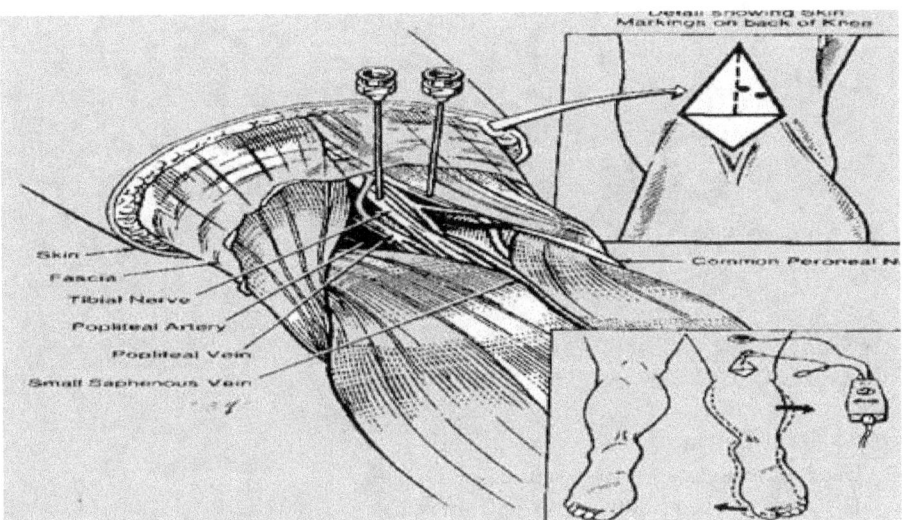

Fig 4: Nerve blocks at the knee

Ilio-inguinal / Iliohypogastric Nerve Block:
- Used in hernia repair, hydrocele, orchiopexy & p.o. analgesia.
- Simple infiltration of abd. Wall medial to Ant. Sup. Iliac spine.
- A 25 gauze needle 1.5 cm medial & inferior to Ant. Sup. Iliac spine punctures skin, Ext. & Internal oblique fascias.
- 3 to 5 ml of 0.25 to 05% of bupivacaine.
- Wound edge infiltration also provides analgesia.

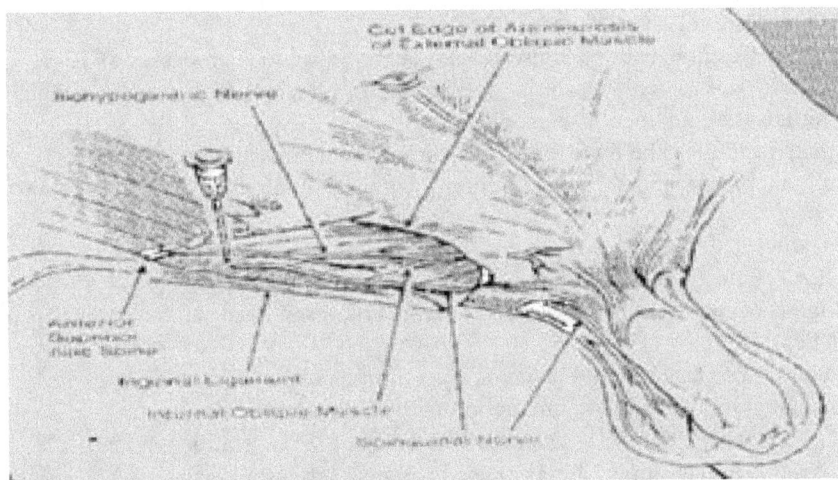

Fig 5. Ilio-inguinal / Iliohypogastric Nerve Block

Penile Block (Dorsal N. of penis (S2,3,4)):
- Use in hypospadias repair, circumcision.
- At the base of penis 0.5 cm on either side of midline.
- Through A 25 gauze needle at 70° angle, 0.1 mg/kg of 0.25% bupivacaine used.

Ring Block: Subcutaneous infiltration at the base of penis.
- Topical lignocaine can also provide analgesia.

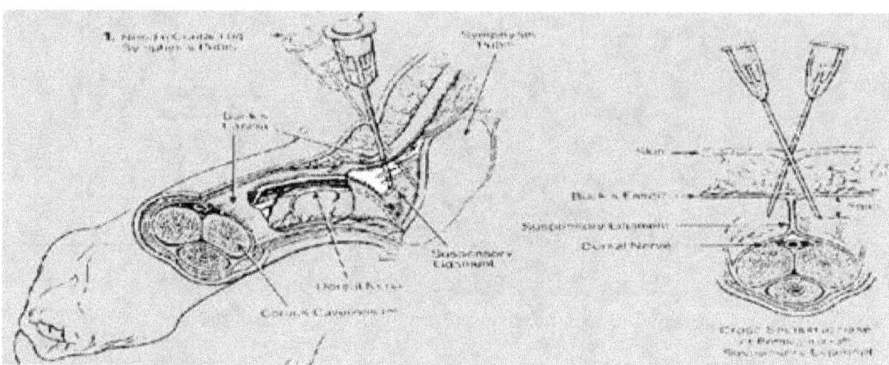

Fig 6: Ring Block

Intercostal Nerve Block:
- Used for analgesia for rib fracture & P.O. pain.
- Distance between rib margins to pleura is 2 mm.
- Bupivacaine (0.5%) 2-5 mg/kg with or without Adrenaline.
- A 25 gauze needle enters lower margin of rib and made to walk past the edge for 1 – 2 mm posteriorly.

Interpleural Block:
- Used in Analgesia for thoracotomy or upper abd. Surgery & trauma.
- Continuous injection with 0.25% bupivacaine 0.25ml/kg/hr.
- Caution – high doses, posture dependant analgesia & pneumothorax

Paravertebral Block:
Used in p.o. analagesia following thoracotomy
- -In lateral position, skin puncture 1-2 cm lateral to spinous processes of T7-9.
- Sup. Border of transverse process is walked past till a loss of resistance occurs after costotransverse ligament is pierced.
- Catheterisation can be done 0.25 ml/kg/hr bupivacaine.
- Caution – pneumothorax, vessel injury & high dose toxicity.

Topical Anaesthesia:
- EMLA – Eutectic mixture of 5% Lignocaine & Prilocaine.
- A high concentration (80%) in water soluble unionised form achieves transdermal spread upto 5 mm depth.
- Used for Venepunctre, circumcision, lysis of prepucial adhesions.
- Methemoglobinemia due to interaction with sulphonamide etc.
- JAC Tetracaine 5% Adr. 1:2000, cocaine 1% used for laceration wounds.
- Lignocaine topical spray (2m/1kg) used for bronchoscopy.
- Lignocaine Jelly applied to urethra as adjunct to cystoscopy.
- Local infiltration 0.5% of L.A. for venous puncture, cutdown and p.o. pain.

References
1. Textbook of Pain, 2nd Ed, CBS Pub New Delhi 2008.
2. Kumar Pramod - Terminal cancer care 2nd Edition, CBS Medical Pubs, New Delhi 2005
3. Kumar Pramod - Guide to Peripheral Nerve Blocks 1st Edition CBS Medical Pubs, New Delhi 2008
4. Kumar Pramod - A Handbook of pain management & related symptoms in cancer, Samvedana, Indraprastha Apollo Hospital New Delhi, 2003
5. Kumar Pramod - Illustrated Atlas on peripheral nerve blocks Anaesthesia Dept. Jamnagar 2002.

Chapter 16.

POST OPERATIVE PAIN RELIEF

Acute Pain Services -
More Pain-Abdominal, Intrathoracic surgery
Complications: Respiratory distress, Hypoxia.
Origin- Skin, Tendons, Bone, Muscle and Viscera.
Increased by coughing, straining, anxiety,andpsychological fear.

Assessment and Management of Pain

Patient Education:
1. Explain the patient's right to have pain assessed and managed.
2. Discuss potential post operative/ procedural pain.
3. Explain that effective pain relief is part of Tt plan
4. Explain the patient's report of unrelieved pain is essential & instruct in how to report pain.
5. That staff will respond quickly to reports of pain
6. Provide information about potential treatments including risks/ benefits/ side effects/ limitations

SCREENING
1. Confirm presence/absence of pain & intensity of pain.
2. Ask "Do you have pain that you would like us to address? And have you had pain in the recent past that concerns you?"
3. Performed at- inpatient – outpatient visit – post procedures – with the routine nursing assessment, unsolicited patient report of pain – time of discharge

Guidelines
1. Choose a pain assessment scale appropriate for patients age/condition.
2. Complete documentation including pain, intensity/quality, location, characteristics, and aggravating/relieving factors.
3. Set a real time patient comfort goal, with patient input- goal may relate to other factors – functional status, quality of life.

Assessment of Pain
1. Visual Analogue Scale (VAS), Facial Expressions.
2. Type of Pain – Burning, Stabbing, Aching.
3. Intensity – Mild, Moderate, Severe.
4. Location – Dermatomal Mapping.
5. Quality – McGill Pain Questionnaire.
6. Unpleasant, Distressing, Awful, Agonizing.
7. Pediatric Pt. – Facial expressions, Oucher, CRIES
   FRACC, Million/BECK Behavior Inventory Types of pain
1. Somatic Pain – Cutaneous, Muscle, Joint, Tendon, Fascia.
2. Viscral – Sympathetic from viscra. Diffuse, Less localised : BP, Pulse changes.
3. Refered – Deep Pain, Viscral /Somatic. Felt in same dermatome.
4. Psychosomatic – No Anatomical Pattern, Psychotherapy.

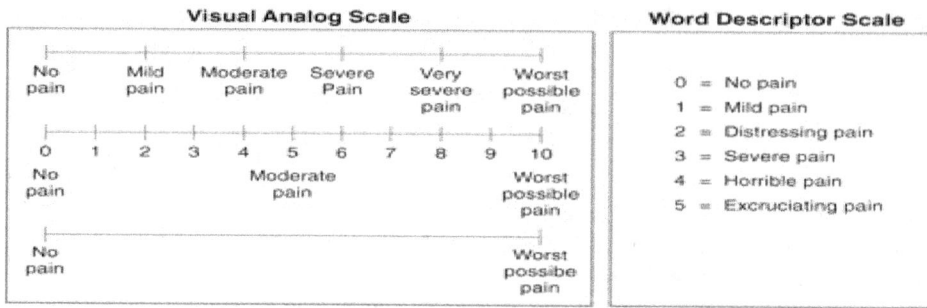

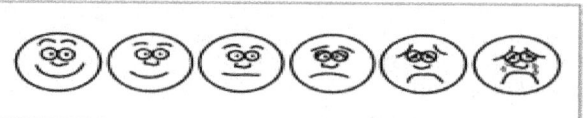

Fig 1. Various types of Pain scales

Acute Post operative pain –
PHYSIOLOGICAL RESPONSE
- Tissue damage – actual or potential
- Release of algesics – Prostaglandins, 5 HT, substance P, bradykinins
- Generation of noxious stimuli
- Increased muscle and sympathetic tone
- Increased metabolism and oxygen consumption

Pathophysiology
- Inflammation produces prostaglandins at the dorsal horn
- Prostaglandins sensitize primary afferent by
  - Activation of silent nociceptors at Na^+ channels
  - Interfering with glycinergic inhibitors
- NSAIDs inhibits production of prostaglandins

- **EFFECTS OF PEPTIDES-** INFLAMMATION, HYPERAEMIA .PLASMA, EXTRAVASATION, LEUCOCYTE ADHESIONS.
- **AXON REFLEX FLARE-** Contraction of smooth muscles in Airways, Urinary bladder, Iris and other tissues
- Leads to Increase in blood flow, Increase in immune cell response.
- **CALCITONIN GENE RELATED PEPTIDE (CGRP)-** Released from sensory nerve endings by antidromic firing
- Local reflex trigger by increase intracellular Ca^{++} leads to inflammation

CARDIOVASCULAR EFFECTS
- Pain stimulates sympathetic neurones
- Tachycardia
- Increased stroke volume
- Increased myocardial oxygen consumption

FEAR OF AGGRAVATION PAIN
- Reduced physical activity
- Venous stasis and platelet aggregation
- It leads to

- o Myocardial ischemia
- o Infarct
- Deep vein thrombosis

GASTROINTESTINAL EFFECTS
- Impulses from viscera and somatic
    - o (e.g. Surgical)
    - o Nausea and vomiting
    - o Ileus
    - o Epidural analgesia reduces ileus

URINARY RETENTION IN PAIN
- Reduces motility of urethra
- Reduced motility of bladder

STRESS RESPONSE TO PAIN
- Tissue injury
    - o Neuroendocrine
    - o immunological
    - o Intercellular biochemical

NEUROENDOCRINE RESPONSE TO PAIN
- Hypothalamic pituitary endocrinal and sympathoadrenal interactions
- Leads to
    - o Increased sympathetic tone
    - o Hypothalamic stimulation
    - o Increased catabolic secretion (cortisol, ACTH, ADH, GH, Glucagon, cAMP)
    - o Decreased anabolic hormone secretion (e.g. insulin, testosterone)

PEDIATRIC PATIENTS
- Physiological abnormalities similar to adults
- Assessment of pain difficult due to developmental, cognitive and emotional difference

ELDERLY PATIENTS
- More systemic disease – e.g. cardiac, pulmonary, endocrine
- Different attitude
- Different expectations about treatment
- Pain is reported less in elderly (Altered pain threshold?)

TREATMENT
Systemic Analgesics –
1. Opioids- Fentanyl
2. Tranquilizers (Midazolam)
3. NSAIDS-No sedation, Cardio respiratory Depression.
4. Dissociative (Ketamine)
5. Adjuvants (Clonidine)

Table: Doses of opioids

Drug	Dose iv/id/PCA	Duration (mts)
1.Sufentanil	10 to 20 µg	20 – 45
2.Morphine	5/10 – 15 mg	30-60 / 120-180
3.Fentanyl	25-50/ 100 µg 10-25 µg PCA	20-40/ 30-60
4.Nalbuphine	10-20/1-3µg PCA	120-240
5.Butorphanol	1-2 µg/kg	120-240
6.Remifentanyl	0.1-0.5µg/kg PCA	2 - 3
7.Tramadol	100 µg/ kg	180

Post Assessment Implementation of Treatment Plan
1. Initiate within one hour of pain identification and assessment.
2. Include patient's comfort goal in plan.
3. Use population- specific guidelines where applicable.
4. Use pharmacology and/or non pharmacologic modalities as indicated.
5. Continue treatment until patient comfort goal is reached.

REASSESSMENT
1. Perform within one hour of any pain intervention.
2. Include intensity, quality, location, characteristics, aggravating & alleviating factors.
3. Use same pain rating scale for all assessments, if scale is changed, note in medical record.
4. Reassess comfort goal as appropriate.

Table 2: COMPARISON OF ANALGESICS

• MILD ANALGESICS	OPIATES
1. Less effective in large dosages- ceiling	1. Dose related analgesia
2. Used orally-less effective No dependence	2. Parentrally SC,I/th,IM,IV
3. Used in chronic low grade pain	3. Used in Acute pain
4. Diverse Mech. of action, Treat cause	4. Opiate Receptors
5. Less side effects. Gastric	5. Resp N,V, Addiction
6. Used in combination	6. Administered alone
7. Aspirin,NSAID,Codeine, Paracetamol	7. Morphine, Buprenorphine

TABLE 3: Opioids in Analgesia

Drug	Dose iv/id/PCA	Duration (mts)
1.Sufentanil	10 to 20 µg	20 – 45
2.Morphine	5/10 – 15 mg	30-60 / 120-180
3.Fentanyl	25-50/ 100 µg 10-25 µg PCA	20-40/ 30-60
4.Nalbuphine	10-20/1-3µg PCA	120-240
5.Butorphanol	1-2 µg/kg	120-240
6.Remifentanyl	0.1-0.5µg/kg PCA	2 - 3
7.Tramadol	100 µg/ kg	180

Patient Controlled Analgesia (PCA) is a method of pain control that gives the patient the power to control their pain.
- Pain medication is administered through a computerized pump.
- The pump contains a syringe of pain medication as prescribed by a doctor that is connected directly to a patient's intravenous (IV) line.
  - The pump is set to deliver a small, constant flow of pain medication.
  - Additional doses can be self-administered as needed by the patient pressing a button.

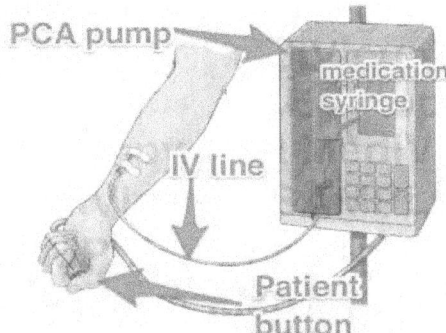

Fig 2. PCA Pump

Table 4: Intravenous PCA Opioids

Agent	Bolus	Lockout Interval	4 h Maximum Dose	Infusion Rate[a]
Fentanyl (10 µg/mL)	10-20 µg	5-10 min	300 µg	20-100 µg/h
Hydromorphone (Dilaudid) (0.2 mg/mL)	0.1-0.2 mg	5-10 min	3 mg	0.1-0.2 mg/h
Meperidine (10 mg/mL)[b]	5-25 mg	5-10 min	200 mg	5-15 mg/h
Morphine sulfate (1 mg/mL)	0.5-2.5 mg	5-10 min	30 mg	1-10 mg/h

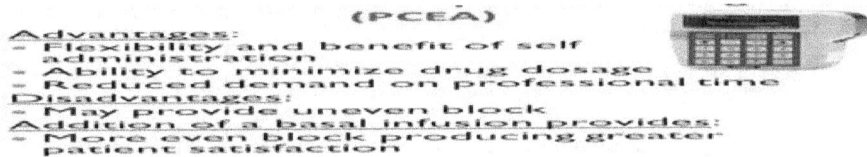

Fig 3: Patient controlled epidural analgesia

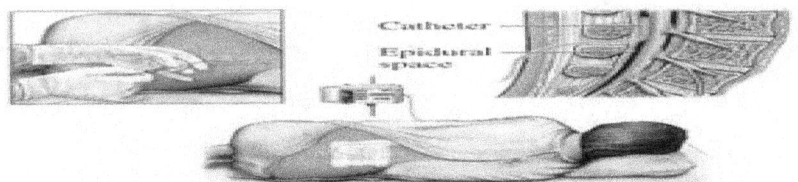

Fig4: CI-PCEA (Computer Integrated Patient Controlled Epidural Analgesia)

Smart pumps: Highly sophisticated infusion technology used with both epidural & intravenous infusions. Incorporate multiple comprehensive libraries of drugs, usual concentrations, dosing units and dose limits, to avoid medication errors.

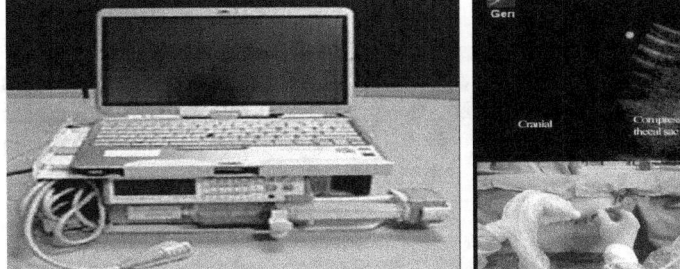

Fig 5a. Smart pump .   Fig 5b. Ultrasound-guided neuraxial technique:

Ultrasound imaging aid for neuraxial blockade:

- It helps to identify the midline, localize the Nerve/ epidural space, measure the skin-to-PN/epidural space distance and estimate the angle of needle insertion
- Facilitates the placement of needles not only in healthy parturient but also in obese pregnant women and patients with scoliosis, malignancy.
- Can be used as a teaching tool, improves the peripheral Nerve block/epidural placement learning curve, In ICU.

Problems: Increased procedural time, cost, need of expertise.

Table 5: Discharge from hospial

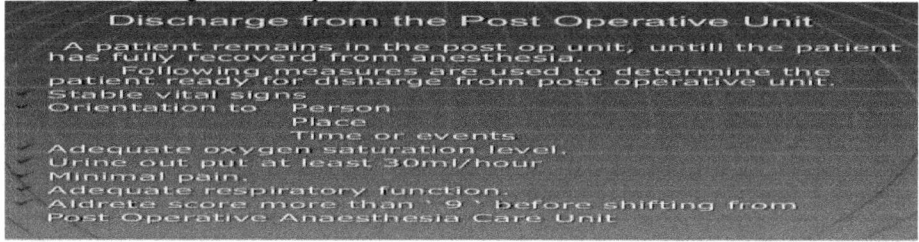

Discharge from the Post Operative Unit

A patient remains in the post op unit, untill the patient has fully recoverd from anesthesia. Following measures are used to determine the patient ready for disharge from post operative unit.
- Stable vital signs
- Orientation to Person
  - Place
  - Time or events
- Adequate oxygen saturation level.
- Urine out put at least 30ml/hour
- Minimal pain.
- Adequate respiratory function.
- Aldrete score more than '9' before shifting from Post Operative Anaesthesia Care Unit

Table 6: Aldrete score

ALDRETE SCORE

Post-Anesthesia Score
A total discharge score of 8-10 is necessary

Post-Anesthesia Score											
PRE-ANESTHESIA VITAL SIGNS/SOURCE		TIME	ADM	15"	30"	45"	1'	2'	3'	4'	DISCHARGE
CIRCULATION	SYSTOLIC BP 20% OF PRE-ANESTHETIC LEVEL 2										
	20-50% 1										
	> 50 0										
CONCIOUSNESS	FULLY AWAKE 2										
	AROUSABLE ON CALLING 1										
	NOT RESPONDING 0										
COLOR	WARM, DRY SKIN W/ PREPROCEDURAL COLORING 2										
	PALE, DUSKY, BLOTCHY, JAUNDICED, OTHER 1										
	CYANOTIC 0										
RESPIRATION	ABLE TO DEEP BREATHE & COUGH FREELY 2										
	DYSPNEA OR LIMITED BREATHING APKEIC 1										
	0										
ACTIVITY	ABLE TO MOVE 4 EXTREMITIES 2										
	ABLE TO MOVE 2 EXTREMITIES 1										
	ABLE TO MOVE 0 EXTREMITIES 0										
COMMENTS		TOTAL									

Teaching self care
  Explain to the patient about expected outcomes
  Immediate postoperative changes
  Written instructions like wound care, activity, dietary recommendations.

References

1. Textbook of Pain, 2nd Ed, CBS Pub New Delhi 2008.
2. Kumar Pramod - Terminal cancer care 2nd Edition, CBS Medical Pubs, New Delhi 2005
3. Kumar Pramod - Guide to Peripheral Nerve Blocks 1st Edition CBS Medical Pubs, New Delhi 2008

Chapter 17:

Trigeminal Neuralgia

It is one of the most painful Conditions:
Treatment is done by medications, surgical skills
There is a lack of knowledge of natural history and
Erroneous claims for various therapies

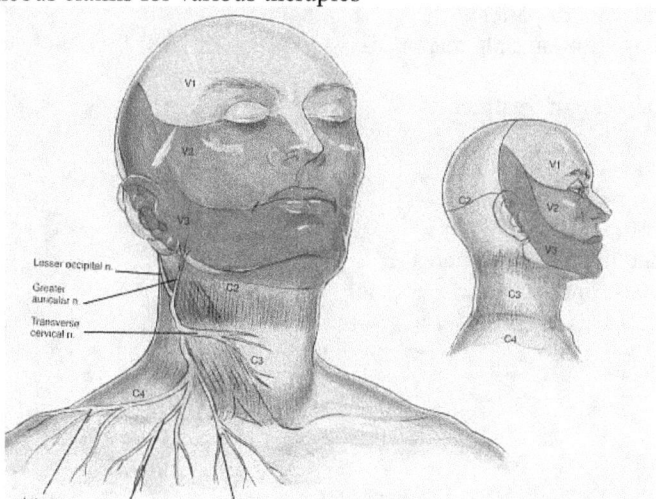

Fig 1: Distribution of branches of trigeminal N

Signs and symptoms

> Electric shock like, brief stabbing pains
> Pain free intervals between attacks
> Abrupt onset and abrupt termination
> Pain restricted to trigeminal nerve distribution
> Minimal and no sensory loss
> Trigger – eating, drinking, tooth brush etc.

Differential diagnosis

Vascular headache –
Intermittent, burning
Lasts for hours, dysaesthetic, rhinitis
Lacrimation, sweating, in clusters
No sensory loss.
Myofascial pain –
> Originates in TM joint, muscles of mastication
> Lateral, aching, cramping local tenderness
> Sensory loss
Local pathology
> Site – paranasal, sinus, jaws, teeth, pharynx
> No sensory loss, local tenderness
> No trigger points
> Throbbing, aching, and burning.

Assessment

Visual analogue scale

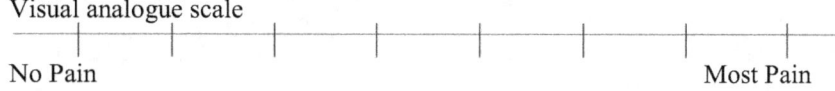

No Pain   Most Pain

Fig 2. Visual analogue scale Score 0 – 10
> Advantages
>> Easily administered and stored

Low cost

Disadvantages
Assumes pain to be a unidirectional experience

Behavioral profile
Severe even suicidal depression high levels of super imposed anxiety

General health questionnaire (GHQ)
Assesses psychological state of patients
Consists of 28 questions with multiple responses
Score : 0 – 28
Score > 8/9 start antidepressant treatment
Advantages:
Simple to understand and administer
Useful for non psychiatric patients.
i. based on physical functions firstly
ii. secondarily ask about psychiatric states

Table 1. General Health Questionnaire

GENERAL HEALTH QUESTIONNAIRE:

It is a questionnaire to assess the psychological status of patient. It consists of 28 questions with multiple responses. A score above 8/9 is considered for start of antidepressant treatment

Minimum score   0
Maximum score   28

We would like to know if you have had any medical complaints and how your health has been in general. Over the past few weeks. Please answer All the questions on the following pages simply by under lining the answer, which you think most nearly, applies to you. Remember that we want to know about present and recent complaints, not those that you had in the past.

It is important that you try to answer all the questions.

Thank you very much for your co-operation.

HAVE YOU RECENTLY					
A1	been feeling perfectly well and in good health ?	Better than usual	Same as usual	Worse than usual	Much worse than usual
A2	been feeling in need of a good tonic ?	Not at all	No more than usual	Rather more than usual	Much more than usual
A3	been feeling run down and out of sorts ?	Not at all	No more than usual	Rather more than usual	Much more than usual
A4	felt that you are ill ?	Not at all	No more than usual	Rather more than usual	Much more than usual
A5	been getting any pains in your head ?	Not at all	No more than usual	Rather more than usual	Much more than usual
A6	been getting a feeling of tightness or pressure in your head ?	Not at all	No more than usual	Rather more than usual	Much more than usual
A7	been having hot or cold spells ?	Not at all	No more than usual	Rather more than usual	Much more than usual
B1	lost much sleep over worry ?	Not at all	No more than usual	Rather more than usual	Much more than usual
B2	had difficulty in staying a sleep once you are off ?	Not at all	No more than usual	Rather more than usual	Much more than usual
B3	felt constantly under strain ?	Not at all	No more than usual	Rather more than usual	Much more than usual
B4	been getting edgy and bad tempered ?	Not at all	No more than usual	Rather more than usual	Much more than usual
B5	been getting scared or panicky for no good reason ?	Not at all	No more than usual	Rather more than usual	Much more than usual
B6	found everything getting on top of you ?	Not at all	No more than usual	Rather more than usual	Much more than usual
B7	been feeling nervous and strung-up all the time ?	Not at all	No more than usual	Rather more than usual	Much more than usual
HAVE YOU RECENTLY					
C1	been managing to keep yourself busy and occupied ?	More so than usual	Same as usual	Rather less than usual	Much less than usual
C2	been taking longer over than things you do ?	Quicker than usual	Same as usual	Longer than usual	Much loner than usual
C3	felt on the whole you were doing things well ?	Better than usual	About the same	Less well than usual	Much less well

Laboratory tests
Clinical examination

Neurological – CT scan, MRI (arterial loop impinging upon trigeminal nerve at pons, multiple sclerosis, angiomas, tumor).

Angiography
Myelography

Prognosis
- Old age – 40-60 years
- Intermittent with spontaneous remissions
- Responds to medical and surgical treatment

Etiology
- Compression of central axon of trigeminal nerve by vessel or tumour at root entry zone
- Demyelination: multiple sclerosis
- Infarction

Anatomical lesions
- Skin, dental
- Blood supply to trigeminal nerve, ganglion, posterior root, brain stem nuclei of trigeminal nerve

Mechanical compression of ganglion
- Carotid artery, bony structures,
- Jaw pathology
- Arteriovenous malformations
- Neuroma, malignancy
- Multiple sclerosis plaque

Pain mechanism
- Excessive attempts by nervous system to regulate the abnormal activity resulting in pain.

Therapy
- Central pain-tranquillizers, antidepressants.
- Opioids and anticonvulsants- no role (acts on local tissue injury area)

Table 2. Medications used in trigeminal neuralgia

Generic name	Dose (mg)	Side effects
Carbamazepine(90%)	600-1200	Nausea, dizziness, hepatic and haemopoitic suppression
Phenytoin(25%)	300-1500	Nausea, dizziness, ataxia
Mephenesin	5-15	Nausea, dizziness, somnolence
baclofen	40-80	Nausea, dizziness

Table 3. Newer drug trial in trigeminal neuralgia

Name	No. of patients	Good results	comment
gabapentin	100	100/100	Failed CBZ & DPH
oxcarbazepine	13	13/13	Failed CBZ &DPH
Pimozide	48	48/48	Better than CBZ
GP47779	11	11/11	Some intolerable

			side effects
L-baclofen	15	11/15	Better than racemic baclofen

Trigeminal neuralgia –nerve blocks
- Block of central & trigeminal division
- LA,alcohal,glycerol,phenol
- Good initial success, low complication rate
- Relief –months to one year (varies)
- No efficacy of steroid injections
- Block of individual branches,supraorbital,infraorbital
- Anaesthesia dolorosa, parasthesia, keratitis.
- Use of nerve locator-accuracy increases.

Trigeminal neuralgia-surgical procedures
- Failed pharmacotherapy
- Gangliolysis
- Craniectomy & decompression

Technique of trigeminal nerve block
- ECG electrode of PNS placed distal to site of block
- Negative electrode attached to 8 cm 22 G needle
- Needle inserted below midpoint of zygomatic arch till lateral pterygoid plate (5cm) is hit
- Reinsert needle cephalad either Anteriorly (maxillary) or posteriorly (Mandibular)
- Muscle twitch elicited with PNS at 5 mAmp
- 1 -1.5 ml 5%phenol injected

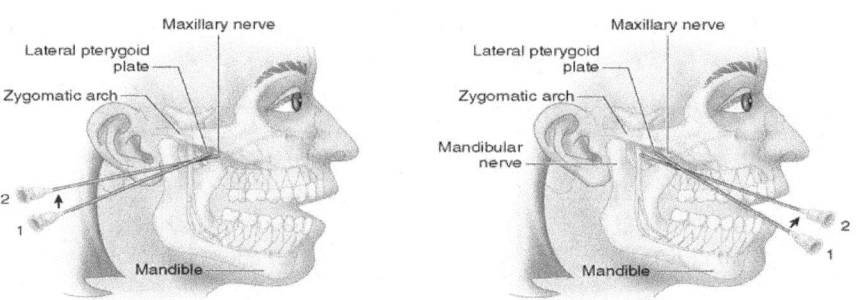

Fig 2. Technique of trigeminal nerve block

Adjuvant drugs used in trigeminal neuralgia
  Carbamazepine   100 mg per day
  Phenytoin   100 mg per day
  Gabapentine   900 mg per day
  Imipramine   50-150 mg per day
                           (as per GHQ score)

Surgical procedures-
Cryotherapy-cooling probe
    Damage the nerve/ganglion
    Relief >1year
    Anaesthesia dolorosa, parasthesia, keratitis

Gangliolysis
    Lowest rate of complication –parasthesia
    Better control over extent of sensory loss
    Long term relief, low cost.

Procedure- fluoroscopic control, G A, Needle 2.5 cm to corner of the mouth in occlusal plane into foramen ovale, 60 Hz current – elicit paresthesia

Radiofrequency lesion in ganglion
Fogarty balloon catheter (#4) into Meckel's cave and inflate for 1-10 min (80%) success

Microvascular decompression
85% success – 5year
Suboccipi8tal craniotomy under GA
Visualize Trigeminal nerve under microscope near pons
Repositioning of offending artery
Coagulating a vein
no sensory loss

Trigeminal Nerve Retrogasserian Neurectomy
Sectioning of trigeminal nerve root between the ganglion and pons
Approach posterior fossae
Partial rhizotomy – reduces anesthesia dolorosa

Stereotactic radiosurgery
Lesion made in trigeminal nerve root near pons
Linear accelerator
Gamma knife – cobalt 60
Intersection of 210 beams used
CT, MRI, contrast cisternography
Pain relief – 77%
No risk surgical infection, GA, hematoma, CSF leak, facial weakness, brain stem injury or hearing loss
Side effects – facial parasthesia, sensory loss.

References

1. Textbook of Pain, 2nd Ed, CBS Pub New Delhi 2008.
2. Kumar Pramod - Terminal cancer care 2nd Edition, CBS Medical Pubs, New Delhi 2005
3. Kumar Pramod - Guide to Peripheral Nerve Blocks 1st Edition CBS Medical Pubs, New Delhi 2008
4. Kumar Pramod - A Handbook of pain management & related symptoms in cancer, Samvedana, Indraprastha Apollo Hospital New Delhi, 2003
5. Kumar Pramod - Illustrated Atlas on peripheral nerve blocks Anaesthesia Dept. Jamnagar 2002

Chapter 18.

Neuropathic Pain

Neuropathic Pain is produced by an injury to the peripheral nerve and/ or central nervous system having associated sensory sign and symptoms.[1] Various aetiological factors are direct trauma, ischaemia, infections, metabolic disease, tumor invasion, surgery, chemotherapy, irradiation, neurotoxins, inherited neuro degeneration. [2, 3, 4] It is associated with (a) spontaneous paresthesia, dysasthesia and pain (b) Pain evoked by movement and (c) tenderness over partly denervated body part.

Types of Neuropathic Pain-

Most commonly following types of Neuropathic Pain are found[3, 4].

1. **Traumatic neuropathy** due to axotomy distal to dorsal root ganglion associated with ongoing pain, hyperalgesia. Apart from post surgical causes, these often affect most productive age groups and young populations, causing often devastating incapacities due to significant neurologic deficits with high percentage of persistent pain. Incidence varies according to peace and armed conflict periods and also according to the level of economic development. In general, injuries are caused by car and labor accidents, by cutting and penetrating objects, crushing, fractures, stretching and gunshot wound. Professional or amateur sportsmen injuries are also common. Several professional or amateur sports activities are associated to peripheral nervous system (PNS) injuries. Although some of these injuries are specific for an individual sport, other peripheral nerve injuries occur in several sports activities. Most commonly sports associated to peripheral nerve injury are soccer, hockey and baseball, but many other sports have unique associations with peripheral nerve injury. Traumatic nervous injuries may be devastating, leading to functional morbidity and psychological stress, and even in case of surgical treatment with motor function recovery, pain may induce deficiency and poor quality of life (QL), even preventing recovery and return to previous life, being difficult to foresee which patients shall develop persistent pain. The incidence of traumatic peripheral nerve injury varies from 2.8 to 5% in the population, according to the type of survey.

2. **Diabetic neuropathies** are length dependent, sometime affecting small fibers only; associated with burning pain & paresthesia in the feet. These are nerve damaging disorders associated with diabetes mellitus. These conditions are thought to result from a diabetic microvascular injury involving small blood vessels that supply nerves (vasa nervorum) in addition to macrovascular conditions that can accumulate in diabetic neuropathy. Relatively common conditions which may be associated with diabetic neuropathy include third, fourth, or sixth cranial nerve palsy[1]; mononeuropathy; mononeuropathy multiplex; diabetic amyotrophy; a painful polyneuropathy; autonomic neuropathy; and thoracoabdominal neuropathy.

3. **Trigeminal Neuralgia** due to compression of trigeminal nerve near brain stem and is associated with mechanical or stimuli evoked lightening attacks of pain.

4. **Phantom limb pain** occurs after limb amputation. There is a very severe pain felt in the ghost limb. Phantom pain sensations are described as perceptions that an individual experiences relating to a limb or an organ that is not physically part of the body. Limb loss is a result of either removal by amputation or congenital limb deficiency.[1] However, phantom limb sensations can also occur following nerve avulsion or spinal cord injury.

Sensations are recorded most frequently following the amputation of an arm or a leg, but may also occur following the removal of a breast, teeth, or an internal organ. Phantom limb pain is the feeling of pain in an absent limb or a portion of a limb. The pain sensation varies from individual to individual.

Phantom limb sensation is any sensory phenomenon (except pain) which is felt at an absent limb or a portion of the limb. It has been known that at least 80% of amputees experience phantom sensations at some time of their lives. Some experience some level of this phantom pain and feeling in the missing limb for the rest of their lives

5. **Post herpetic Neuralgia** is caused by herpes zoster virus, associated with an intense burning pain and hyperalgesia along affected dermatomes of the peripheral nerve involved.

6. **Sciatica** is a shooting pain in the leg along the line of distribution of sciatic nerve caused by inflammation compression of its spinal nerve roots.
7. **Carpal tunnel syndrome** is due to compression of nerve in the wrist leading to a pain in proximal area of wrist & fingers.
8. **Chronic pain** disorders include disc degeneration causing damage to the spinal nerves.
9. **Pudendal neuralgia** is due to a pressure over Pudendal nerve leading to pain in pelvis.
10. **Central pain syndrome** caused by adamage to nervous system e.g. posts stroke pain and neurological diseases.
11. **Complex regional pain syndrome** has sympathetic system related pain after nerve injury, responding fully to sympathetic blocks[2]. Complex regional pain syndrome (CRPS), also known as reflex sympathetic dystrophy (RSD) or algodystrophy, is a disorder of a portion of the body, usually the arms or legs, which manifests as **pain**, swelling, limited range of motion, and changes to the skin and bones. It may initially affect one limb and then spread throughout the body; 35% of affected people report symptoms throughout their whole bodies. There are multiple names for this disease, as well as two subtypes. Type I (also called reflex sympathetic dystrophy) refers to CRPS without evidence of a specific peripheral nerve injury. Type II refers to when there is specific evidence of a nerve injury.

    The cause of CRPS is unknown. This typically occurs after an injury to the area in question such as a fracture or after surgery.[3] It is proposed that inflammation and alteration of pain perception in the **central nervous system** play important roles. It has been suggested that persistent pain and the perception of non-painful stimuli as painful may be caused by inflammatory molecules (IL-1, IL2, TNF-alpha) and neuropeptides (substance P) released from peripheral nerves. This release may be caused by inappropriate cross talk between sensory and motor fibers at the affected site.[4] CRPS is not believed to be caused by psychological factors, yet pain can cause psychological problems, such as **depression**. There is often impaired social and occupational function.
    Treatment involves a multidisciplinary approach involving medications, **physical and occupational therapy**, psychological treatments, and **neuromodulation**. Despite this, the results are often unsatisfactory, especially if treatment is delayed.
12. **Failed back surgery syndrome** after discectomy or spinal fusion may be due to pain generator produced because of recurrent spinal stenosis, degeneration of next level, in adequate decompression, nerve damage or epidural fibrosis.

Neuropathic pain may be classified according to its peripheral or central nervous system involvement.

Table 1: Types of Neuropathic Pain[4]

Peripheral	Central
Traumatic neuropathy	Compression myelopathy (spinal canal stenosis)
Trigeminal neuralgia	HIV myelopathy
Diabetic neuropathic pain	Multiple sclerosis pain
Nerve compression/infiltration by tumors	Ischaemic myelopathy
Herpetic neuralgia	Pain after stroke
Complex regional pain syndrome (CRPS)	Pain after spinal cord injury
Chemotherapy / Radiotherapy induced neuropathy	Radiation myelopathy
Entrapment neuropathy (carpal tunnel syndrome)	Syringomyelia
Radiculopathy	Parkinson disease pain
Phantom limb pain	
Toxic exposure related neuropathies	
Inflammatory demyelinating polyradiculoneuropathy	
Alcoholic polyneuropathy	
HIV sensory neuropathy	
Nutritional deficiency related neuropathies	
Iatrogenic neuralgias (post mastectomy / Thoracotomy pain)	
Idiopathic sensory neuropathy	

Mechanism of Neuropathic Pain-

Peripheral Mechanism –
1. **Abnormal sodium Channels and Ectopic neural activity:**
   There is an ectopic and spontaneous discharge due to neuroma formation, at injury site or in dorsal root ganglion (DRG) [2]. Such ectopic activity may be caused by abnormal or dysfunctional sodium channels and explain the benefit of sodium- channel blockers e.g. lignocaine, mexiletine, phenytoin, carbamazepeine and tricylic antidepressants[5, 6, 7].
2. **Symapathetic Dysfunction:**
   The damaged primary afferent fibers developing adrenergic sensitivity and surviving afferents acquiring noradrenergic sensitivity has been shown in animal studies. Complex regional pain syndrome has sympathetic system related pain after nerve injury, responding fully to sympathetic blocks[2].
3. **Neurogenic inflammation:**
   Neuropeptides e.g. substance P and prostaglandins (PGE_2) having inflammatory action are released at the site of primary afferent nociceptors and sympathetic post ganglionic neurons following a neural trauma. This explains the pain relief in response to NSAIDS, lignocaine and capsaicin[3]. The connective tissue sheath is supplied by primary afferents (Nervi nervorum) which may enter the nerve trunk with endo vascular bundle. The compression and inflammation of the sheath leads to pain and tenderness. There is a sprouting of afferents and sympathetic neurons in DRG[2].

Central Mechanisms-
1. **Central sensitization:**
   This occurs with intense and long term C fibers input e.g. post herpetic neuralgia (PHN) leading to pain. Further, with central sensitization large diameter and low threshold Aβ mechanoreceptors become capable of generating pain. At NMDA receptor sites, the substance P and glutamate activity leads to central sensitization[4].
2. **Deafferentation hyper activity in dorsal horn cells:**
   After peripheral nerve damage or dorsal rhizotomy there is a spontaneous firing in many dorsal horn cells e.g. brachial plexus avulsion pain[8, 9].
3. **Central reorganization:**
   Peripheral nerve damage leads to loss of central terminals of unmyelineted primary afferents; however large diameter Aβ afferents start responding intensely to mild stimulation and sprouts to innervate the deafferented nociceptive neurons of dorsal horn[3, 4].
4. **Loss of inhibitory large diameter myelinated fiber afferents** in nerve injury leads to pain as per Gate control hypothesis. Pain relief after Transcutaneous electrical nerve stimulation (TENS) in mononeuropathies in trauma and dorsal column stimulation induced selective activation of the central branches of large afferents explains it[3].

Various changes at different sites in sensory neurons after an injury to spinal nerve can be summarized as under[5]:

a. Spontaneous neural discharge ectopic sensitivity at nerve injury site. **b.** The expression in DRG is re-regulated due to loss of trophic support and development of spontaneous neural activity. **c.** The development of Wallerian degeneration distal to injury leads to release of cytokines and growth factors at uninjured portions of the nerve. **d.** Partial denervation at peripheral tissues causes release of trophic factors leading to primary afferent's sensitization. **e.** The molecular expression in DRG of uninjured nerve is reregulated, due to increased trophic support. **f.** Postsynaptic dorsal horn cell sensitization, leading to an increased cutaneous stimuli response. **g.** Activation of microglial cells leads to sensitization of dorsal horn. **h.** Descending modulation of DRG neurons leads to its enhanced response. These site are depicted in figure 1 below:

Assessment:

It involves assessing the pain and other associated symptoms for diagnosis and planning the treatment. A detailed history of neuropathic pain may reveal a delay in onset of pain following injury / disease, localization of pain and sensory loss, paroxysms of unprovoked spontaneous pain leading to disturbed sleep / or a change in character of pain. The pain may be constant / intermittent and stabbing, burning, sharp, shooting, electrical, numbness or tingling. Pain may be caused or relieved by applying pressure[3].

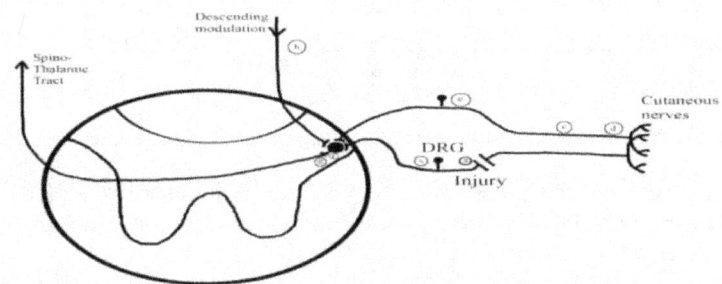

Figure 1: Spinal nerve injury changes at different sites in sensory neurons.

Pain intensity can be rated and validated with verbal, numerical or visual analogue scales[10]. The assessment of unusual abnormal sensations is done by Neuropathic Pain scale[11] and Neuropathic Pain Questionnaire[12]. However the former is still not validated while later differentiates neuropathic from nociceptive pain. Chronic Pain negatively affects quality of life so measuring physical and emotional function is used in evaluating the response to treatment[5, 13]. The assessment of psychological co-morbidity (anxiety/ depression), disturbed sleep, and work related issues, treatment expectations, rehabilitation needs and family support is performed[14].

Clinical examination of somatosensory system:
1. Any positive sensory features without evidence of inflammation.
2. Allodynia / hyperalgesia with pain in response to light touch / temperature. Dynamic allodynia with evoked pain worsened by light touch than with pressure or pain relieved by pressure.
3. Hyperpathia with an increased pain threshold in response to normal stimulus e.g. pinprick / temperature but summation spread and / or prolonged pain after sensation[3].

Quantitative sensory testing (QST):
This standardizes the sensory function measurement in controlled clinical trials to supplement neurological examination.
The nerve conduction velocity test[5] and electromyography are useful to study large myelinated peripheral nerve function. Magnetic resonance imaging detects anatomical integrity of thermonociceptive sensory processing regions of brain e.g. brainstem, thalamus, sensory cortex etc, so as to assess their role in pain[3].

Treatment:
1. **Pharmacotherapy:** Includes specific drugs e.g. anticonvulsants, antidepressants, antiarrythmics, GABA receptor blockers and NMDA receptors.
   The first line medications This list includes gabapentin, lignocaine patch, opioids, tramadol and tricyclic antidepressants (TCA) which are being used as initial treatment in neuropathic pain. Opioids & TCA require greater caution due to their side effects. Gabapentin has been used in phantom limb pain, herpes, spinal cord injury and Guillain-Barre syndrome[3, 15].

Table 2: First line drugs used in neuropathic pain[3].

Drug	Initial Dose	Maximum Dose
Gabapentin	100-300 mg at night or 3 times / day	3600 mg/d in 3 divided doses
5% Lignocaine patch	1- 3 patches daily up to 12 h	Maximum of 3 patches daily in 12 h
Opioid analgesics	5-15 mg every 4 h	120-180 mg/d

Tramadol hydrochloride	50 mg once / twice daily	400 mg/d (100 mg 4 times daily)
Tricyclic antidepressants (nortriptyline, desipramine)	10-25 mg at night	75-150 mg/d

Second line Drugs are considered when first line medications are not effective[4].

Lamotrigine has been used in clinical trials for HIV sensory neuropathy[16], diabetic neuropathy[17] central post stroke pain[9] and spinal card injury[18].

Carbamazepine is most effective drug for trigeminal neuralgia pain. There are other anticonvulsants like oxcarbazepine, tiagabine, topiramate & zonisamide which are also awaiting result of controlled trials. Selective serotonin reuptake inhibitors are tolerated better have fewer side then TCA. Drugs like paroxetine, citalopram, fluoxetine, bupropion and venlafaxine are prescribed to patients not responding to nortryptiline[4,19].

Beyond second line Medications: 1 Drugs which are often found effective in individual circumstances. This includes capsaicin, clonidine, dextromethorpham and mexiletine[4].

2. **Stimulation techniques:** TENS, dorsal column stimulation and deep brain stimulation are being used in intractable neuropathic pain. The limitations of later invasive procedures include infection, bleeding or dislocation of electrodes[2,3].
3. **Chemical Neurolysis** is being used in gassarian ganglionlysis, using glycerol successfully. The patients with complex regional pain syndrome respond to sympathetic block using alcohol or local analgesics[3].
4. **Neurosurgical Procedures:** Neurectomy, rhizotomy, dorsal root entry lesioning, cordotomy and thalamotomy are used for chronic intractable pain relief. These destructive pain procedures may lead to increased deafferentation and more severe pain. So these procedures may not be used in neuropathic pain except trigeminal neuralgia. Micro vascular decompression of transposition and vascular compression is effective in trigeminal neuralgia[3].

Conclusion:

The diagnosis and management of Neuropathic Pain remains highly challenging because of complex pathophysiology and both peripheral & central mechanisms involvement. The pain is refractory to commonly used analgesics while available drugs in current use have limitations. Therefore a proper clinical assessment, careful planning & monitoring are essential.

REFERENCES:
1. Backonja M. Defining neuropathic pain. Anesth Analg. 2003; 97:785-790.
2. Bennett GJ. Neuropathic pain. In: Wall PD, Melzack R. Textbook of Pain. 3rd Ed. Edinburgh, Scotland: Churchill Livingstone; 1994:201-224.
3. Kumar P. Management of neuropathic pain. In: A textbook of pain. 2nd Ed, CBS publishers, New Delhi, 2008: p 254-257
4. Dworkin RH Backonja M, Rowbotham MC et al. Advances in neuropathic pain. Diagnosis, Mechanisms and Treatment Recommrendations. Arch Neurol. 2003; 60(11): 1524-1534
5. Campbell JN, Meyer RA. Mechanisms of neuropathic pain. Neuron. 2006, 52(1): 77-92

6. Dellemijn PLI, Fields HL, Allen RR et al. The interpretation of pain relief and sensory changes following sympathetic blockade. Brain, 1994; 117:1475-1487.
7. Devor M, Keller CH, Deerinck TJ et al. Sodium channel accumulation on axolemma of afferent endings in nerve ending neuromas in Apteromotus. Neuro Sci. Lett 1989; 102: 149-154.
8. Rowbotham MC, Petersen KL, Fields HL. Is postherpetic neuralgia more than one disorder? Pain Forum. 1998; 7:231-237.
9. Fields HL, Rowbotham MC, Baron R. Post-herpetic neuralgia: irritable nociceptors and deafferentation. Neurobiol Dis. 1998; 5:209-227.
10. Dworkin RH, Nagasako EM, Galer BS. Assessment of neuropathic pain. In: Turk DC, Melzack R, eds. Handbook of Pain Assessment. 2nd Ed. New York, NY: Guilford Press; 2001:519-548.
11. Galer BS, Jensen MP. Development and preliminary validation of a pain measure specific to neuropathic pain: the Neuropathic Pain Scale. Neurology. 1997; 48:332-338.
12. Krause SJ, Backonja MM. Development of a neuropathic pain questionnaire. Clin J Pain. 2003 Sep-Oct; 19(5):306-14.
13. Dworkin RH, Nagasako EM, Hetzel RD, Farrar JT. Assessment of pain and pain-related quality of life in clinical trials. In: Turk DC, Melzack R, eds. Handbook of Pain Assessment. 2nd Ed. New York, NY: Guilford Press; 2001:659-692.
14. Haythornthwaite JA, Benrud-Larsen LM. Psychological aspects of neuropathic pain. Clin J Pain. 2000; 16:S101-S105.
15. Backonja M, Beydoun A, Edwards KR, et al, for the Gabapentin Diabetic Neuropathy Study Group. Gabapentin for the symptomatic treatment of painful neuropathy in patients with diabetes mellitus: a randomized controlled trial. JAMA.1998; 280:1831-1836.
16. Simpson DM, Olney R, McArthur JC, Khan A, Godbold J, Ebel-Frommer K, for the Lamotrigine HIV Neuropathy Study Group. A placebo-controlled trial of lamotrigine for painful HIV-associated neuropathy. Neurology. 2000; 54:2115-2119.
17. Eisenberg E, Luria Y, Braker C, Daoud D, Ishay A. Lamotrigine reduces painful diabetic neuropathy: a randomized, controlled study. Neurology. 2001; 57:505-509.
18. Finnerup NB, Sindrup SH, Bach FW, Johannesen IL, Jensen TS. Lamotrigine in spinal cord injury pain: a randomized controlled trial. Pain. 2002; 96:375-383.
19. McQuay HJ, Carroll D, Jadad AR, Wiffen P, Moore A. Anticonvulsant drugs for management of pain: a systematic review. BMJ. 1995; 311:1047-1052.

Chapter 19.

Low Back Pain and Myalgia

LOW BACK PAIN

Low back pain is a common health problem. About 65% to 80% of the world's population develops back pain at some point during their lives[1] Careful clinical evaluation helps separate patients with mechanical back pain from those with non-mechanical pain[2].

The clinical history is an essential step in evaluating patients with low back pain. The age of a patient is helpful in determining the potential cause of back pain. The sex of the patient may also help select potential cause of low back pain.

The duration and location of pain help decide the kinds of questions that the evaluating physician will ask. Mechanical low back pain tends to have an onset associated with a physical task and is usually of short duration (days of weeks). Medical causes of low back pain tend to have a more gradual onset with no identifiable precipitating factor.

Most back pain is limited to the lumbo-sacral area of the low back. Radiation of pain in the thighs or the knee may be related to referred pain from elements of the spine (muscle, ligaments or apophyseal joints). Pain that radiates from the low back to below the knees is usually neurogenic in origin and support a pathologic process effecting spinal nerve roots.

The history is directed towards understanding the chronologic developments of low back pain, its character and response to therapy. The anatomic structures of the lumbosacral spine receive specific types of sensory innervations that are associated with distinct qualities of pain. The major categories of pain include superficial somatic, deep somatic (spondylogenic) radicular, neurogenic, visceral, referred and psychogenic.In patients with a history suggestive of mechanical low back pain, the physical examination should concentrate or the evaluation of musculoskeletal and neural tissues of the lumbosacral spine.[3]

There are many causes of backache. The common causes are PID, facet joint degeneration, arachnoiditis, pelvis lesions and tuberculosis, where as uncommon causes are cauda equina tumours, arteriovenous malformations (AVM), primary and secondary spinal tumours, ankylosing spondylitis and osteomyelitis.

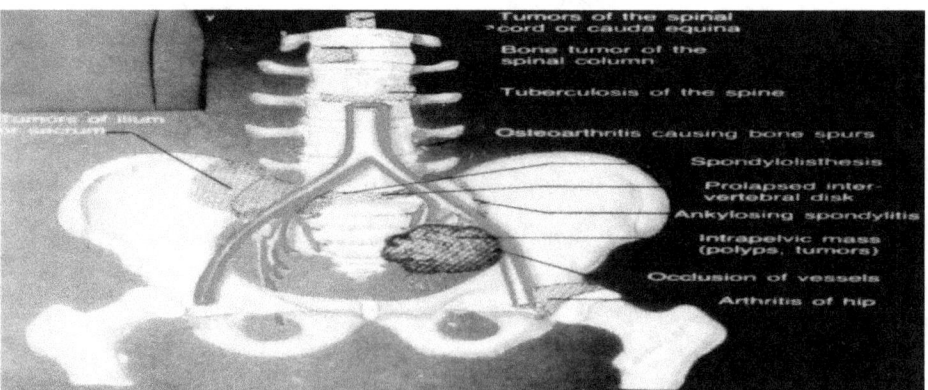

(Fig.1). Causes of low back pain

The cause of backache is detected by ruling out the causes one by one. This is done by proper history, clinical examination and investigations.

Among neurological examination, SLR test, motor-sensory deficit, examination of deep tendon reflexes and Babinski reflex are the main cardinal points to be seen carefully.

As far as investigation is concerned plain X-ray particularly lateral view is the basic requirement, whereas myelogram, CT scans, myelography is further necessiry according to the need. MRI has a number of advantages compared to other radiological techniques. MRI is able to define bony and soft tissue structures without intrathecal contrast. The entire length of the spinal cord and canal may be evaluated in multiple planes.

MRI has become the primary imaging modality for the study of the spine. MRI is an excellent technique to view the spinal cord. MRI identified syrinx, cord infarctions, cord injury, multiple sclerosis, demyelination and intramedullary tumours. The development of contrast media (Gadolennium) has improved the characterization of spinal cord tumours. MRI can detect infection of the spine very well. It's a very useful technique for mechanical disorders of the spine like disc prolapse, spondylolisthesis, various spondylitic changes and fractures. Thus a consensus is growing that MRI is the most useful technique for lumbar spine imaging.

But MRI findings are only significant in patients with correlating clinical symptoms and signs. One may find substantial abnormalities of herniated disc and spinal stenosis, whereas actual clinical findings are minimal. Therefore, the finding of an abnormal disc is more reliable in symptomatic individual.

A number of other radiographic techniques are available for the evaluation of lumbosacral spine. These are spinal angiography, discography, thermography etc. These are used infrequently compared to the X-ray, CT or MRI. Similarly majority of patients don't require laboratory studies with their initial evaluation.

Electrodiagnostic studies are extension of the neurologic examination and provide a means to identify nerve and muscle damage. These tests can confirm the clinical suspicion of nerve root compression, define the distribution and severity of involvement and document or exclude other illness of nerves or muscles that contribute to the patient's symptoms and signs. These tests include evaluation of electrical activity generated by muscle fibres at rest and during contraction (electromyography and speed of conduction of impulses electrically generated in peripheral nerves–nerve conduction studies).

Electrodiagnostic tests are most helpful in documenting objectively the neurophysiologic abnormalities in a patient where clinical examination (pain radiation, sensory changes, and muscular weakness) does not necessarily indicate nerve root dysfunction.

Electromyography (EMG) is the test most commonly ordered to document the presence of a radiculopathy. EMG findings are based upon the interpretation of the observer. The experience of the examiner is very important in obtaining the most accurate information from the EMG evaluation. As opposed to EMG, nerve conduction tests become abnormal as soon as nerve damage occurs.

The limitations of electrodiagnostic studies must be considered when evaluating patients with low back pain. These studies do not determine a specific diagnosis. Localization of the lesion is not easy since most muscles in the lower extremity are innervated by two or more nerve roots.

Despite these limitations, electrodiagnostic tests remain an important part of the investigation of low back pain patients. An abnormal EMG is corroborative evidence of organic disease and helps the physician determine who is a potential candidate for surgical intervention. Electromyography changes may recede with resolution of the nerve impingement. However, patients with a good operative decompression with relief of symptoms may have EMG abnormalities persist 1 year after surgery. In patients without neurologic dysfunction, EMG and nerve conduction tests are normal.

After investigating such patient of low back pain (LBP) utmost care should be taken in deciding the treatment. First of all decision should be made between conservative and operative line of treatment. It depends on the aetiology of LBP, age of patient, clinical findings, radiological investigations, associated medical condition and obesity. Spinal endoscopic procedures are also in use for diagnostic and therapeutic purposes.

Conservative therapy includes rest, physiotherapy, simple analgesics and vitamine B_1, B_6 and B_{12}. Candidates with acute pain without neurological deficit can be very well treated with bed rest and analgesics, whereas those with chronic history needs supervised physiotherapy. The need of analgesics should be restricted as far as possible. Simple, tolerated and non- toxic analgesics would be worthwhile to use rather than sophisticated research product having inadequate trials. Opioids are useful in a patient with psychosocial factor.

Patient with obesity requires dietary restriction and weight reduction. The use of steroid should be reversed only for emergency situation or while deciding conservative treatment in acute cases with neurological deficit.

Role of Physiotherapy

The aim of physiotherapy is to restore function and to educate patient in their biomechanical capabilities. The modalities used include moist heat, traction, diathermy, electrical nerve stimulation and massage.

Maintaining the lumbar spine in a reduced lordotic curve (supine with slight knee flexion) is usually comfortable and the pelvic tilt position increases nutrition and circulation to the spine. Patients should be cautioned not to lift heavy and bulky objects without assistance.

Decision for operative line of treatment is a challenging task to a neurosurgeon or orthopaedic surgeon particularly in a borderline case. Patient of LBP without neurological deficit should be treated conservatively as far as possible.

Principles of operation depend on the aetiology. Those with mechanical compression having benign aetiology (disc prolapse, listhesis etc.) needs to be decompressed adequately, whereas mechanical compression with aggressive disease can be operated conservatively.

Several different factors may lead to persistent pain following lumbar spine surgery. This is classically known as failed back surgery syndrome (FBSS). There are several different causes of FBSS, includes misdiagnosis, in appropriate operation, surgical complication and psychosocial problems. The best treatment of FBSS is prevention. Proper selection of patients for surgery is the primary determinant of successful outcome.

EPIDURAL MEDICATIONS FOR BACK PAIN

Low back pain and sciatica continues to challenge the physician in the areas of a aetiopathogenesis, diagnosis and therapy. Epidural steroids have been used with varying success rate for the treatment of low-backache. Lack of controlled trials, protocols and identification of various factors, which influence ultimate outcome raises doubts regarding the efficacy of the use of steroids, Study of various factors like aetiopatho-genesis, chronicity of pain, route of medication, the volume and dose of methyl prednisolone and lastly evolving an appropriate index for evaluation of pain relief (Pain Relief Score) [6] has tremendously improved the management of low backache. Further more, the use of image intensifier or CT guidance resulted in accurate localisation and deposition of depomedrol close to the site of pathology.

INDICATIONS

Patients with compressive myelopathy with or without radiculopathy respond well to the epidural steroids[8]. Best results are seen in patients having LBP or acute onset followed by sub acute origin[9]. Patients with chronic LBP show poor response with epidural steroids. Indications are as follows:

    Acute PID
    Spondylolisthesis
    Post herpetic
    Fracture of spine
    Coccidynia
    Idiopathic
    Lumabr spondylosis
    Ankylosing spondylitis

Poor or no Response: Lumbar canal stenosis (LCS) Facet joint involvement.

MANAGEMENT

The principles of management include an accurate diagnosis based on clinical, radiological or electro-physiological investigations. The basic aim of clinical examination and investigation is to arrive at the nature of the disease as well as the site of lesion.[9] Epidural steroids are contraindicated in patients with tubercular pathology. After the diagnosis is confirmed and after explaining the procedure and prognosis to the patients the epidural drug is deposited close to the site of pathology preferably under image intensifier or CT with or without radio-opaque dye. Or else the catheter tip may be placed close to the site of pathology by approximately measuring distance from the skin.

Methyl prednisolone when injected epidurally stays for more than 2 weeks and thereby exerting slow sustained effect. Dictum is that the epidural should be repeated at least for three times at an interval of 10-15 days provided there is some improvement following first injection. If there is no response following first few injections revise the diagnosis and consider for other modalities of treatment (Facet Rhizotomy or Laminectomy)

Epidural injections have been recommended to delivery drug to the area of the affected nerve roots, there by decreasing the systemic effect of the administered steroid. White and colleagues[9] showed that epidural steroid was most effective in the presence of nerve root irritation as evidenced clinically by signs of root irrigation (positive SLR), radicular pain, and dermatomal hyperaesthesia, weakness of muscle groups innervated by the involved nerve roots, decreased deep tendon reflexes or electrophysiologically by changes in H-reflex or NCV. While Keeps and Duncalf[10] concluded that its use was not scientifically proven. On other hand several studies demonstrated success rate ranging from 67% to as 87%[2-6]. There are several prospective, randomized controlled studies on the use of epidural steroid injections with disc pathology[2, 11, 12].

Table 1: Epidural steroids Indications
- Selection of patients
  Compressive myelopathy
  L_5–S_1 Radiculopahty
  PID/Post herpetic/Spondylolisthesis
  Coccyxidinia/Sec. spine
  Post laminectomy
- Ischaemic myelopathy—LCS
- Facet joint involvement
- Idiopathic

For the sake of uniformity Rastogi et al (1994)[5, 6] proposed pain Relief Score (PRS) (Table2) based on pain relief, duration of pain relief and improvement in neurological status.

Table 2: Pain relief Score (PRS)

Pain relief Percentage	Improvement in neurological Deficit	Duration of pain relief months	Score
0	No change	0	0
1-25	Improvement	0-3	1
26-50	Normal	4-6	2
51-75	–	7-11	3
76-100	–	> 12	4

Maximum score: 10
0–5: Poor/unsatisfactory pain relief
6–8: Good
8–10: Excellent

Recently, cervical and lumbar epidural steroids injections have been used successfully in the treatment of Bechterew's syndrome[8] (Ankylosing spondylitis). Use of thoracic or lumbar epidural steroids in secondaries spine is limited. Rastogi ET al[6] showed good relief of pain 4/7 patients and complete reversal of neurological deficit (paresis, bladder and bowel involvement) in 1/7 cases. Patients with post laminectomy syndrome are also benefited with epidural depormedrol as 7/8 patients showed good relief of pain.

Epidural triamcenalone and methyl prednisolone depot has definit value in the management of chronic low back pain. Long-term relief of pain and improvement in mobility can be achieved using epidural steroid provided emphasis is laid on proper selection of patients[12, 13]. Thi also involves understanding of the underlying pathology and last but not the least the placement of drug in the proximity of the lesion using image intensifier or CT guidance. The possible neurological irritation by oil base, solutions lead to the use of water soluble triamcenalone epidurally[14].

Transcutaneous Nerve Stimulation -Conventional TENS should be tried first in naturopathic pain, neuralgia, causalgia and nociceptive pain from bone and joints. A suitable stimulation frequency is 80 – 100 Hz and the stimulation intensity should be 2-3 times that at the sensory threshold. To be effective the stimulation should always evoke electrical paresthesiae in the painful area[9].

In some pts, the underlying pathology or previous treatment has destroyed the afferent nerve fibres to the extent that electrical paresthesiae cannot be evoked. Acupuncture like TENS should then be tried. This mode is further the primary choice in irradiating pain such as in sciatica and in deep myogenic pain. Here, short trains of 8-16 stimuli are given at a low repetition rate of 1-2 Hz. The intensity should be 3-5 times that at the sensory threshold to evoke visible muscle contractions in myotomes segmentally related to the painful area. The pt may feel muscle fatigue the first few days of treatment but this does not present a problem in the long run.

Myalgia

Myalgia or muscle pain, is a symptom of many diseases and disorders. The most common causes are the overuse or over-stretching of a muscle or group of muscles. Myalgia without a traumatic history is often due to viral infections. Longer-term myalgias may be indicative of a metabolic myopathy, some nutritional deficiencies or chronic fatigue syndrome.

Causes

The most common causes of myalgia are overuse, injury or strain. However, myalgia can also be caused by diseases, disorders, medications, or as a response to a vaccination. It is also a sign of acute rejection after heart transplant surgery.

The most common causes are:
- Injury or trauma, including sprains, hematoma
- Overuse: using a muscle too much, too often, including protecting a separate injury
- Chronic tension

Muscle pain occurs with:

Rhabdomyolysis, associated with:
- Viral
- Compression injury leading to crush syndrome
- Drug-related
- Commonly fibrates and statins
- Occasionally ACE inhibitors, cocaine, and some retro-viral drugs
- Severe potassium deficiency
- Fibromyalgia
- Ehlers-Danlos syndrome

Auto-immune disorders, including:
- Mixed connective tissue disease
- Systemic lupus erythematosus
- Polymyalgia rheumatica
- Polymyositis
- Dermatomyositis
- Multiple Sclerosis (this is neurologic pain localised to myotome)

Infections, including:
- Influenza (the flu)
- Lyme disease
- Babesiosis
- Malaria
- Toxoplasmosis
- Dengue Fever
- Hemorrhagic fever
- Muscular abscess
- Compartment syndrome
- Polio
- Rocky Mountain spotted fever
- Trichinosis (roundworm)
- Ebola

Other
- Postorgasmic illness syndrome (POIS)[1,2,3]

Overuse
Overuse of a muscle is using it too much, too soon and/or too often.[4] Examples are:
- Repetitive strain injury.

Injury
The most common causes of myalgia by injury are: sprains and strains.[4]

Autoimmune
Multiple sclerosis (neurologic pain interpreted as muscular), Myalgic Encephalomyelitis (chronic fatigue syndrome), Myositis, Mixed connective tissue disease, Lupus erythematosus, Fibromyalgia, syndrom, Familial, Polyarteritis nodosa, Devic's disease, Morphea, Sarcoidosis

Metabolic defect
Carnitine palmitoyltransferase II deficiency, Conn's syndrome, Adrenal insufficiency, Hyperthyroidism, Hypothyroidism, Diabetes, Hypogonadism, postorgasmic illness syndrome(POIS).[1,2,3]

Other
Chronic fatigue syndrome a.k.a. Myalgic Encephalomyelitis, Channelopathy, Ehlers Danlos Syndrome, Stickler Syndrome, Hypokalemia, Hypotonia (Low Muscle Tone), Exercise intolerance, Mastocytosis, Peripheral neuropathy, Eosinophilia myalgia syndrome, Barcoo Fever, Herpes, Hemochromatosis a.k.a. Iron Overload Disorder, Delayed onset muscle soreness, AIDS, HIV, Tumor-induced osteomalacia, Hypovitaminosis D, infarction.[5]

Withdrawal syndrome from certain drugs
Sudden cessation of high does corticosteroids, opioids, barbiturates, benzodiazepines, caffeine or alcohol can induce myalgia in many respects.

Treatment
When the cause of myalgia is unknown, it should be treated symptomatically. Common treatments include heat, rest, paracetamol, NSAIDs and muscle relaxants, peripheral nerve blocks, trigger point injections.

Upper back pain
The most common upper backache is in the region of Trapezius or Levator scapuli (Fig 2) muscle at the back. There is associated referred pain and neck stiffness. This is a life style problem specially in office workers in computer professionals. It can be treated by physiotherapy and trigger point injection with local analgesics and steroids.

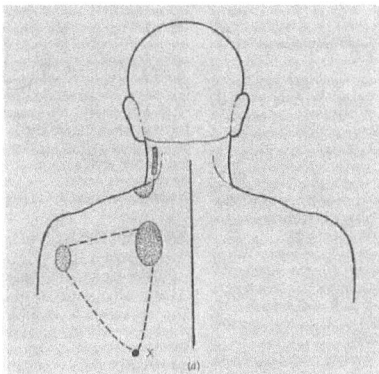
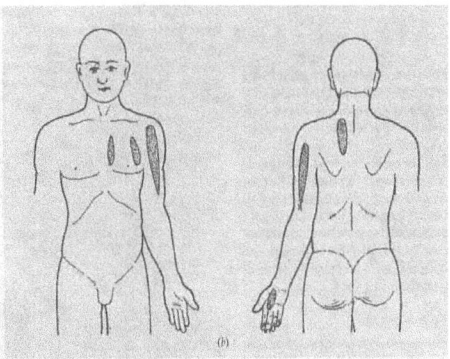

Fig 2 a & b: Distribution of Myofacial pain affecting Levator scapuli. X indicate trigger points, dark and stippled area shows radiation of pain.

REFERENCES

1. Goeberg HW, Jillio, SJ, Gordener WJ, et al. Pain radiculopathy treated with epidural injection of procaine and hydrocortisone acetate. Results in 113 patients. Anesth Analg 40: 130–4.
2. Brevik H, Helsa PE, Molnar I, et al: Treatment of chronic low back pain and sciatic: Comparison of caudal epidural injection of bupivacaine and methylprednisolone with bupivacaine followed by saline. Adv. Pain Res Ther 1976; 1:927–31.
3. Winnie AP, Hartman, JI, Meyers, HI, et al. Pain clinic and extradural corticosteroid for sciatica. Anesth Analg 1972; 51L990–9.
4. Swerdlow M Sayle-Cree, WA Study of extadural medication in the relief of the lumbosciatic syndrome. Anaesthesia 1970; 25:341–5.
5. Rastogi V, Murthy, BVS, Bhattacharya P, et al. Caudal and lumbar epidural methyl prednisolone depot in chronic low back pain—A comparison Indian Journal of Pain 1991; 27:30.
6. Rastogi V, Krishna M, Saraf SK, et all Factors influencing the pain relief obtained with methylprednisolone in low back pain and sciatica. The Pain Clinic 1994;7:291–95.
7. Kumar P. Socio-individual predictory in low back pain in relation to epridural steroids versus interferential therapy. Indpain, 2004, 18(2), 21–26.
8. Stav A, Ovadia L, Stemberg; A, et al. Cervical and lumbar epidural steroid injections for pain relief in patients with Bechterew';s syndrome ; Preliminary study. The pain Clinic 1994; 7:283–89.
9. White AH, Derby R, Wynne GS. Epidural injections for diagnosis and treatment of low back pain. Spine 1980; 5:78–86.
10. Kepes ER, Duncalf D. Treatment of backache with spinal injections of local anesthetics, spinal and systemic. Pain 1985; 22:33–47.
11. Green PWD et al. The role of epidural cortisone injectin in the treatment of discogenic low back pain. Clin Orthop 1980; 153:121–125.
12. Kumar P, Seema Parekh. Epidural steroids in low back ache; Dissertation for M.D Anesthesiology, Saurashtra University, Rajkot. 2001.
13. Kumar P, A Text book of Pain, 1st Edn, New Delhi, Modern Publishers, 2005.
14. Adarsh and Kumar P. Epidural triamcinolone vs physiotherapy modes in low backache Asian Arch, Anaesth Rescues 2005, LXIII (2), 1261–1266

Chapter 20:

LABOUR ANALGESIA

History of Labour pain: Valmiki **Ramayan**- in Ashok vatika Sita said to her maid that "whenever Ravan is tourchering me, I feel a pain which is intolerable, similar to the pain which a lady feels when a vaidya is cutting her abdomen to remove a child from her womb.

Bible- Old Testament-Genesis-3.16

Garden of Eden – Eve persuades Adam to eat apple
God curses her "Unto women, I will multiply thy, sorrow and thy conception, in sorrow though shall bring forth children

Chinese Medicine: Acupuncture, Moxibustion

Mediavel period- Europe-Methods for labour pain relief: Deep suggestion, Alcohol, Opium, Hemp, Suspending mother to a tree, Mandrake.

"A BLACK DAY IN THE HISTORY OF MANKIND" -1591 Edinburgh - A young woman named Euphanie Macalyane got the punishment for seeking pain relief during labor. She was burnt alive on direct order from King of Scotland James VI

Sir J.Y.Simpson -Ether –19 Jan 1847, Chloroform –8 Nov 1847

Sir .John Snow 1857- Father of General Anaesthesia. Queen Victoria received Chloroform for labour pain during the birth of prince Leopold. John Snow gave anaesthesia to her at the birth of Prince Leopold (8th child) in 1853 and in 1857 at the birth of Princess Beatrice

Father of Pain Relief- Dr. John Bonica Wrote Text Book on Pain

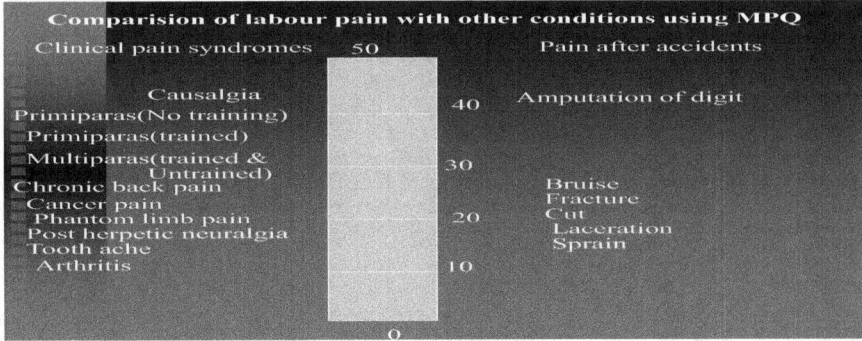

Fig 1. Pain Pole

Labour Pain – Noxious & unpleasant stimulus leads to Fear, anxiety which in turn causes stress leading to Decrease in Uterine flow, fetal HR & O_2, utero placental blood flow.

Increases – Metabolic acidosis, O_2 demand, hyperventilation & hypocapnea (tetany) later respiratory alkalosis → O2 dissociation curve shifted to left.

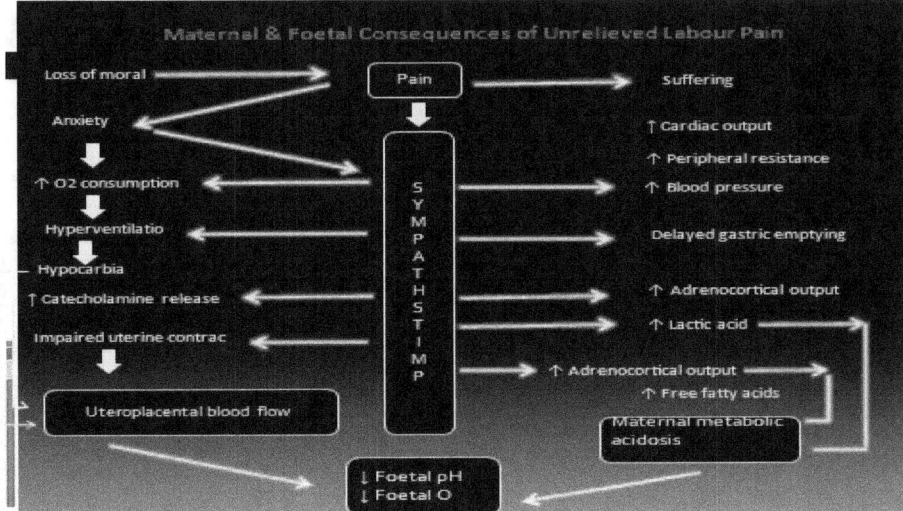

Fig 2. Consequences of labour pain

Labour Analgesia –
Non Pharmacological Methods
Emotional support, Massage, Biofeed back, TNS, Hypnosis
Pharmacological Methods
Inhalationals – Ether, Entanox, Trilene, Iso & Desflurane

Systemic Analgesics –
1. Opioids (Fentanyl)
2. Tranquilizers (Midazolam)
3. NSAIDS
4. Dissociative (Ketamine)
5. Adjuvants (Clonidine)

Table 1 : Opioids in Labour Analgesia

Drug	Dose iv/id/PCA	Duration (mts)
1. Sufentanil	10 to 20 µg	20 – 45
2. Morphine	5/10 – 15 mg	30-60 / 120-180
3. Fentanyl	25-50/ 100 µg 10-25 µg PCA	20-40/ 30-60
4. Nalbuphine	10-20/1-3µg PCA	120-240
5. Butorphanol	1-2 µg/kg	120-240
6. Remifentanyl	0.1-0.5µg/kg PCA	2 - 3
7. Tramadol	100 µg/ kg	180

Patient Controlled Analgesia (PCA) is a method of pain control that gives the patient the power to control their pain.
* Pain medication is administered through a computerized pump.
* The pump contains a syringe of pain medication as prescribed by a doctor that is connected directly to a patient's intravenous (IV) line.
  * The pump is set to deliver a small, constant flow of pain medication.
  * Additional doses can be self-administered as needed by the patient pressing a button.

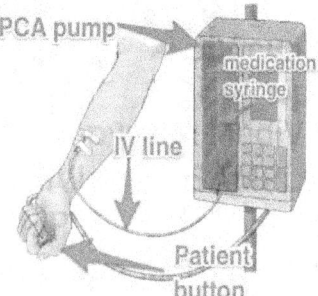

Fig 2. PCA Pump

Various Routes of Nerve blocks in labour pain relief-
Epidural, Intrathecal, CSE, Spinal catheter, Caudal, Pudendal and Walking epidural.

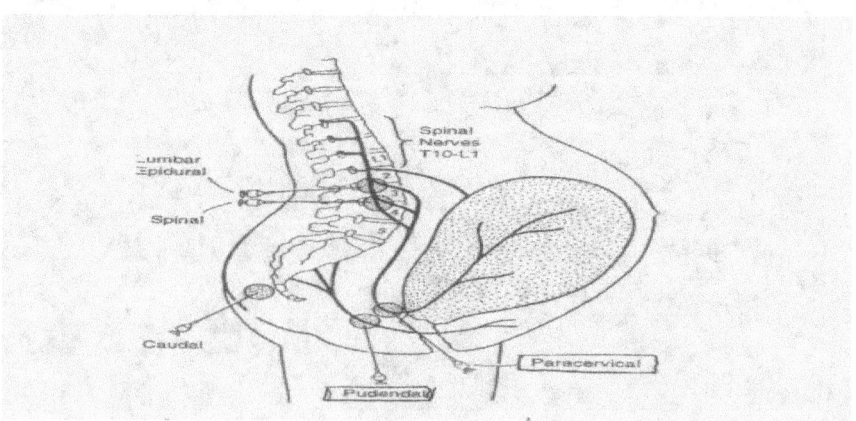

Figure 3: Various Routes of nerve blocks in labour pain.
Drugs used- Local Analgesiics, opiates, adjuvents.
LA drugs-Bupivacaine (0.03-0.5%), Lignocaine, Bupiva+Fentanyl, Ropivacaine, L-bupivacaine.
Side effects:- Motor block, Cardiotoxicity.

Epidural - Opioids, Adjuvents

Indications – Same as spinal, Labour pain, Postop.
For long lasting pain relief – catheter, infusion pumps.
Advantages –Easy, Segmentl, No Complication of SA
Disadvantages: – Less precise, dural puncture, Neurological problems.

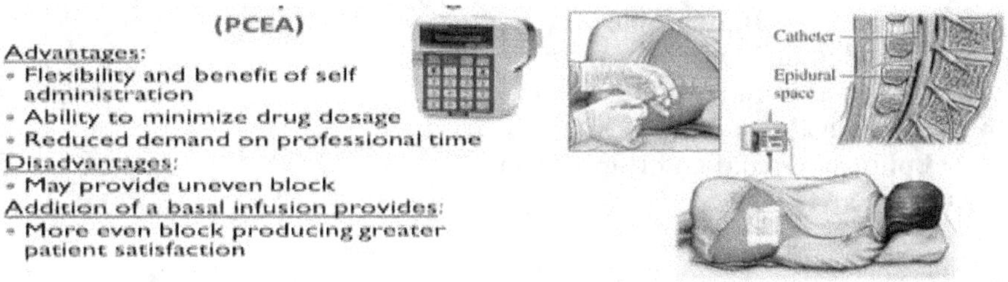

(PCEA)
Advantages:
- Flexibility and benefit of self administration
- Ability to minimize drug dosage
- Reduced demand on professional time
Disadvantages:
- May provide uneven block
Addition of a basal infusion provides:
- More even block producing greater patient satisfaction

Figure 4: Epidural PCA

Table 2: Continuous epidural LA/opioid infusion

Loading dose(8-10 ml)	Infusion rate(8-14 ml/h)
Bupivacaine 0.25%	Bupivacaine 0.125%
Bupivacaine 0.25% + Fentanyl 50-100mcg	Bupicaine 0.125% +Fentanyl 1-2mcg/ml
Bupivacaine 0.25%	Bupiva 0.3-0.06% +Sufenta 0.2-0.5mcg/ml
Bupivacaine 0.25%	Bupiva 0.08% + Diamorphine 25-50mcg/ml

Table3: Combined Spinal Epidural (CSE)/Intrathecal Labour Analgesics

Route	LA Drug	Opioids
CSE-Intrathecal	Bupivacaine 1-2.5 mg (0.1- 0.25%)	Fentanyl 20-25mcg Sufentanyl 3-5mcg
CSE-Epidural Top-ups	Bupivacaine 0.1-0.125% 10 – 5 mg	Fentanyl 20 – 25mcg Sufentanyl 5-10mcg
Intrathecal	Bupivacaine 3-5mg Ropivacaine 2-4mg Lignocaine 20-40mg	Fentanyl 15-25mcg Sufentanyl 5-10mcg Clonidine 30mcg

Labour Pain – Lack of awareness in India
    Patients, relatives & obstetricians- normal part of joyous occasion of new birth by the family
    Obstetricians divert attention to safe birth only
    Mother's pain is a necessary evil or a curse of god to the eve
    Depriving the mother of having the right to have pain relief
    Changing scenario, safe modalities, demand from mother, gradual acceptance.
PAINLESS LABOUR – WALKING EPIDURALS-

Requirements:-
It needs a barely perceptible sensory block T_{10}-S_2, retention of sensation without pain and maintenance of motor power.

Walking Epidurals in Labour – Why?
  Increases Maternal Satisfaction.
  Reduces long term maternal backache.
  Possible reduction in forceps delivery.
  No loss of motor power during Labour.
WALKING EPIDURALS – HOW?
  Analgesia without - Anaesthesia.
                  - Loss of Motor Power.
                  - Bupivacaine dose Reduction.
Bupivacaine dose Reduction Technique-
  (1) **Combined Spinal Epidural – 50% reduced.**
  (2) **Spinal or Epidural Opioids.**
  (3) **CSE or Epidural Opioid and Bupivacaine.**
SUBARACHNOID ANALGESIA
  Less bupivcaine used.
  Rapid reliable analgesia.
  Headache.
MOBILE EPIDURAL
  Mother's Preference: - Ability to move legs. - Bed bladder catheterization, Better nursing care.
ADVANTAGE -Woman can sit on chair.
              - Ability to walk about.
              - Avoids 18-24 hrs. Of recumbency
              - Hyper coagulable women with Pulmonary Embolism.
UPRIGHT Vs RECUMBENT POSITIONS(Nikodemi, 1993 – Cochraine Database).
Less Pain, shorter labours,better foetal heart rate patterns, bearing down-less difficult, greater maternal preference.
WALKING ABOUT DURING LABOUR-m Medicolegal Consequence of falls:
              - Hypotension – High doses bupivacaine.
              - Dizziness – Opiates.
              - Loss of Motor Power.
              - Loss of Proprioception – Neurological.

PRECAUTIONS- Motor **loss : Straight leg raising test, Knee bending, hip flexions.**
          Foetal Monitoring: Telemetery.
          Accompanying adult – to Labour area, toilet.
          Mobility to be retained, walking not desirable.
          ROMBERG Sign

Table 4: MOTOR BLOCK – Modified Bromage Scale

Scale	Criteria	Degree of Block
0	Free movement of lags, feet, ability to raise legs.	- None
1	Inability to raise extended legs, flex knee Full flexion of feet or ankle present.	- Partial 33%
2	Inability to raise lag or flex knee, flexion of ankle and feet present.	- Partial 66%
3	Inability to raise leg; flex knee, ankle or move toes.	- Complete paralysis

BREEN T.W. (1993)-Epidural for Labour in Ambulatory Pts. Gr. 1(n=53) – Epidural fentanyl in 75 mcg bolus+Infusion 37.5 mcg Fentanyl/Hr. Gr II (n=77) – Bupivacaine (0.04%), 15 ml bolus+Fentanyl 14 mcg + Adrenaline 14 mcg, repeated hourly.

Table 5: BREEN T.W. (1993)

Breen at all – 1993	Gr I (Fent)	Gr II(FBA)
Analgesia - Adequate	90.8%	92.2%
Ambulation	70%	68%
Duration of Analgesia	287 min	156min
Additional supplements -	21%	52%
Hip flexion weakness -	Nil	17%
Orthostatic Hypotension -	Nil	9%
Neonatal Outcome -	Safe	Safe

Table 6. Comparison of Fentanyl with Epidural bupivacain+ fentanil (P.Kumar -2000)

Parameters	Fentanyl 50mcg (N=50)	Bupiva-10mg+Fentanyl 50mcg(n=50)
Analgesia	242 min	240 min
Hip flexion weakness	None	20%
Knee Bending	100%	10%
Hypotansion	None	10%
Leg. Weakness	10%	30%
Retention of Urine	10%	10%
Good neonatal outcome	100%	100%
Delivery Normal	40%	40%
Ambulation	100%	70%

Double catheter technique: A lumbar epidural catheter placed at the first- or second-lumbar interspace can be used to provide analgesia during the first stage of labor, followed by the use of a caudal epidural catheter to provide analgesia during the second stage. This increases the likelihood of providing a true segmental block. This technique is most useful in cases in which an extensive sympathectomy must be avoided (e.g., aortic stenosis, primary pulmonary hypertension).

Ultrasound-guided neuraxial technique: Ultrasound imaging is becoming an increasingly popular aid for performing neuraxial blockade due to the following advantage-

It helps to identify the midline, localize the epidural space, measure the skin-to-epidural space distance and estimate the angle of needle insertion

Facilitates the placement of epidural needles not only in healthy parturient but also in obese pregnant women and patients with scoliosis

Can be used as a teaching tool, improves the epidural placement learning curve .

However, problems with ultrasound-guided neuraxial techniques are increased procedural time, increased cost of the procedure and need of expertise

Novel LOR (loss of resistance) methods: The loss of resistance technique is most frequently used to detect the epidural space. As LOR is a subjective feeling, higher failure rates occur with inexperienced anesthesiologists. Various methods have been developed to facilitate epidural space detection of which the following are worth mentioning:

a. **EPIDRUM®:** This is a recently developed air operated, LOR device for identifying epidural space. It is placed between the epidural needle and the syringe and has a thin diaphragm on the top. The diaphragm deflates once the needle tip enters the epidural space

b. **EPISURE® AutoDetect syringe:** The Episure syringe is a unique spring-loaded LOR syringe. It has a coaxial compression spring within a Portex Pulsator™ LOR syringe. This syringe supplies a constant pressure while the operator is advancing the Tuohy epidural needle .

Advantages of novel LOSS Of Rrsistance methods

Enables the anesthesiologist to control the Tuohy needle with both hands, and therefore passage through ligamentum flavum can be controlled better.

Visual observation of LOR overcomes operator subjectivity and variability, thus, their use might offer a more precise end point compared with the standard LOR syringe.

c. **Novel epidural needles: Needle-shaped Ultrasound probe:** This is simply an optically guided insertion of epidural needle. Three optical fibers are embedded in Tuohy needle shaft, one emits light; two absorb light and the optical spectra are analyzed to identify the various tissue planes

d. **Smart pumps:** Highly sophisticated infusion technology can be used with both epidural as well as intravenous infusions. They are called "smart" because they incorporate multiple comprehensive libraries of drugs, usual concentrations, dosing units and dose limits, to avoid medication errors.

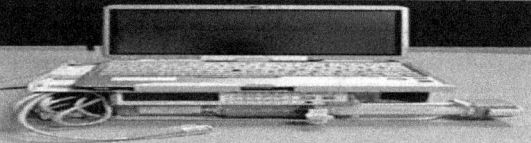

Fig 5. CI-PCEA (Computer Integrated Patient Controlled Epidural Analgesia) pump

References

1. Textbook of Pain, 2nd Ed, CBS Pub New Delhi 2008.
2. Kumar Pramod - Terminal cancer care 2nd Edition, CBS Medical Pubs, New Delhi 2005
3. Kumar Pramod - Guide to Peripheral Nerve Blocks 1st Edition CBS Medical Pubs, New Delhi 2008
4. Kumar Pramod - A Handbook of pain management & related symptoms in cancer, Samvedana, Indraprastha Apollo Hospital New Delhi, 2003
5. Kumar Pramod - Illustrated Atlas on peripheral nerve blocks Anaesthesia Dept. Jamnagar 2002.

Chapter 21:

Interventional pain management

Interventional pain management or interventional pain medicine is a super – specialty of the medical specialty pain medicine, devoted to decrease or eliminate pain with use of invasive & non invasive techniques. This can be accomplished in following ways:
- Interrupting the pain signal along a neural pathway.
- Remodeling anatomical source of pain.
- Neuroaugmentation (SCS, PNS).
- Implantable drug delivery system.

Table 1: Medical Conditions treated-

Type of Treatment of Treatment	Indications of Treatment
Epidural Steroid Injections	Used to relieve pain caused by nerve irritation that is the result of spinal stenosis, herniated or torn discs. Also, epidural steroid injections are commonly administered to reduce pain caused by enlarged facet joints.
Joint Injections	Used as a diagnosis and treatment procedure for conditions of the joints, including but not limited to, facet joint syndrome, arthritis, and sacroiliitis.
Trigger Point Injections	Administered to alleviate painful areas of muscle, like that of myofascial pain.
Intrathecal Pump Implantation	Applicable for instances of chronic and intractable pain, cancer pain, and severe spasticity.
Lumbar Sympathectomy	Indicated for pain caused by peripheral vascular disease or complex regional pain syndromes.
Percutaneous Disc Decompression	Administered to patients who are experiencing pain that is a result of a bulging or contained herniated disc.
Nerve Blocks	Deployed for instances of neuralgic pain caused by injury or disease, including neuropathy, surgical injuries to nerves, and other conditions.
Kyphoplasty	Used to treat recent vertebral compression fractures due to osteoporosis, myeloma, metastasis, and vertebral angioma with intractable pain and no neurological symptoms.
Stellate Ganglion Block	Indications for referral include shingles and reflex sympathetic dystrophy/causalgia of the face and arms.
Radiofrequency Lesioning	Appropriate for a number of conditions such as pain of the facet joint, disc, sympathetically mediated pain, sacroiliac joint pain, and nociceptive radicular pain.
Spinal Cord Stimulation	Applied to reduce pain that is the result of back- related disorders like failed back syndrome, degenerative disc disease, lumbar adhesive arachnoiditis, complex regional pain syndrome.

Interventional Techniques for Cancer Pain:
Neurolytic celiac plexus block for pancreatic cancer, abdominal malignancies; vertebroplasty, pathologic vertebral compression fracture and spinal analgesics.

Neurosurgical Pain Therapies

Table 2: Neurosurgical Pain Therapies

Augmentative	Ablative
• Peripheral nerve stimulation • Spinal cord stimulation • Thalamus (PVG-PAG)	• Neurectomy • Sympathectomy • Ganglionectomy

stimulation • Motor cortex/deep brain stimulation • Intrathecal/epidural drug infusion • Intraventricular drug infusion	• Rhizotomy • Spinal DREZ lesioning • Cordotomy • Myelotomy • Nucleus caudalis DREZ lesioning • Trigeminal tractotomy • Mesencephalotomy • Thalamotomy • Cingulotomy • Hypophysectomy

Interventional Tecniques
Spinal & Epidural Opioid & Steroids
1. PNS,SCS & DBS
2. Neurolysis-Chemical neurolysis, Radiofrequency thermo coagulation Cryo analgesia
3. Vertebroplasty & Kyphoplasty
4. Dry Needling, Infiltration, Prolotherapy, TPI
5. Acupuncture
6. Radiotherapy
7. Ozone therapy
8. Caudal Epidural Decompressive Neuroplasty (Lysis Of Adhesions)
9. Percutaneous Management Of Visceral Pain
10. Neurosurgical Procedures

EQUIPMENTS USED ARE
- Fluoroscopic Guided
- Ultrasound Guided
- CT Guided
- MRI Guided

SPINAL CORD STIMULATION
- Relieves pain by applying sufficient electrical stimulation to cause paresthesias covering or overlapping the area(s) of pain without discomfort or motor effects
- Mechanism Of Action- "gate control theory of pain,"

SPINAL CORD STIMULATION
- SCS is minimally invasive and reversible.
- A typical SCS system has four components.
1. A neurostimulator that generates an electrical pulse (or receives radio frequency pulses) – this is surgically implanted under the skin in the abdomen or in the buttock area.
2. An electrode(s) implanted near the spinal cord either surgically or percutaneously (the latter via puncture, rather than through an open surgical incision, of the skin).
3. A lead that connects the electrode(s) to the neurostimulator.
4. A remote controller that is used to turn the neurostimulator on or off and to adjust the level of stimulation.

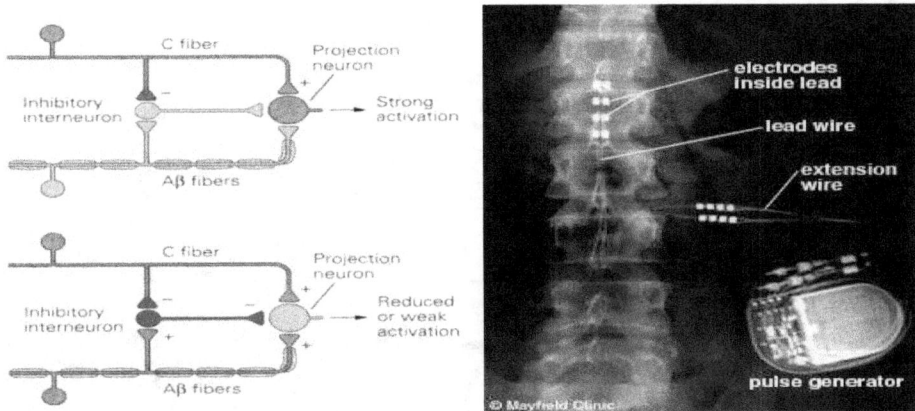

Fig 1 & 2: Stimulation of Spinal cord

INDICATIONS-
- Failed back surgery syndrome,
- Ischemic pain of peripheral vascular disease
- Postcordotomy dysesthesias,
- Reflex sympathetic dystrophy
- Phantom limb and stump pain.

CONTRAINDICATIONS-
- Coagulopathy, Sepsis,
- Serious drug behavior problems,
- Inability to cooperate or to control the device
- Demand cardiac pacemaker (without ECG monitoring or changing the pacemaker mode to a fixed rate).

COMPLICATIONS-
- Electrode fatigue fracture, Electrode migration/malposition
- Exposure to electromagnetic fields (e.g., diathermy, security systems)
- Spinal cord or nerve injury,
- CSF leak
- Infection
- Bleeding

RADIOFREQUENCY ABLATION

ACTION-
- Destruction of the nerves that signal pain
- The effect of RF on tissue depends on the temperature generated:
- >45°C, irreversible tissue injury occurs;
- Between 42 and 45°C, temporary neural blockade occurs.

INDICATIONS-
- Head and neck pain ,
- Spine pain ,
- Neuropathic pain

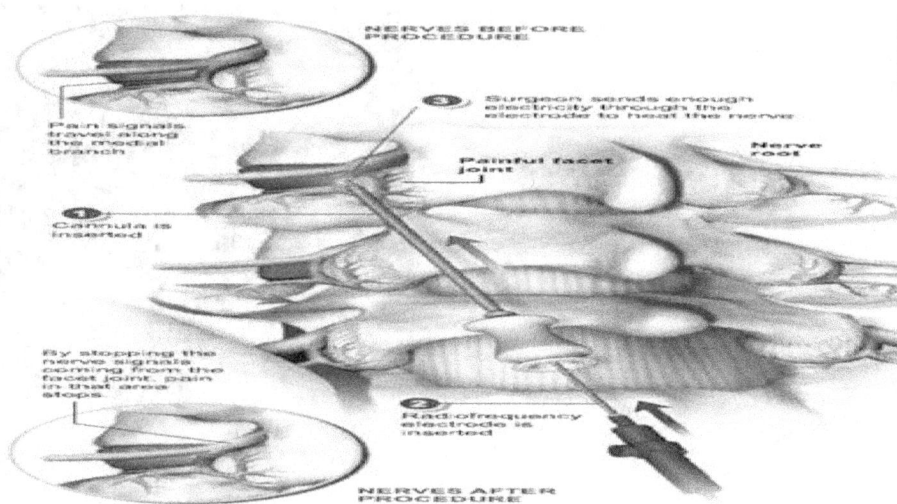
Fig 3: Procedure of spinal cord stimulation

COMPLICATIONS-
- Neurologic deficits from the intended target or nearby neural structures,
- Deafferentation pain,
- Neuritis,
- Burn injury at breaks in the needle insulation,
- Hematoma
- Infection

CRYONEUROLYSIS
Temporarily destroys a nerve through the application of extreme cold. The extreme cold degenerate the nerve axons without damaging surrounding connective tissue. Larger myelinated fibers cease conduction at 10°C. At 0°C, all nerve fibers entrapped in the ice ball stop conduction. Can be cooled upto -70 degrees. Pain relief lasts upto 3 months.

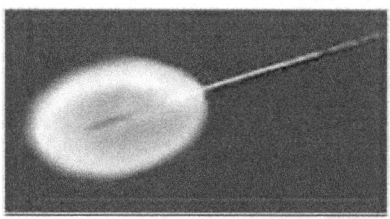 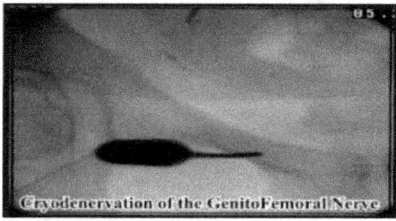
Fig 4 & 5: Showing Cryoneurolysis

INDICATIONS-
- Postthoracotomy Pain, Postherniorrhaphy Pain
- Intercostals Neuralgia, Painful Neuroma
- Cervical And Lumbar Facet And Interspinous Ligament Pain
- Coccydynia, Perineal Pain
- Ilioinguinal, Iliohypogastric, And Genitofemoral Neuropathies
- Superior Gluteal Nerve Neuralgia
- Cranial Neuralgia, Supraorbital Nerve Neuralgia
- Infraobital Neuropathy, Mandibular Neuropathy

VERTEBROPLASTY

Bone cement is injected percutaneously into a fractured vertebra with the goal of relieving back pain caused by vertebral compression fractures

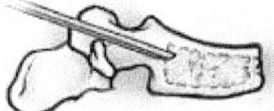 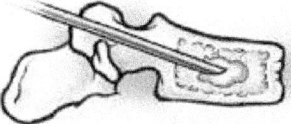

Fig. 6 & 7: Percutaneous vertebroplasty using bone cement.

Recent research has demonstrated that percutaneous vertebroplasty can relieve pain from vertebral compression fractures for up to nearly three years following the procedure.

Kyphoplasty
The center of vertebral body accessed with a tube, a balloon is inserted through it, a cavity is formed and balloon removed. The cavity is filled with cement.

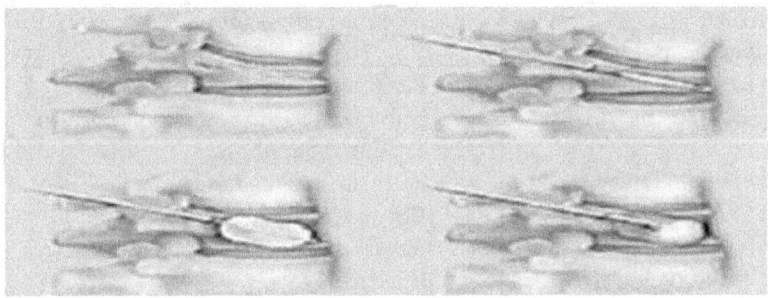

Fig. 8(1-4): Kyphoplasty Technique

Joint Interventions
Other joint intervention techniques involve Facet Joint RF ablation, cervical facet injection (RFA) and Socroiliac joint injection.

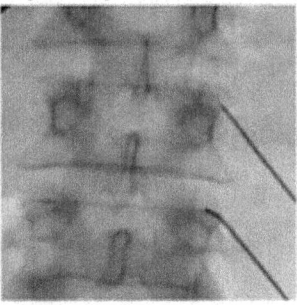 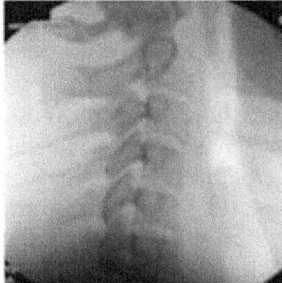 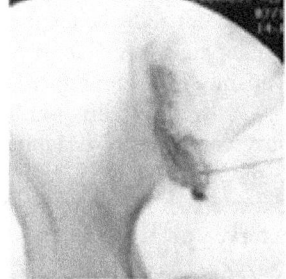

Facet Joint RF Ablation   Cervical Facet Injection (RFA)   Sacroiliac Joint Injection (Arthrogram)

Fig 9: Joint Interventions

CAUDAL EPIDURAL DECOMPRESSIVE NEUROPLASTY (LYSIS OF ADHESIONS)

Indications-
- Failed back surgical
- Disc disruption
- Mets of spine compression fracture
- Multilevel degenerative arthritis
- Epidural scarring following infection or meningitis
- Pain unresponsive to spinal cord stimulation

- Pain unresponsive to spinal opioids

Contraindications-
- Sepsis
- Coagulopathy
- Local infection at the site of the procedure
- Patient refusal

Neuroplasty is done to repair nerve damage. It is a procedure that is used to break up scar tissue that has formed around the nerve in the epidural space of the spine, so medications such as the steroid can reach the affected nerve/nerves so pain and other symptoms will lessen or go away. The actual procedure is similar to a caudal steroid injection in that a thin catheter is inserted from very low in the spine and it runs up to the point where there is scarring.

Table 3: Complications of Caudal Epidural Decompression Neuroplasty.

Immediate Complications	Late complications
<ul><li>Bleeding in the epidural space</li><li>Bending of the tip of the needle</li><li>Penetration of the Dura</li><li>Subdural insertion of the catheter</li><li>Shearing of the catheter</li><li>Hypotension</li></ul>	<ul><li>Penetration of the Dura</li><li>Numbness in the dermatomal distribution</li><li>Temporal anesthesia</li><li>Permanent paresthesias</li><li>Bowel and bladder dysfunction</li><li>Sexual dysfunction</li><li>Headache</li><li>Infection at the site of penetration</li><li>Epidural abscess</li><li>Arachnoiditis</li></ul>

COELIAC PLEXUS BLOCK

Neurolytic celiac plexus blockage can be beneficial interventional technique.
Principal: the celiac plexus is primarily a sympathetic central nervous system structure mediating transmission from upper abdominal viscera.

Effective palliation has been shown to improve quality of life and has been suggested to improve survival. Neurolysis achieved by percutaneously injecting phenol in to celiac plexus can be helpful for 3-6 months. Alternate nociceptive pathway also exist which requires continued use of opioids. Useful in patients who develop intolerable side effects or whose pain is inadequately controlled with the non interventional approaches. Complications are rare (gangrene of bowel, pneumothorax and paraplegia).

INDICATIONS-
To control pain of the epigastric viscera, especially due to
Primary or metastatic upper abdominal cancers
Chronic pancreatitis
Intra abdominal surgery

Drugs Used-
For a sensory block: 0.25% Bupivacaine with or without 1:200,000 epidurally.
For a neurolytic block-50% - 100% Alcohol diluted with sterile water or local anesthetic.
Total volume: not more than 15-20 ml for each injection.
Overfilling the space may cause the alcohol to leak and spread posteriorly, resulting in alcohol neuritis.

Anatomy
Celiac Ganglia are two seats of ganglia. The average numbers are one to five.
Left side ganglia are lower than right side on average less than a vertebral level.

Sizes on both sides vary between 0.6 – 0.9 cm below the celiac artery.
Size of ganglion varies between 0.5 – 4.5 cm.

Technique of Celiac Plexus Block

Posterior approach (Kappis)
Anterior approach
Tran's aortic approach
Trans – intervertebral disc approach
Intra – abdominal
Retrocrural
Transcrural celiac plexus block
Continuous block via catheter

PROCEDURE-

Prone position: Lines are drawn connecting the spine of T12 with points 7-8 cm lateral at the edges of the 12th ribs. Performed with a 15-cm, 20-22 G needle. Advance the needle at a 45 angle from the horizontal plane toward the body of T12 or L1. Bony contact should be made at an average depth of 7-9 cm. withdraw the needle and reinsert it at an increased angle of 5-10 degrees to allow the tip to slide off the vertebral body anterolaterally.

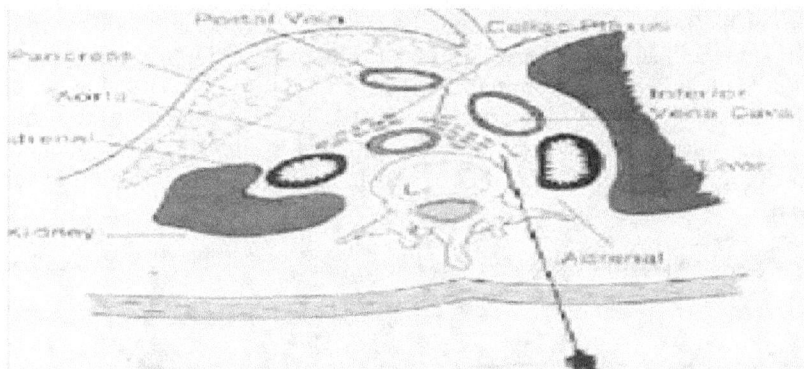

Fig. 10: Posterior approach (Kappis).

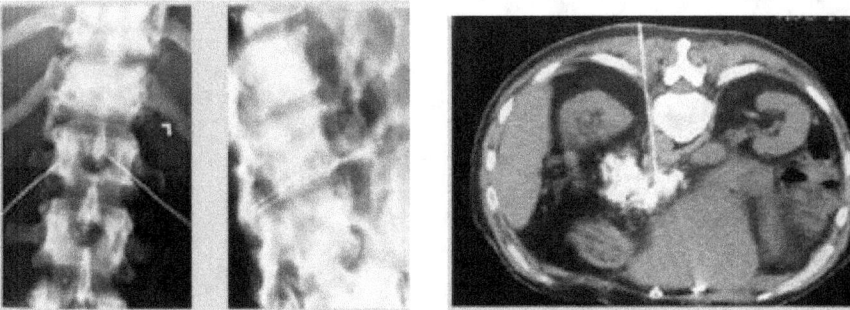

Fig.11: Caeliac plexus: AP & Lateral view Fig.12: CT guided Tran's thoracic approach.

Complications
- Hypotension
- Related to needle insertion/technique
  Pneumothorax
  Needle placed too far cephalad
  Puncture of surrounding structures, mainly kidneys
- Due to puncture of the aorta or vena cava- bleeding
- Related to sympathetic block/neurolytic agent
- Systemic toxicity
- Transient mild diarrhea (lasting up to 2 weeks)

- Paraplegia (rare but most serious) - related to use of alcohol damaging the artery of Adamkiewicz.

Neurolytic celiac plexus blockage can be beneficial interventional technique.
The celiac plexus is primarily a sympathetic central nervous system structure mediating transmission from upper abdominal viscera. Effective palliation has been shown to improve quality of life and has been suggested to improve survival. Nurolysis by percutaneously injecting phenol in to celiac plexus can be helpful for 3-6 months. Alternate nociceptive pathway also exist which require continued use of opioids. Useful in patients who develop intolerable side effects or whose pain is inadequately controlled with the non interventional approaches. Complications are rare (gangrene of bowel, pneumothorax and paraplegia).

HYPOGASTRIC PLEXUS BLOCK

This block is used for painful conditions of distal ureterus, gonads, sigmoid colon, vagina, rectum, bladder, perineum, vulva, prostate, uterus, and the major pelvic blood vessels.

Procedure
After sterile preparation of the area, a 15 cm 20 or 22-G needle is positioned by means of fluoroscopy (tunnel vision) at the front of the intervertebral space of L5/S1. It is important to aspirate in order to avoid injection into the iliac blood vessels. From an anterior posterior view, the tip of the needle must be paravertebral at the level of the intervertebral space of L5/S1. From a lateral view, the tip of the needle must be at the anterior border of the vertebra of L5/S1. In order to confirm the needle position and to avoid intravascular injection, it is wise to inject a contrast agent. The contrast agent should not spread beyond the lateral borders of the vertebral body of L5 or in a dorsal direction towards the nerve roots (Figure 2 and 3).

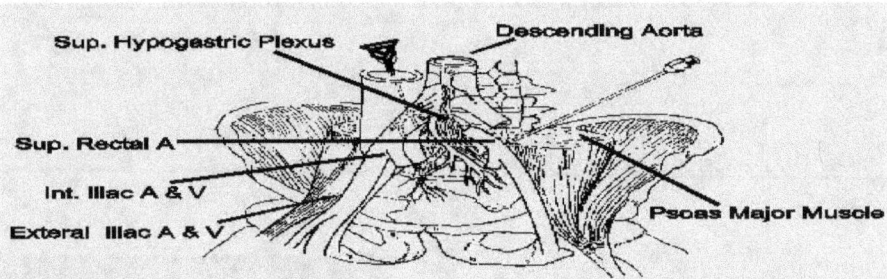

Fig. 13: Superior Hypogastric plexus block.
For hypogastric plexus test block procedures, 6-8 ml bupivacaine 0.25-0.5% can be used.
For therapeutic purposes, 6-8 ml 10 % phenol in telebrix solution injected at each side of the vertebra can be used. Fractionated injection, using continuous fluoroscopy control of the contrast spreading, will increase the safety of the procedure.

Complications
- Neurolysis of somatic nerves.
- Intravascular injection of neurolytic solution.
- In bilateral hypogastric superior plexus block, male sexual dysfunction can occur.

Advanced Interventional Pain Treatments
   Intraspinal opioid administration
   Radiofrequency ablation
      Intralesional
      Specific nerves / ganglion
   Vertebroplasty / kyphoplasty
   Neurolytic blocks
Others:
- Dry needling,
- Infiltration,
- Prolotherapy,

- Acupuncture
- Radiotherapy
- Ozone therapy

Radiofrequency Leisoning

Ionic heating of tissue with cooled radiofrequency is very accurate procedure. Internal cooling doubles the leison radius and increases the leison volume by a factor of 8.

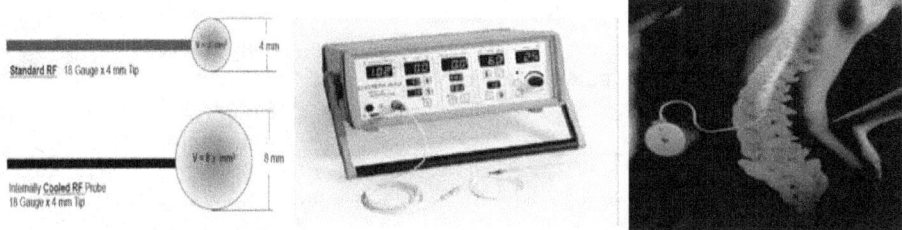

Fig. 14, 15 & 16: Radiofrequency Leisoning; Principle, COBMAN equipment & Medtronics Pump.

Neurosurgical Pain Therapies

Table 4: Neurosurgical Pain Therapies

Augmentative	Ablative
<ul><li>Peripheral nerve stimulation</li><li>Spinal cord stimulation</li><li>Thalamus (PVG-PAG) stimulation</li><li>Motor cortex/deep brain stimulation</li><li>Intrathecal/epidural drug infusion</li><li>Intraventricular drug infusion</li></ul>	<ul><li>Neurectomy</li><li>Sympathectomy</li><li>Ganglionectomy</li><li>Rhizotomy</li><li>Spinal DREZ lesioning</li><li>Cordotomy</li><li>Myelotomy</li><li>Nucleus caudalis DREZ lesioning</li><li>Trigeminal tractotomy</li><li>Mesencephalotomy</li><li>Thalamotomy</li><li>Cingulotomy</li><li>Hypophysectomy</li></ul>

Intrathecal Drug Delivery Systems

AKA: Pain pump

Mechanism of Action:
Drug delivered directly to the intrathecal space.

Drugs Used:
- Morphine
- Baclofen
- Bupivacaine
- Clonidine
- Ketamine

Table 5: Intrathecal Drug Delivery Systems

PROS	CONS
<ul><li>Short reversible trial</li><li>Delivery of drug directly to the site of action</li><li>1mg IT Morphine = 300 gm oral Morphine</li><li>Cancer Pain: pain, toxicity, survival 6mo</li></ul>	<ul><li>Short reversible trial</li><li>opioid benefit with time (40% failure with time)</li><li>Contraindications to placement</li><li>Complications (granuloma)</li></ul>

Common Types of Diagnostic and Therapeutic Spinal Injections
Epidural steroid injections
Selective nerve root blocks (selective transforaminal injections)
Medial / lateral branch nerve blocks and facet joint intra – articular injections
Neurolytic and radiofrequency nerve ablation procedures
Sacroilic joint and other intra – articular joint injections
Sympathetic ganglion nerve blocks
Diagnostic discographic injections
Intradiscal therapeutic procedures (percutaneous disc decompression)

Epidural steroid injection
Strong evidence for short term pain relief and moderate evidence for long term pain relief up to in 68% patients for one year.

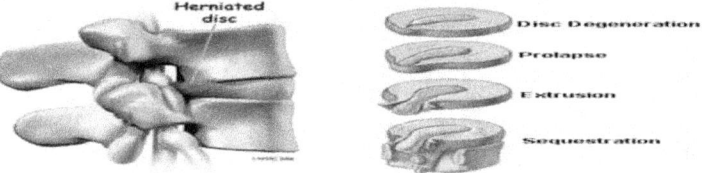

Fig17: Vertebral disc herniation

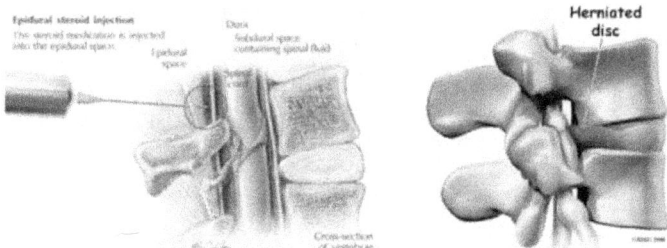

Fig 18: Epidural steroid injection

Conclusion:
- Pharmacological management of pain will continue to have to rely on a multimodal approach with old medications finding new uses and indications.
- Many factors must be considered before deciding on the type of pain therapy to be provided to the surgical patient.

References

1. Textbook of Pain, 2nd Ed, CBS Pub New Delhi 2008.
2. Kumar Pramod - Terminal cancer care 2nd Edition, CBS Medical Pubs, New Delhi 2005
3. Kumar Pramod - Guide to Peripheral Nerve Blocks 1st Edition CBS Medical Pubs, New Delhi 2008
4. Kumar Pramod - A Handbook of pain management & related symptoms in cancer, Samvedana, Indraprastha Apollo Hospital New Delhi, 2003
5. Kumar Pramod - Illustrated Atlas on peripheral nerve blocks Anaesthesia Dept. Jamnagar 2002
6. Staats PS, et al. Pain Med 2001; 2:28-34.
7. Lillemoe KD, et al. Ann Surg 1993; 217:447-55.
8. Cruccu et al. Evidence Based Guidelines for Interventional Pain Medicine. (EFNS guidelines on neurostimulation therapy for neuropathic pain. Eur J Neurology 2007; 14:952-70.)
9. Ward et al., Anesth. Analgesia 58:461; 1978.
10. http://www.medtronic.com/IN/images/intro_intrathecal1.gif.
11. Manchikanti L et al. Pain Physician 2000; 3:7-42.
12. Stav A et al. Acta Anaesthesiol Scand. 1993; 37:562-6.

Chapter 22.

Orofacial Pain and Migraine

ACUTE AND CHRONIC OROFACIAL PAIN:
Acute orofacial pain is primarily associated with an inflammatory process within the teeth and their periodontal structures.[1] acute and chronic manifestations of pain in the orofacial region, as in other body parts, differ from one other in their time course, etiological mechanisms, response to therapy and behavioral reactions. The most prevalent chronic orofacial pain is musculoskeletal and originates from muscles, tendons and the temporomandibular joint. Primary vascular type orofacial pain (VOP) is another prevalent diagnostic entity typified by severe episodic, pulsatile pain accompanying autonomic signs and symptoms. Variable temporal patterns necessitate abortive or prophylactic modalities of treatment for VOP. Neuropathic orofacial pain (NOP) can be of the neuralgic paroxysmal type, as in trigeminal neuralgia, or of a continuous chronic nature, often associated nerve injury, as in deafferentiation pain.

PRIMARY VASCULAR TYPE CRANIOFACIAL PAIN
Primary vascular type craniofacial pain includes migraine, cluster headache (CH), and paroxysmal crania (PH)[1] (Headache Classification committee of the international headache society 1988;. The etiology of these headaches and facial pains is considered to be neurovascular, and they share signs and symptoms[2]. Common diagnostic features are: episodic pain that is unilateral, Pulsatile, severe and may wake the patient from sleep. Accompanying phenomena include local autonomic signs (e.g. tearing, rhonirrhea) in PH and CH, and systemic signs (e.g nausea, photophobia) in migraine. Atypical odontalgia has been described as a possible example of primary vascular-type pain in the mouth.[3], but recently vascular orofacial pain has been defined[4] which may represent an orofacial equivalent of primary vascular-type headaches. Although presenting similar signs and features, different entities of vascular-type craniofacial pain respond distinctively to therapy, stressing the importance of correct diagnosis.[5]

Table 1: Signs and symptoms common to vascular-type craniofacial pain
  Pain is
  a) periodic
  b) severe
  c) unilateral
  d) pulsatile
  e) wakes the patient from sleep
  Accompanied by:
  a) local autonomic signs
      i) ocular: tearing, redness
      ii) nasal: rhinorrhea, congestion
      iii) local swelling or redness
  b) systemic signs
      i) nausea, vomiting
      ii) photo/phonophobia

MIGRAINE
Migraine with or without aura is a periodic, unilateral headache occurring mostly in the forehead and temple areas. Pain intensity is moderate to severe, usually throbbing, sometimes accompanied by photo- and phonophobia, and associated with nausea and occasional vomiting. The two forms of migraine—migraine with and without aura—are interrelated; one form may transform into the other, and both respond equally well to 5-hydroxytryptamine (5-HT) receptor agonists. Dilatation of large intra- and extracranial arteries occurs in both forms during an attack, but regional cerebral blood flow changes occur only in migraine with aura.

Table 2: Differential diagnosis of primary vascular type craniofacial pain

	Migraine headache	Cluster headache	Paroxysmal hemicrania	Vascular orofacial pain
Age and sex				
Age of onset (years)	20-40	30-40	30-40	40-50
Male : female ratio	1:2	5:1	1:2	1:2.5
Location				
Laterality	unilateral, may change sides	unilateral, rarely changes sides	unilateral, rarely changes sides	mostly unilateral
site	forehead, temple	orbital and periorbital	temporal and periauricular	intraoral and lower face
time course attack duration periodicity frequency of pain attacks	hours to days periodic 1-6 /month	15-120 min periodic/chronic in clusters, 1-2/day	minutes chronic/periodic daily, 6-15/day	minutes to hours periodic/chronic daily, varies in frequency.
character	throbbing, deep	paroxysmal, boring	paroxysmal, lancinating	Throbbing, may be paroxysmal
type of pain	moderate to severe	severe	severe	Moderate to severe
pain intensity	stress, hunger, menstruation	alcohol	movement of head	Sometimes cold foods
precipitating factors	nausea, photophobia. Visual aura	Lacrimation, rhinorrhea, ptosis, miosis.	Lacrimation, rhinorrhea, eye redness.	Cheek swelling and redness, tearing.
associated signs				

MIGRAINE WITHOUT AURA

An idiopathic, recurring headache disorder lasting 4-72 hours, migraine without aura is typically unilateral, Pulsating in quality, of moderate to severe intensity aggravated by physical activity, and associated with nausea and sometimes vomiting and with photo- and phonophobia. Certain diagnostic criteria must be met to fulfill the definition of migraine without aura. (Headache Classification committee of the international headache society 1988)[1] These include at least five attacks that have at least two of the following characteristics: (a) unilateral location, (b) pulsating quality, (c) moderate to severe intensity, and (d) aggravation by physical activity.

MIGRAINE WITH AURA

An idiopathic, recurring headache disorder, migraine with aura typically is associated with neurological symptoms (migraine with typical aura) and consists of one or more of the following: visual disturbances, unilateral paresthesia and/or numbness, unilateral weakness, and aphasia or unclassifiable speech difficulty. The aura lasts less than one hour and will be usually followed by the migraine without aura.

Epidemiology: based on many studies a 1 year prevalence in adults o about 10-15% has been suggested for migraine, including migraine both with and without aura[6]. The male to female ratio is about 1 to 3, with a prevalence of 5-8% in males and 15-25% in females. The female preponderance in migraine is more consistent across studies than the overall prevalence figure of migraine. The age of onset is early, and about half of cases start before the age of 20 years. Interestingly, no sex differences are apparent until age 11, after that age a female preponderance appears which may be linked to female hormones.[7] The 1 year prevalence of migraine with aura is approximately 2-4% which s lower than that of migraine without aura.

Precipitating factors: there are many precipitating factors, including emotional or psychological stress, menstruation, contraceptive medication, sleep (usually too long), fasting and fatigue. Other precipitating factors are associated with various foods and beverages such as chocolate, diary products, alcohol, fruit, fried foods, tea, coffee, and seafood. Food additives such as nitrites, nitrates, and sodium glutamates are among ewll-known trigger factors.

Treatment: Migraine headaches can be treated either prophylactically or abortively. Frequency of attacks is the most important consideration for treatment approach. Abortive treatment, aimed at stopping the pain attack once it has started, is used when there are no more than three attacks per month. When four or more attacks occur per month, prophylactic treatment should be considered. Analgesics and anti-inflammatory drugs are to be considered first, and if these are not effective the recently introduced 5-HT agonists such as sumatriptan should be utilized. On rare occasions opioids, preferably as an intranasal spray, may be considered. Combination drugs are also available, some of which contain ergotamine combined with other medications such as caffeine, codeine, and an antiemetic. Drug efficacy is greater when abortive therapy is initiated as early in the course of the attack as possible, and when a full dose is used.

In contrast to abortive treatment, which is used during the attack, prophylactic medication is taken on a daily basis in order to reduce the severity and frequency of potential migraine attacks. Three main groups are presently considered as most effective, with relatively few and minor side effects. These include β-adrenoceptor blocking drugs, tricyclic antidepressants, and anticonvulsants.

Table 3: Treatment of primary vascular-type craniofacial pain

	Migraine Headache	Cluster headache	Paroxysmal hemicrania	Vascular orofacial pain
Abortive	Triptans (sumatriptan, rizatriptan, zolmitriptan); NSAIDs (COX-1 or COX-2 inhibitors)	Oxygen (100%, 6 liters/min for 15 min); sumatriptan; ergot	Indomethacin	NSAIDs (COX-1 or COX-2 inhibitors); other non-narcotic analgesics
Prophylactic	Amitriptyline; β blockers; valproates	Ergot, methysergide, lithium carbonate	Indomethacin	Amitriptyline; β blockers

Table 4:

Class/Substances	Attack Frequency	Adverse Events	Contraindications
Beta-Adrenoceptor Antagonists			
Propranolol: 80–160 mg per day	50% reduction	Bradycardia	Asthma
Metoprolol: 100–200 mg per day	50% reduction	Hypotension	Bradycardia
Atenolol: 50–100 mg per day	50% reduction	Fatigue	Cardiac failure
		Sleep disturbance	Hypoglycemia
		Dyspepsia	
		Depression	
Calcium Channel Antagonists			
Flunarizine: 5–10 mg × 1 per day	50% reduction	Sedation	Depression
		Weight gain	Parkinson disease
		Depression	
		Sleep disturbance	
(Verapamil): 120–240 mg × 2 per day	50% reduction	Constipation	Bradycardia
		Bradycardia	Conduction defect
5-HT Antagonists			
Pizotifen: 0.5–1 mg × 1–3 per day	50% reduction	Increased appetite	Narrow-angle glaucoma?
		Weight gain	Prostatic hypertrophy?
		Drowsiness	
Cyproheptadine: 4 mg tablet × 2–4 per day	50% reduction		
5-HT Agonists			
Methysergide: 1–2 mg × 1–3 per day (Should be given for 4–6 months, stopped for 4–6 weeks, and then restarted)	50–75% reduction	Nausea	Pregnancy
		Sleep disturbance	Cardiac and peripheral vascular disorders
		Peripheral vasoconstriction	Impaired kidney or liver functions
		Retroperitoneal/pleuro-pulmonary fibrosis	Collagen diseases
Anti-Epileptics			
Sodium valproate: 300–500–600 mg × 1–3 per day	50–75% reduction	Nausea, vomiting	Pregnancy
		Alopecia	Thrombocytopenia
		Tremor	Liver disease
		Weight gain/loss	
Tricyclics			
Amitriptyline: 10–100 mg per day (bedtime)	50% reduction	Sedation	Narrow-angle glaucoma
		Weight gain	Prostatic hypertrophy
		Dry mouth	Recovery phase after myocardial infarction
		Blurred vision	

Comparison of effect, adverse events and contraindications for different classes of drugs used in the preventive treatment of migraine

CLUSTER HEADACHES

Cluster headache (CH) is characterized by attacks of severe unilateral pain in the orbital and periorbital area. Pain lasts from 15 to 180 minutes and occurs from once every other day to as often as 8 times a day. Episodic CH refers to a temporal pattern consisting of a series of pain attacks, or "active" episodes, occurring in succession (hence clustering) over period of 4-12 weeks with "inactive" periods that lasts from 6-18 months. In the active period pain occurs daily or almost daily. About 10% of patients have a continuous on constantly active pattern known as chronic cluster headache[8].

Pain pattern. Pain is unilateral, excruciatingly severe, and paroxysmal, occurs in the ocular, frontal, and temporal areas. Most cases, the pain starts in the orbital area, but as it continues and becomes more severe it radiates to the forehead, temporal region, upper and lower jaws, and, in some cases, to the neck and shoulder. Five pain attacks of this type are necessary to fulfill the diagnostic criteria for cluster headache.[1] (headache classification Committee of the international headache society 1988). Nocturnal attacks are typical and account for about 50% of attacks, with the highest frequency occurring toward early morning. Attacks tend to be shorter and less severe in intensity at the beginning and towards the end of each cluster period. However, the duration of each attack tends to lengthen during the course of the disease.[8]

Fig. Showing ascending and descending pathways of migraine

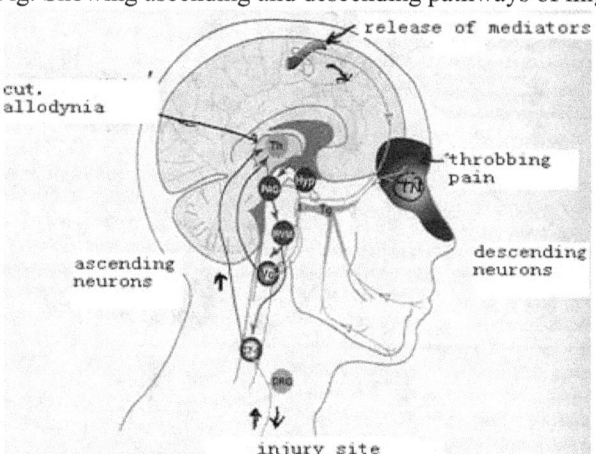

Accompanying phenomena: pain attacks are accompanied by ipilateral conjunctival injection, lacrimation, stuffiness of the nose, and rhinorrhea. Forehead and facial sweating and eyelid edema also occur. Ipsilateral ptosis and miosis may be associated with some attacks; occasionally, they persist after attacks and may remain permanently.

Precipitating factors. Alcohol precipitates attacks in the active period but not during the remission period. Histamine, administered intravenously or subcutaneously, and sublingual nitroglycerine also may precipitate an attack, and can be used as diagnostic tools.

Treatment: treatment consists of abortive and prophylactic approaches. The most effective abortive treatment is the administration of 100% oxygen, through a loosely applied face mask, at a rate of 7-8 L/minute for 15 minutes.[9] ergot preparations and subcutaneously administered sumatriptan have a beneficial effect.

Prophylactic treatment is administered during the active period. Ergot preparations should not exceed 10 mg per week, as higher doses may produce peripheral arterial spasm and necrosis. Methysergide can be administered only for short periods (weeks) to avoid retroperitoneal fibrosis. Lithium carbonate is utilized for the chronic type of cluster headache, but blood levels should be carefully monitored.[10]

PAROXYSMAL HEMICRANIA:

Paroxysmal hemicrania (PH) is a vascular-type headache characterized by very frequent, short bouts of severe unilateral pain around the orbit and temple. Chronic and episodic forms, similar to cluster headache (CH), have been described. Associated signs include ipsilateral conjunctival injection and tearing with nasal congestion and rhinorrhea. The absolute response of PH to indomethacin therapy differentiates from CH.

Location: pain occurs typically in the temporal, periauricular, and periorbital areas.[11] hence the term hemicrania. Referral to the shoulder, neck, and arm has been reported. Unlike CH, which may change sides, the vast majority of cases of PH do not. Most cases is PH are unilateral and do not become bilateral, but strong pain may cross the midline.[12]

Accompanying phenomena: As in other primary vascular-type headaches, PH is accompanied by a number of usually ipsilateral autonomic phenomena. These may occur bilaterally, but are more pronounced on the symptomatic side. The most commonly seen are lacrimation (62%), nasal congestion (42%), and conjunctival changes and rhinorrhea (36% each). Heart rate changes (bradycardia, tachycardia, or extrasystoles) [11], increased local sweating and salivation are not common but have been reported in PH.

Treatment and prognosis: treatment is prophylactic with a consistent response to indomethacin that clearly distinguished it from cluster headache, which is nonresponsive. Most cases report a positive response within 24 hours, but 3 days at 75 mg followed, if needed, by 150 mg for a further 3 days is recommended as trial therapy[13]: on discontinuation, symptoms usually reappear within 12 hours to a few days, but long-lasting remission for months to years has been described. Persistently high dosage requirements may indicate underlying pathology. Indomethacin-resistant cases have been reported and successfully treated with calcium channel blockers[14] and acetazolamide (a diuretic with anticonvulsant properties also known to reduce intraocular pressure)[15]. Although amitriptyline has not been reported to be even partially effective in PH, it has been found useful as an adjunctive drug to enable indomethacin dose reduction (and thus reduce side effects) and to aid in sleep.[16]

Primary vascular type craniofacial pain:

There is unequivocal evidence for the evidence of sensory axons innervating cephalic blood vessels. Together they have been termed as trigeminovascular system[17]. These trigeminal axons relay nociceptive information to the central nervous system (CNS); when stimulated antidromically, they promote neurogenic inflammation. Because this inflammation takes place within the restricted space of the cranium, the pain of migraine may be more severe than if it occurred in a more flexible space. Such pain mechanisms are possible in other craniofacial structures with confined spaces. Thus, the pain in cluster headache may be associated with a perivascular inflammatory process of the carotid artery in its bony canal or with increased intraocular pressure.[2] it is not surprising that such a neurogenic inflammatory process, when confined to antoher limited space, i.e., the tooth-pulp chamber or inferior alveolar canal, may cause strong intraoral pain that mimics pulpitis. Evidence for a neurogenic inflammatory process within the tooth pulp may support possible mechanisms for a vascular-type dental orofacial pain. Nerve fibers exhibiting positive immunoreactivity to substance P and calcitonin gene-related peptide have been demonstrated in the dental pulp and oral mucosa in several species, including humans.[ ] Neurogenic inflammation in the trigeminovascular system seems to play a central role in the genesis of vascular type headaches, and the same mechanism could function in the oral mucosa and teeth. It is possible that pressure build-up plays a role in intrapulpal pain sensation.

NEUROPATHIC OROFACIAL PAIN:

Pain initiated by a primary lesion or dysfunction of the nervous system is defined as neuropathic pain. The appearance of neuropathic pain signifies some abnormal process in the peripheral or central nervous system. This process may be ongoing (e.g., symptomatic trigeminal neuralgia) or may have healed, but leaving the nervous system in a pathological state. (e.g.,. deafferentation pain). When affecting the orofacial region it is termed as neuropathic orofacial pain (NOP)[19.] NOP may be primary or secondary, and its differential diagnosis includes trigeminal neuralgia, deafferentation pain, SUNCT syndrome (defined below), and neuritis, among others. Clinically, neuropathic pains may be divided into two broad categories: paroxysmal and continuous. These characteristics are diagnostically and therapeutically important. At times NOP is difficult to diagnose, but because some entities are therapeutically straightforward with a good response (e.g., trigeminal neuralgia), accurate diagnosis is essential. Others are notoriously difficult to treat (e.g., deafferentiation pain), and adequate patient management and support are essential. Some threatening conditions may be associated with these pain entities, such as CNS tumors, systemic disease, or pressure on a peripheral nerve by space-occupying lesions.

SUNCT syndrome

Shortlasting, unilateral, neuralgiform headache attacks with conjunctival injection and tearing (the SUNCT syndrome) are considered to belong to the neuropathic pain entities. SUNCT is a unilateral craniofacial pain characterized by brief paroxysmal pain accompanied by ipsilateral local autonomic signs, usually conjunctival injection and lacrimation. Nasal stuffiness

COMBINATION SYNDROMES:

Cluster-tic syndrome and hemicrania-tic syndrome can occur in combination with trigeminal neuralgia. Neuropathic craniofacial pain secondary to trauma

A total of 2% of all neuralgias in the orofacial region are thought to be secondary to pathological lesions. For example, TN occurring in young patients (especially 20-4- years) or presenting bilaterally may signify underlying disease, i.e., multiple sclerosis or tumor. Accompanying phenomena such as sensory changes, muscle weakness, and autonomic signs should alert the clinician. Secondary neuropathic pain may also develop after trauma or viral infection.

DEAFFERENTATION

Mechanical injuries to peripheral nerves may ultimately lead to a variety of painful condition. Various factors will determine the quality of the pain and accompanying sensory changes. These factors include the severity and type of injury, the time elapsed since injury and the group of nerve fibers damaged. Involvement of the sympathetic nervous system may cause interaction and pain that is sympathetically "maintained".

PHANTOM TOOTH PAIN (ATYPICAL ODONTALGIA)

IASP has defined atypical odontalgia as a severe throbbing pain in the tooth without major pathology. The high incidence of pain that is pulsatile and episodic, with pain that migrates and even changes sides, makes it likely that this may be a vascular phenomenon. Indeed, the term vascular toothache has been interchangeably used to describe this pain entity. However, this condition has also been referred to as phantom toothache, implying mechanism. The question whether atypical odontalgia is a vascular or neuropathic syndrome is a source of controversy. Indeed, many cases present with continuous pain that is contrary to a classical vascular-type pain. When the pain displays a constant, burning quality a neuropathic-type mechanism is likely to exist, and the term neuropathic orofacial pain is used instead of atypical odontalgia. It is possible that cases of atypical odontalgia metamorphose into, or coexist with, neuropathic-type pains in response to repeated dental interventions aimed at pain relief.

CRANIOFACIAL MACROTRAUMA:

Peripheral nerve injury has been implicated in post traumatic headache and facial pain. This may take the form of paroxysmal neuralgic pain or chronic deafferentation pain seen in more severe injuries. Even in relatively minor head trauma, widespread shearing may cause extensive axonal injury that is commonly known as diffuse axonal injury and may contribute to central mechanisms of post traumatic pain

Nerve entrapment in scar tissue or direct nerve injury with aberrant regeneration and abnormal nerve activity due to neuroma formation, as seen in other traumatic neuropathic conditions, may be the peripheral pathological basis. Trigeminal nerve axons are less prone to developing ectopic hyperexcitability, suggesting that post-traumatic pain in the trigeminal region may be more infrequent than in other regions of the body.

SYMPATHETICALLY MAINTAINED PAIN

Sympathetically mediated pain (SMP) refers to a group of disorders in which, as the name suggests, the sympathetic component of the autonomic nervous system is involved. IASP considers SMP to be a feature of complex regional pain syndromes, which include syndrome previously named reflex sympathetic dystrophy and causalgia. Local interaction at the injury site between sensory and sympathetic fibers initiates a positive feedback system that serves to maintain pain. Continued peripheral input probably results in central sensitization and peripheral sensory changes such as hyperesthesia, allodynia, and hyperpathia. Essentially, SMP is a descriptive term that is used for any pain condition that is sympathetically dependent and therefore relieved by sympatholytic procedures. It has not been widely studied in the head or face and mostly appears in case reports.

OTHER CLINICAL SYNDROMES ASSOCIATED WITH NEUROPATHIC OROFACIAL PAIN:

Multiple sclerosis, tumour of the brain and branches of trigeminal nerve, diabetes, herpes and geniculate neuralgia respond to treatment of cause.

Table 5: Primary and secondary neuropathic orofacial pain

Primary	Secondary
Idiopathic neuralgias: 　Trigeminal 　Glossopharyngeal 　Geniculate	Post traumatic: 　Sympathetically independent 　Sympathetically mediated
Pretrigeminal neuralgia	Viral: 　Postherpetic 　Geniculate
SUNCT syndrome	Neural tumours 　Central 　Peripheral
Combinations: 　Cluster-tic 　Chronic paroxysmal 　Hemicrania-tic	Systemic disease: 　Multiple sclerosis 　Mixed connective tissue disease 　Diabetes

REFERENCES:

1. Headache Classification Committee of the International Headache Society. Classification and diagnostic criteria for headache disorders, cranial neuralgias and facial pain. Cephalgia 1988;7:1-96.
2. Pareja JA, Pareja J, Palomo T, Cabarello V, Pamo M. SUNCT syndrome: repetitive and overlapping attacks. Headache 1994;34:114-116.
3. Rees RT, Harris M. atypical odontalgia. Br. J. Oral Surg 1978;16:212-218.
4. Benoliel R, Elishoov H, Sharav Y. The diagnosis and treatment of persistent pain following trauma to the head and neck. J oral maxillofacial surg 1994;85:158-161.
5. Sharav Y, Benoliel R. Primary vascular-type craniofacial pain. Compendium cont educ dent 2001; 22:119-132.
6. Rasmussen BK, Breslau N. Migraine, epidemiology. In: Olesen J, Tfelt-Hansen P, Welch KMA (Eds). The headaches, New York: Raven press, 1993, pp 169-173.
7. Bille B. Migraine in school children. Acta Paediatr 1962; 51 (suppl 136.)
8. Nappi G, Russell D. Cluster headache clinical features. In: Olesen J, Tfelt-Hansen P, Welch KMA (Eds). The headaches, New York: Raven press, 1993, pp 97-104.
9. Ekbom K, Sakai F. Cluster headache, management. In: Olesen J, Tfelt-Hansen P, Welch KMA (Eds). The headaches, New York: Raven press, 1993, pp 591-599.
10. Kudrow L. Lithium prophylaxis for chronic cluster headache. Headache 1977; 17:15-18.
11. Haggag KJ. Russell D. Chronic paroxysmal hemicrania. In: Olesen J, Tfelt-Hansen P, Welch KMA (Eds). The headaches, New York: Rraven press, 1993, pp 601-6-8.
12. Kudrow DB, Kudrow L. Successful aspirin prophylaxis in a child with chronic paroxysmal hemicrania. Headache 1989; 29; 280-281.
13. Pareja J, Sjaastad O. Chronic paroxysmal hemicrania and hemicrania continua. Interval between indomethacin administration and response. Headache 1996, 36:20-23.
14. Shabbir N, McAbee G. Adolescent chronic paroxysmal hemicrania responsive to verapamil monotherapy. Headache 1994; 34: 209-210.
15. Warner JS, Wamil AW, McLean MJ. Acetazolamide for the treatment of chronic paroxysmal hemicrania. Headache 1994; 34:597-599.
16. Benoliel R, SharavY. Trigeminal neuralgia with lacrimation or SUNCT syndrome? Cephalgia 1998a; 18:85-90.
17. Moskowitz MA. The trigeminovascular system. In: Olesen J, Tfelt-Hansen P, Welch KMA (Eds). The headaches, New York: Raven press, 1993, pp 97-104.
18. Wakisaka S. Neuropeptides in the dental pulp: distribution, origins, and correlation. J Endodontics 1990; 16:67-69.
19. Benoliel R, Sharav Y. Neuropathic orofacial pain. Compendium Cont Educ Dent 1998c; 19:1099-1116.

Chapter 23:

PAIN CLINIC

Issues: Trained Doctors from established Pain Clinic.
Persuade Hospital Colleagues.
Investigate legal Practices involved.
Inform Specialists, Family physicians, Public.

Types of PAIN CLINIC
Uni disciplinary – Single Specialist.
Multi discipinary Clinic – 2-3 Specialists.
Regional Pain Clinic - University / Metros.
Outpatient Facility :-
- Consultation Room.   - Procedure Room.
- Examination Room.   - Changing Room.
- Office, Library.

In patient Facility: - Hospital Beds, Specialists, Jr. Doctors, Nurses, Trained Staff.

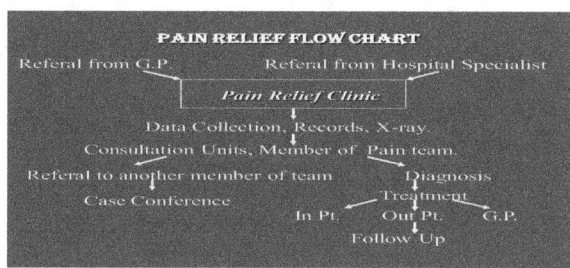

Fig 1. Flow chart of Pain Clinic

Pain Clinic - Management
1. Detailed History
2. Examination, Investigation
3. Dermatomal Mapping.
4. Records. diagnosis

Objectives Of Treatment
1. Pain Relief - Sleep at night - Alert in day time.
2. Mild Analgesic, narcotics – Regularly.
3. Adjuvants- Laxatives, Anti depressant

Pain full conditions referred:
1. Traumatic – Neuroma, Muscle tendon, Painful scars.
2. Musculoskeletol – Backache, Protrusion of I.V.D. Disc Degeneration, Spondylosis.
3. Neurological – Trigeminal/ glossopharyngeal Neuralgia, Nerve lesion, Entrapment, Dental, Headache.
4. Autonomic – Peripheral vascular insufficiency, causalgia.
5. Neoplasitc
6. Diagnostic & Psychosomatic problems.
7. Miscl.– Restless leg, Shoulder hand synd; fracture, Herpes.

Types of pain
1. Somatic Pain – Cutaneous, Muscle, Joint, Tendon, Fascia.
2. Viscral – Sympathetic from viscra. Diffuse, less localised: BP, Pulse changes.
3. Refered – Deep Pain, Viscral /Somatic. Felt in same dermatome.
4. Psychosomatic – No Anatomical Pattern, Psychotherapy.

Dermatomal Mapping

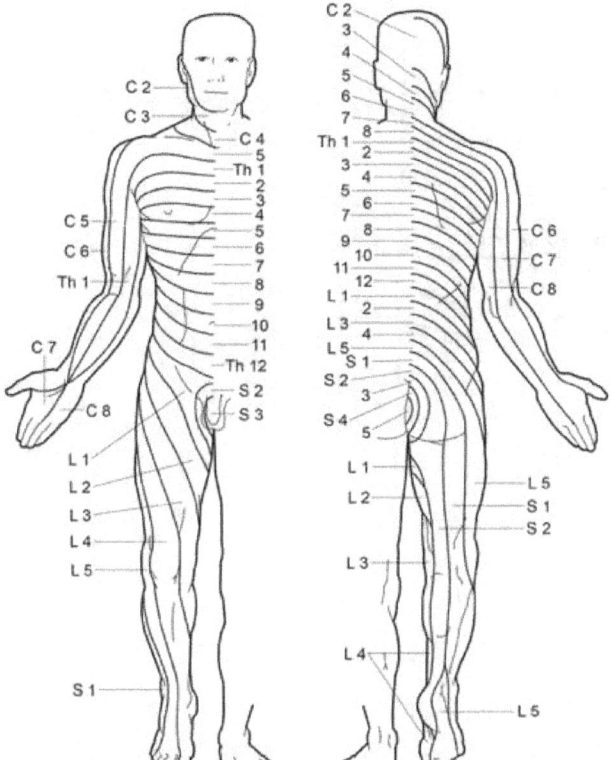

Fig 2. Dermatomal mapping.

Radiology Investigaions:
Plain X-Ray, Brain scans: CT,MRI,PET. f MRI - Noxious-evoked brain activity

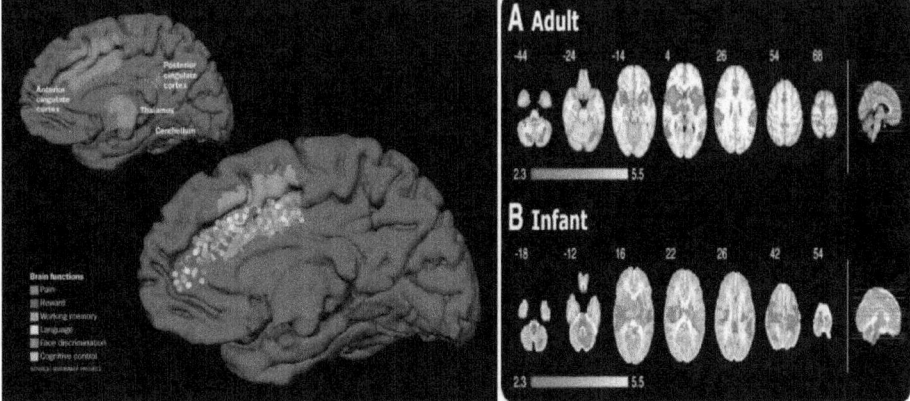

Fig3. f MRI - Noxious-evoked brain activity

Mechanism of aetiology
1. Compression of nerve roots, Trunks, Plexus by Tumor.
2. Obstruction of Viscera – Stomach, Colon, Rectum.
3. Mechanical Obstruction of Vessel – headache, Extremity.
4. Necrosis, Infection, Inflammation- Uterus, Buttock.
5. Infiltration – Tumefaction,
6. Swelling – Fascia, Bone, Peritoneum.
7. Combination of above.

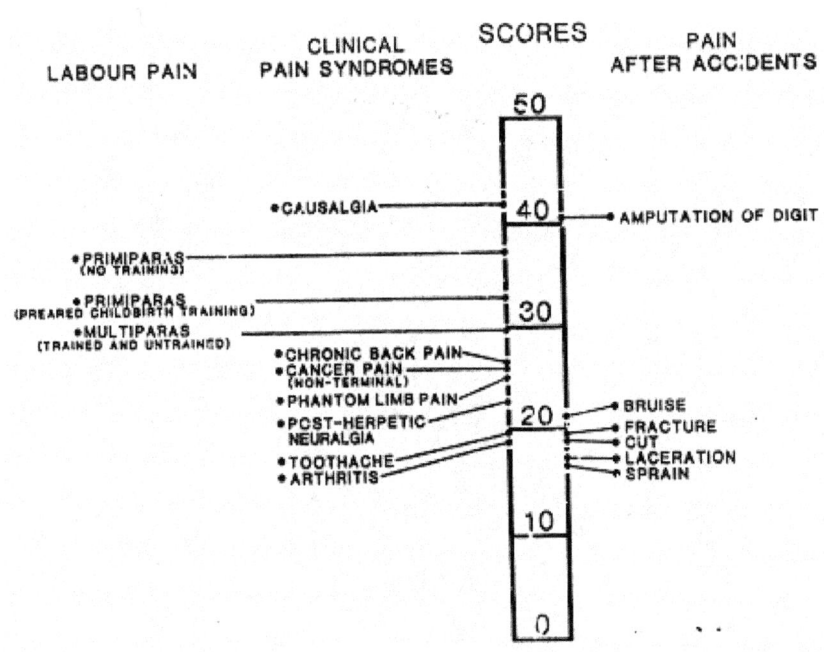

Fig 4: Pain pole

Assessment of Pain
8. Visual Analogue Scale (VAS), Facial Expressions.
9. Type of Pain – Burning, Stabbing, Aching.
10. Intensity – Mild, Moderate, Severe.
11. Location – Dermatomal Mapping.
12. Quality – McGill Pain Questionnaire.
13. Unpleasant, Distressing, Awful, Agonizing.
14. Pediatric Pt. – Facial expressions, Oucher, CRIES
15. FRACC, Million/BECK Behavior Inventory

Acute Pain Services   -
POST OPERATIVE PAIN RELIEF
More Pain-Abdominal, Intrathoracic surgery
Complications-Respiratory distress, Hypoxia.
Origin- Skin, Tendons, Bone, Muscle, Viscera. Increase by coughing, straining, anxiety, psychological fear.
Drugs - IV morphine, buprenorphine, tramadol.
Watch- Regular doses, side effects, addiction.
Children: Aspirin, morphine-.1-.2m/kg, codeine 1m/kg.
Local analgesic blocks – Intercostal N B, cryoprobe
(2) Epidural /Intrathecal -LA. Opiates, ketamine
(4) Continuous infusion-LA: Opiates. (5) Tens. (6) PCA

Table 1: Intravenous PCA opioids

Agent	Bolus	Lockout Interval	4 h Maximum Dose	Infusion Rate[a]
Fentanyl (10 µg/mL)	10-20 µg	5-10 min	300 µg	20-100 µg/h
Hydromorphone (Dilaudid) (0.2 mg/mL)	0.1-0.2 mg	5-10 min	3 mg	0.1-0.2 mg/h
Meperidine (10 mg/mL)[b]	5-25 mg	5-10 min	200 mg	5-15 mg/h
Morphine sulfate (1 mg/mL)	0.5-2.5 mg	5-10 min	30 mg	1-10 mg/h

Patient Controlled Analgesia (PCA) is a method of pain control that gives the patient the power to control their pain.
- Pain medication is administered through a computerized pump.
- The pump contains a syringe of pain medication as prescribed by a doctor that is connected directly to a patient's intravenous (IV) line.
  - The pump is set to deliver a small, constant flow of pain medication.
  - Additional doses can be self-administered as needed by the patient pressing a button.

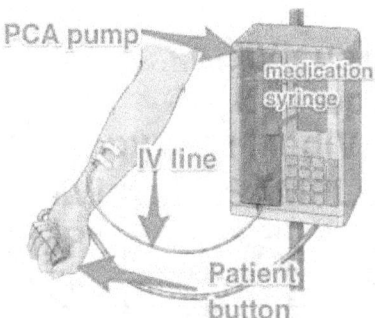

Fig 5. PCA Pump

Chronic Pain-
Peripheral & central sensitization -allodynia, hyperalgesia, and hyperpathia

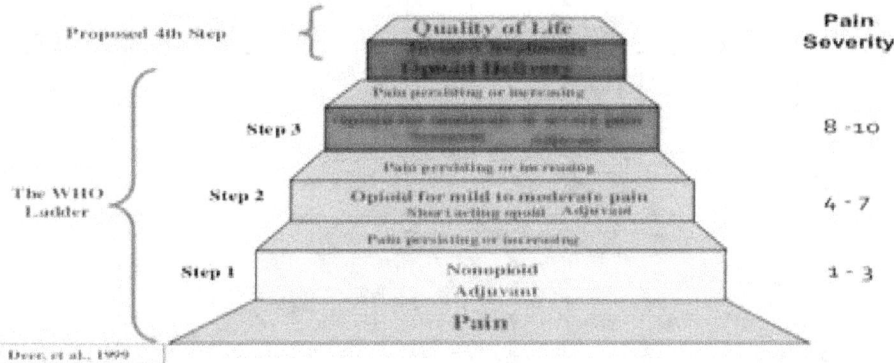

Fig 6: Modified WHO 3 step Analgesic ladder

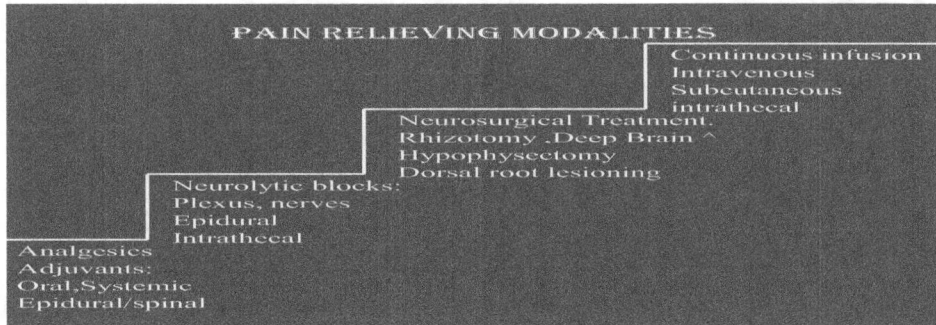

Fig 7: Pain relieving modalities.

Table 2. COMPARISON OF ANALGESICS

• MILD ANALGESICS	• OPIATES
1. Less effective in large dosages- ceiling	1. Dose related analgesi
2. Used orally-less effective No dependence	2. Parentrally SC,I/th,IM,IV
3. Used in chronic low grade pain	3. Used in Acute pain
4. Diverse Mech. of action, Treat cause	4. Opiate Receptors
5. Less side effects. Gastric	5. Resp N,V,addiction
6. Used in combination	6. Administered alone
7. Aspirin,NSAID,Codeine,Paracetamol	7. Morphine,Buprenorphine

Table 3. Opioids in Analgesia

Drug	Dose iv/id/PCA	Duration (mts)
1. Sufentanil	10 to 20 μg	20 – 45
2. Morphine	5/10 – 15 mg	30-60 / 120-180
3. Fentanyl	25-50/ 100 μg 10-25 μg PCA	20-40/ 30-60
4. Nalbuphine	10-20/1-3μg PCA	120-240
5. Butorphanol	1-2 μg/kg	120-240
6. 6. Remifentanyl	0.1-0.5μg/kg PCA	2 - 3
7. Tramadol	100 μg/ kg	180

Table 4: DRUG DELIVERY IMPLANTS

	Days	Weeks	Months	Years	Years
Type I Simple Epi, S.A.Catheter					
Type II Tunneled Catheter					
Type III Reservoir port					
Type IV Manually activated					
Type V Continuous infusion					
Type VI Programmed infusion					

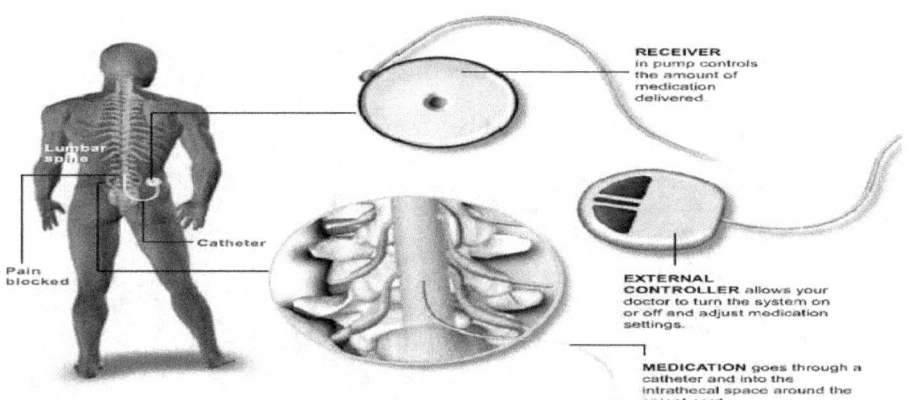

Fig 8: DRUG DELIVERY IMPLANTS

INTRATHECAL INJECTIONS – Opioids, Neurolytics
Accurate Placement of Neurolytic Agents, Indoor patients

- Indications :- Ca cervix, Rectum, Pelvis,
- Agents – Absolute Alcohol – Hypobaric, Diffuses Fast, Relief Shorter, Inflammation, Burning at site.
- Phenol 5% - Hyperbaric, Local analgesic, prolonged relief, effective.
- Chlorocresol 5% in glycerin, hyper baric, effective diffusion.
- Complications – Patchy degeneration, Headache Arachnoidoitis, retention of urine, paresis, N.V.

Epidural –
Opioids, Neurolytics, Adjuvents
Indications – Same as spinal, Sciatica, Ca, Postop, Long lasting Pain relief – Catheter, Infusion Pumps.
Diagnosis & Therapy –Epiduroscopy, Vertebroplasty, Reynaud's, Burger's D, Visceral Pain.
Malignancy-3/5 ml 3/10% Phenol: Ca-rectum, Viscera

Advantages –Easy, Segmentl, No Complication of SA
Disadvantages: – Less precise, dural puncture, Neurological.

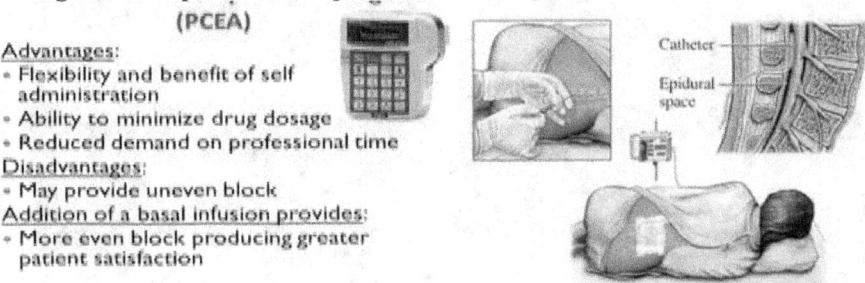

Fig 9. Epidural PCA

PHYSIOTHERAPY

- Massage, Short wave diathermy, Ultrasound, IFT, TNS, Wax Bath, cervical traction,
- Manipulation of joints and bones.
- Manual therapy using hands tools on soft tissue.
- Cold laser therapy to alleviate inflammation and pain and release endorphins.
- Micro current stimulation, which emits alpha waves into the brain and increases serotonin and dopamine to alleviate pain naturally.
- Movement therapy and exercise.
- Trigger Point Dry Needling in the Shoulder – Myofascial.
- Ozone Therapy.

Recent Advances

Visual observation of Loss Of Resistance: overcomes operator subjectivity and variability, offer a more precise end point compared with the standard LOR syringe.

Novel epidural needles: Needle-shaped Ultrasound probe: This is simply an optically guided insertion of epidural needle. Three optical fibers are embedded in Tuohy needle shaft, one emits light; two absorb light and the optical spectra are analyzed to identify the various tissue planes
CI-PCEA (Computer Integrated Patient Controlled Epidural Analgesia)

Smart pumps: Highly sophisticated infusion technology used with both epidural & intravenous infusions. Incorporate multiple comprehensive libraries of drugs, usual concentrations, dosing units and dose limits, to avoid medication errors.

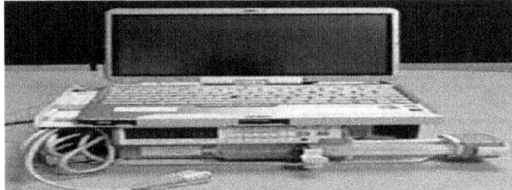

Fig 10. Smart pumps

Ultrasound-guided neuraxial technique:
Ultrasound imaging aid for neuraxial blockade:
- It helps to identify the midline, localize the Nerve/ epidural space, measure the skin-to-PN/epidural space distance and estimate the angle of needle insertion
- Facilitates the placement of needles not only in healthy parturient but also in obese pregnant women and patients with scoliosis, malignancy.
- Can be used as a teaching tool, improves the peripheral Nerve block/epidural placement learning curve, in ICU.

Problems: Increased procedural time, cost, need of expertise.

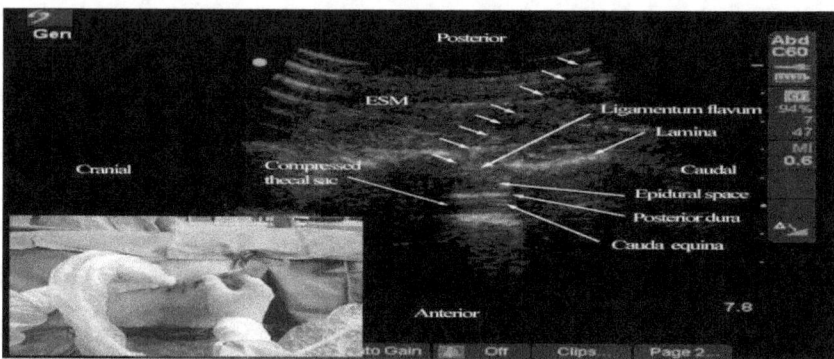
Fig 11. Ultrasound-guided neuraxial technique

Backache-
Upper: Myofacial, Trauma, Positional

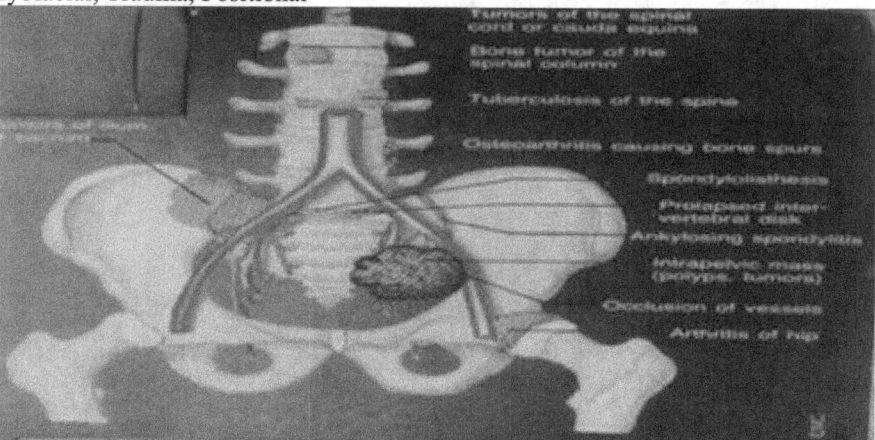
Fig 12. Causes of backache

Chronic Intractable Pain
LOW BACKACHE- EPIDURAL INJECTION
1) Hydrocortisone 50 mg/Depomedrol 80 mg
2) Lignocaine 0.5% / Bupivacaine 0.25%
3) Buprenorphine 0.1 mg
1. Moderate acting- diclofenac, tramadol
2. Long acting- Piroxicam-20 mg
3. Adjuvant- Central muscle relaxant, Ketamine

Management of cancer pain
1) Mechanism Producing it.
2) Localisation and severity of Pain.
3) Physical & Mental Condition of Patient.
4) Type of Neoplasm, Grade of deafferentation.
5) Availability of Modes of therapy: Surgery, Radiotherapy, Chemotherapy, PNB, Radiofrequency leisoning, Analgesics, Psychotherapy, Hospice care. Ozone, Hyperbaric Oxygen Therapy.

Psychological support
May not need psychotherapist services.
Physician provides sympathy, under- standing, kindness, GHQ scoring.
Need- Patient senses his prognosis.
Defeatist attitude by physician towards disease.
Adjuvants: – Nourishing food, Nursing Care, Sleep, Rehabilitation.
Behavioral Therapy.

Spinal Cord stimulation
This can provide in 67% patients up to 50% pain reduction upto a period of 6 months. It is effective in limb ischemia (77%), peripheral neuropathy967%) and post herpetic neuralgia (82%). Various implants e.g. Eon, Bionics are being used in this technique.

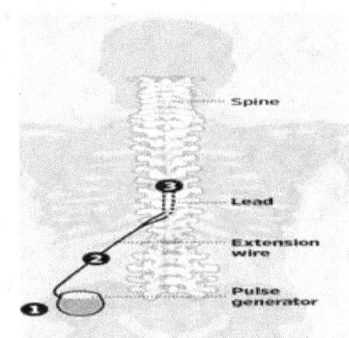

Fig 13. Spinal implants :

NON-INVASIVE BRAIN STIMULATION TECHNIQUES
- Brain stimulation is a technique that can guide brain plasticity and thus be suitable to treat chronic pain-a disorder that is associated with substantial reorganization of CNS activity.
- Therefore, therapies that directly modulate brain activity in specific neural networks might be particularly suited to relieve chronic pain.
- Repetitive transcranial magnetic stimulation (TMS) and Transcranial direct current stimulation (tDCS) are particularly appealing as they can change brain activity in a non-invasive, painless and safe way.

TMS-TRANS CRANIAL MAGNETIC STIMULATION
- Developed in 1985.
- It is based on a time-varying magnetic field that generates an electric current inside the skull, where it can be focused and restricted to small brain areas by appropriate stimulation coil geometry and size.
- This current, if applied repetitively, repetitive TMS (rTMS), induces a cortical modulation that lasts beyond the time of stimulation.

tDCS –TRANS DIRECT CRANIAL STIMULATION
- Induces similar modulatory effects.
- tDCS is based on the application of a weak direct current to the scalp that flows between two relatively large electrodes—anode and cathode electrodes.
- Some studies have shown that the efficacy of tDCS depends critically on parameters such as electrode position and current strength.
- Application of tDCS for 13 min to the motor cortex can modulate cortical excitability for several hours.
- This technique can also be used to obtain clinical gains in neuropsychiatric disorders such as stroke, epilepsy, and tinnitus.

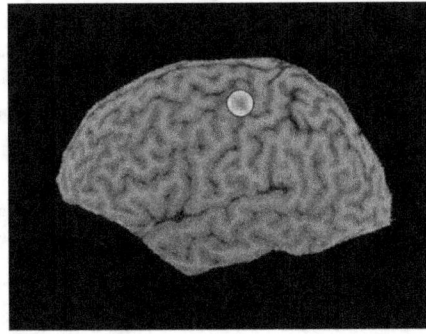
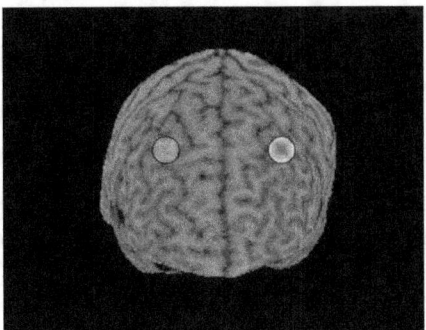

Fig14:.
1. High-frequency rTMS of the primary motor cortex.
2. Low and high-frequency rTMS of dorso lateral prefrontal cortex

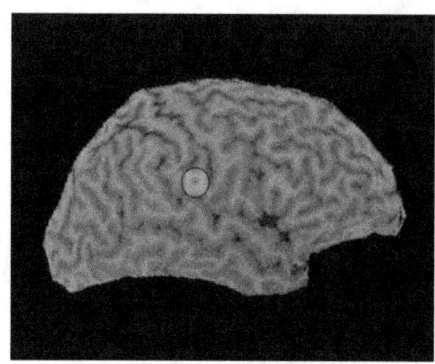 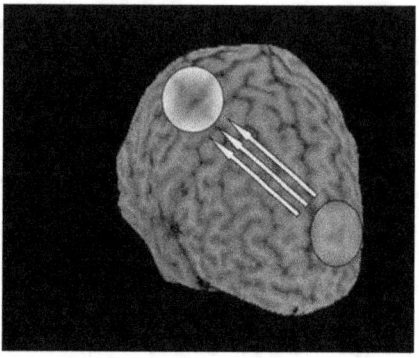

Fig15.
1. Low-frequency rTMS of the secondary somatosensory cortex.
2. Anodal tDCS of the primary motor cortex.

- At the beginning of the 1990s, a new and less invasive strategy of brain stimulation was developed, known as epidural motor cortex stimulation,
- It showed substantial pain improvement and brought new life to the concept of brain stimulation for the treatment of chronic pain.
- Epidural cortical stimulation not only decreased the neurosurgical risks of brain stimulation for chronic pain, but also invited the exploration of non-invasive brain stimulation techniques, tDCS and rTMS.

RESULTS FOR rTMS-
- Right and Left secondary somatosensory cortex stimulation with 1 Hz, 20 Hz.
- The results showed that 1 Hz (of left and right secondary somatosensory cortex) and right somatosensory cortex (with 1 and 20 Hz) stimulation led to a significant pain reduction.

RESULTS FOR tDCS
- Patients with chronic pain due to spinal cord injury were randomized to receive active motor tDCS (2 mA for 20 min for five consecutive days).
- There was a significant pain improvement after active anodal stimulation of the motor cortex.
- tDCS has some advantages over rTMS-
- It has longer-lasting modulatory effects of cortical function.
- Is less expensive.
- Easy to administer.

Deep brain Stimulation

It is an invasive procedure involving stimulation of PAG and sensory thalamus / internal capsule have a success in 79-87% cases. It is effective for nociceptive pain, neropathic and failed spinal surgery syndrome (FBSS).

Small electric current applied to an iontophoretic chamber on skin, containing a charged active agent and its solvent vehicle. Another chamber, a skin electrode carries return current. .

Anode chamber repel a positively charged chemical, cathode repel a negatively charged species into the skin.

Future Trends
Wickens' Multiple Resources Theory - Resources in different sensory systems function independently supporting Virtual Reality technology, based on integrating multimodal (visual, auditory, tactile and olfactory) sensory distractions.

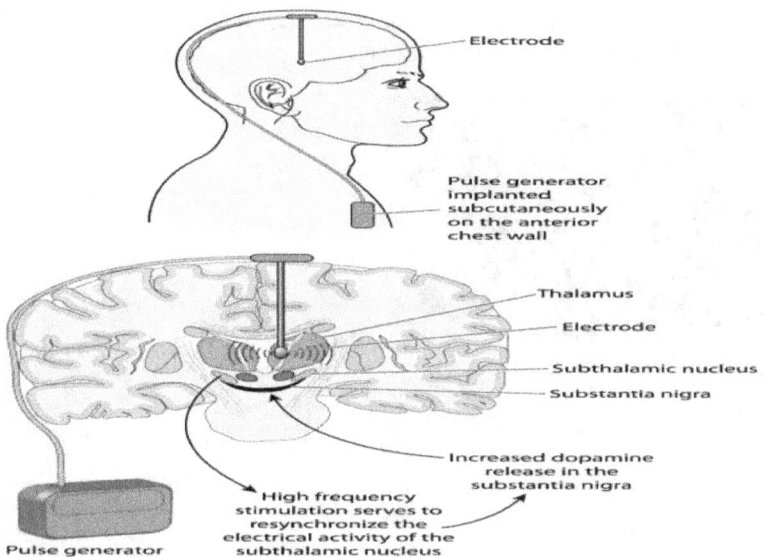

PAG=periaqueductal gray;
PVG=periventricular gray
RVM=rostral ventromedial

Fig 16. Deep brain stimulation

Transcranial magnetic stimulation

Mechanism due to
- inhibition of limbic system -secondary activation of pain and mood regulating regions egcingulategyrus, insula, hippocampus
- Prefrontal rTMS
- Facial pain, FMS, post-gastric bypass
- Motor cortex rTMS

Fig 17: Transcranial Magnetic stimulation

Iontophoresis Transdermal system

- Electrotransport delivery platform technology (E-TRANS/IONSYS)
- Hydrogel reservoir into the skin
- Low-intensity direct current
- Bolus dose 40 ug
- Dose interval 10 min
- Upto 24 hours or a maximum of 80 doses
- Audible beep & LED light indicator

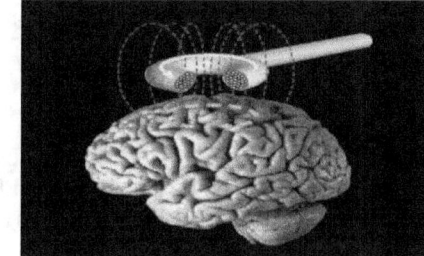

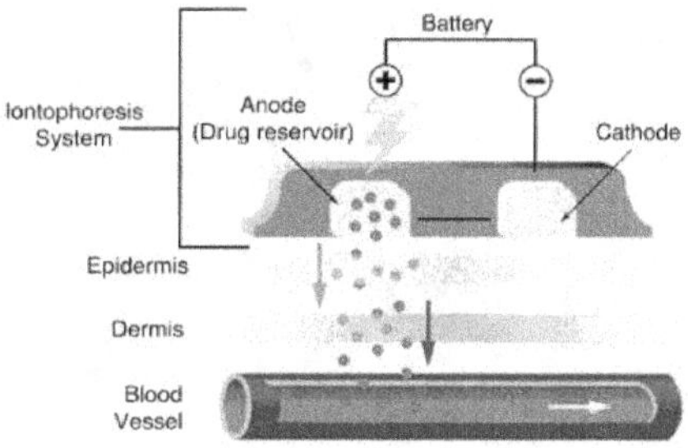

Fig 18. Iontophoresis Transdermal system.

New opiorphin analogue

Human opiorphin QRFSR-peptide protects enkephalins from degradation by human neutral endopeptidase (hNEP) aminopeptidase-N (hAP-N)
Inhibits pain perception in a behavioral model of mechanical acute pain
Activates restricted opioid pathways specifically involved in pain control contributing to a greater balance between analgesia and side-effects than found with morphine
Opiorphin could give rise to new analgesics with fewer adverse effects than opioid agonists

Gold et al – Inter cortical modulation among signalling pathways of the pain matrix through attention, emotion, memory and other senses (e.g., touch, auditory and visual), produces analgesia. An overall decrease of activities in the pain matrix may be accompanied by increases of activity in the anterior cingulate cortex and orbitofrontal regions of the brain.

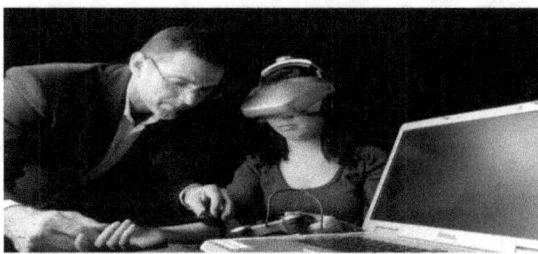

Fig 19: Medoc 30 × 30 mm ATS thermal stimulator

References
1. Textbook of Pain, 2nd Ed, CBS Pub New Delhi 2008.
2. Kumar Pramod - Terminal cancer care 2nd Edition, CBS Medical Pubs, New Delhi 2005
3. Kumar Pramod - Guide to Peripheral Nerve Blocks 1st Edition CBS Medical Pubs, New Delhi 2008
4. Kumar Pramod - A Handbook of pain management & related symptoms in cancer, Samvedana, Indraprastha Apollo Hospital New Delhi, 2003
5. Kumar Pramod - Illustrated Atlas on peripheral nerve blocks Anaesthesia Dept. Jamnagar 2002.
6. Virtual reality and pain management: Current trends and future directions.Agela & Gold. Pain Manag, 2011, 1(2) : 147-157

Chapter 24.

Temporomandibular Disorders and Dental Pain

Pains in the musculoskeletal system are among the most common types of painful disorders in the body, including the orofacial region. The temporo-mandibular disorders (TMD) are currently viewed as a cluster of related pain conditions in the masticatory muscles temporo-mandibular joint (TM|J), and associated structures, i.e., they are considered a form of musculoskeletal pain.

INTENSITY OF SPONTANEOUS TMD PAIN

TMD pain can be persistent and constant, but there can also be substantial variation across time with exacerbations and spontaneous remission. Standard descriptions of persistent TMD pain usually state that the intensity ranges from mild to moderate to strong or even excruciating levels of pain and that the pain is often exacerbated by muscle function[1] of perceived pain intensity requires the use of standardized scales, such as verbal descriptor scales of visual analogue scales (VAS) [2]. A survey of recent clinical studies on persistent TMD pain indicated that the average pain level measured on a 100-mm VAS with the jaws at rest ranges between 30mm and 50mm[3]. VAS scores greater than 30mm probably represents at least moderate pain levels. The perceived pain intensity of TMD generally fluctuates with significant differences between the lowest, highest and average pain VAS scores during a week and between different facial sites. The use of diaries also can be helpful to estimate the pain because the perceived pain intensity of TMD patients can change over time simply due to regression of the mean. Furthermore the memory of pretreatment jaw-muscle pain is significantly dependent on the past and present levels of pain[4] showed that the experimental chewing increased the levels of pain in a majority of patients with persistent jaw-muscle pain.

QUALITY OF SPONTANEOUS TMD PAIN

The usual way to describe persistent TMD pain is as deep, dull ache, sometimes with a boring, pressing or tightening type of pain. The McGill Pain Questionnaires (MPQ), originally introduced as an attempt to provide a detailed description of the quality of pain[5], has become the most frequently used pain questionnaires.

In a sample of 200 patients with persistent facial pain including TMD pain, Turp et al. (1997) found that more than 30% of subjects used the words 'aching', 'tight', 'throbbing', 'tender', 'exhausting', 'nagging', 'sharp' and 'tiring'. The choice of 'radiating' (26%) and 'pressing' (22%) seems rather specific for TMD pain conditions compared to other pain conditions[6]. The quality of pain appears to be markedly different between patients with myofascial TMD pain and pain in the TMJ[7]. It is unclear whether this difference can be explained by activation of different nociceptive fibers in the muscle and joint tissue or by higher-order cognitive-emotional differences. Thus, certain words seem to be specifically related to the description of persistent TMD pain, but no word is specifically indicative of this pain condition in a similar way that 'pulsating' has been tied to migraine and 'pressing' and 'tightening' to tension-type headache.

Pain drawings made by patients are simple, but useful tools to illustrate the localization and extent of pain areas in genera. Pain drawings completed on a systematic basis by patients with pain complaints in the craniofacial region have revealed that only about 19% have pain confined to this region, whereas 66% have widespread referred pain outside the craniofacial and cervical regions[7].

The various theories on referred pain mechanisms have been reviewed recently[3]. There is a general agreement than the diffuse nature and poor localization of muscle pain is related to central convergence of afferent fibers onto common central neurons because this feature will in effect reduce the spatial resolution of somatosensory information. The nociceptive afferents from muscles, joints, skin and viscera converge onto common projection neurons. It is nevertheless unclear why muscle or joint pain can be referred to the skin, whereas the reverse is seldom encountered. Differences between cutaneous and muscular nociceptive afferents in terms of somatotopic organization, sizes of receptive fields, and laminar distribution of their terminals may explain the predominant referral of muscle pain[10]. Other mechanisms than central convergence are also likely to be involved in the expression of referred pain because there is normally a time delay between the onset of local and referred pain. One possibility is that the nociceptive barrage from muscle tissue opens up latent connections, in a form of central divergence[8]. The synaptic connections between neurons that originally had no effective drive from the myositis-induced muscle may now become effective. The neurobiology sub serving such mechanisms is probably related to central sensitization of second-order neurons and the development of hyper excitability.

MANAGEMENT OF OROFACIAL MUSCULOSKELETAL PAIN

Because the underlying mechanism of TMD pain is only partially understood, it is difficult to design therapy to cure the pain. Instead a more realistic goal will be to alleviate pain. Thus, the management strategies for TMD pain follow the same principles of management of other musculoskeletal pain conditions and may be physically, pharmacologically and psychologically oriented (Table).

Table 1: Possible strategies for non-surgical management of teporo-mandibular disorders

Physical	Pharmacological	Psychological
Stretch therapy	Topical NSAIDs	Information
Jaw exercises	Oral NSAIDs	Counseling
Massage	Acetaminophen	Education
Ultrasound	Glucocorticosteroids	Stress management biofeedback
Heat/cold	Muscle relaxants	Relaxation
TENS	Benzodiazepines	Cognitive-behavioral therapy
Soft laser	Tricyclic anti-depressants	Psychotherapy
Acupuncture		
Oral splints	Opioids	

PHYSICAL MANAGEMENT OF TMD PAIN

There may be a significant reduction in perceived pain intensity following the intervention (e.g., acupuncture, biofeedback or splints), but that there may only be marginal or even no difference when the active treatment is compared to a placebo control. Thus, the specificity of many of the proposed treatments appears to be remarkably low. Oral splints have also been used extensively for management or even for 'curing' TMD pain.

PHARMACOLOGICAL MANAGEMENT OF TMD PAIN

Nonsteroidal anti-inflammatory drugs (NSAIDs) like ibuprofen in combination with diazepam provide significantly better pain relief compared to ibuprofen alone or placebo. A short-acting benzodiazepine, triazolam, improved sleep, but failed to provide significant pain relief in TMD patients. A combination of acetaminophen, codeine and doxylamine succinate (antihistaminic) provided significant pain relief than placebo in another study in mixed TMD patients.

PSYCHOLOGICAL MANAGEMENT OF TMD PAIN

Systematic studies on the efficacy of psychological management of TMD pain are rather scarce. A combination of biofeedback, stress management, and oral splints provides significant and long-lasting pain relief in TMD pain patients[2]. It appears to be important to tailor the treatment to each individual patient and not to consider psychological interventions on TMD pain as a treatment of last resort, but rather use it concurrently with biomedical and dental treatments.

SURGICAL MANAGEMENT OF PAIN

In some selected cases with persistent pain in the TMJ and restrictions in movement, which have not responded adequately to conservative treatment, surgical approaches may be recommended to alleviate the symptoms. The procedures range from irrigation of the upper joint space of the TMJ (arthrocentesis), direct inspection, lysis and lavage (arthroscopy), to positional changes in the condyle (modified condylotomy) or removal of the disk (diskectomy). It is clear treat that irrespective of the specific procedure, the success rate is close to 80% or more.

ACUTE DENTAL PAIN

Usually, dental pain is a result of dental caries. Initially, when the carious lesion is confined to the dentine, pain is evoked due to changes in temperature or exposure to sweet substances. As the lesion penetrates deeper into the tooth, the pain produced by these stimuli becomes stronger and lasts longer (hyperalgesia). Eventually, when the carious lesion affects the tooth pulp, an inflammatory process develops (pulpitis), which is associated with acute, intermittent spontaneous pain. Following pulp necrosis, microorganisms and products of tissue disintegration invade the area around the root apex (periapical periodontitis), and the tooth becomes very sensitive to chewing, touch and percussion. At that stage the explosive, intermittent pain, typical of pulpitis, acquires a continuous boring nature and the tooth is no longer sensitive to changes in temperature. In clinical practice the demarcation between these various stages is sometimes indistinct; e.g. the tooth may be sensitive simultaneously to temperature changes and to chewing.

DENTINAL PAIN:

Pain originating in dentine is a sharp, deep, sensation. It is usually evoked by an external stimulus and subsides within a few seconds. Such stimuli are normally produced by food and drinks that are hot, cold, sweet or sour and the pain evoked by such stimuli indicates a hyperalgesic state of the tooth. The pain is poorly localized, and the patient may not be able to distinguish whether it originates from the lower or upper jaw. Duplication of pain produced by control application of cold or hot stimuli to various teeth in the suspected area can aid in identifying the affected tooth. Dentinal pain due to caries is best treated by removal of the carious lesion and restoration of the tooth. Sensitivity usually disappears within a day.

Table 2: Differential diagnosis of dental and periodontal pain

Pain origin	Localization	Character	Intensity	Intensifiers	Associatesigns	Radiology
Dentinal	poor	Evoked, does not outlast stimulus	Mild to moderate	Hot, cold, sweet, Heat, cold, chewing	Caries, exposed defective	Interproximal caries, defective
Pulpal	very poor	Spontaneous, explosive, intermittent	Moderate to severe		Deep caries, extensive restorations	Deep caries pulp exposurely no periapical changes at acute stage
Periodontal	Good	Continues for hours: deep and boring	Moderate to severe	chewing	Periapical tenderness, redness and swelling	
Periapical lateral	Good	Continues for hours: deep and boring	Moderate to severe	Chewing	Periodontal tenderness, redness, swelling, tooth mobility.	Sometimes alveolar bone resorption

PULPAL PAIN

Pain associated with pulp pathology (pulpitis) is spontaneous, strong and often throbbing and is exacerbated by temperature changes, sweet foods and pressure on the carious lesion. When pain is evoked it outlasts the stimulus and can be excruciating for many minutes. Similar to dentine pain, localization of pulpal pain is poor and seems to be even worse when pain becomes more intense. Pain may be described by patients in different ways. It may manifest as a continuous dull ache and can be periodically exacerbated for short or long periods of minutes to hours[9].Ppain may increase and throb when the patient lies down and in many instances it wakes the patient from sleep. The pain of pulpitis is frequently not continuous and abates spontaneously; the precise explanation for such abatement is not clear. Localization of the affected tooth is achieved through hot and cold application and by percussion. Depending on the prognosis of the pulp (reversible or irreversible pulpitis) and that of the tooth, treatment may aim at conserving the pulp, extirpating it, or extracting the tooth. Pulpal pain usually disappears immediately after effective treatment.

PERIODONTAL PAIN:

Periodontal pain usually results from an acute inflammatory process of the gingiva, periodontal ligament, and alveolar bone due to bacterial infection. Pain is readily localized and the affected teeth are very tender to pressure. Two pathological pathways are common with pain resulting from either (1) pulp infection or pulp necrosis that results in periapical inflammation; or (2) Periodontal infection with pocket formation that results in a lateral Periodontal abscess. Although pain characteristics, ability to localize the pain, and pain producing situations are similar in both cases, treatment differs for etiological reasons and these categories are therefore discussed separately.

Table 3: Acute and chronic orofacial pain features

	Acute	Chronic
Time course	Short (hours to days)	Long (months to years)
Aetiology	Peripheral inflammatory	Central neuropathic
Response to: analgesics psychrotopics	Good poor	poor moderate to good
Behavioral response	anxiety, "guarding"	depression, "illness behavior"

ACUTE PERIAPICAL PERIODONTITIS:

Pain is spontaneous and moderate to severe in intensity for extended periods of time (hours). Pain is exacerbated by biting on the tooth and, in more advanced cases even by closing the mouth and bringing the affected tooth in contact with the opposing teeth. In these cases, the tooth feels extruded and is sensitive to touch. Frequently the patient reports that pulpal pain preceded the pain originating from the periapical area. Localization of pain originating from the periapical area is usually precise; in this respect periodontal pain differs from the poorly localized dentinal and pulpal pain. However, although the patient is able to indicate affected tooth, in approximately half the cases that pain is diffuse and spreads into the jaw on the affected side of the face.[9]

During examination the affected tooth is readily located by means of tooth percussion. The periapical vestibular area may be tender to palpation. The pulp of the affected tooth is non vital, and therefore does not respond to thermal changes or to electrical pulp stimulation. In more severe, purulent cases (acute periapical abscess) there is swelling of the face associated with cellulitis, sometimes accompanied by fever and malaise. The affected tooth may be extruded and mobile[10].

Treatment is aimed at the source of irritation in the pulp chamber and the root canal, which are open and debrided to allow drainage. Grinding the tooth to prevent contact with the opposing teeth helps to relieve pain. If cellulitis, fever and malaise are present, systemic administration of antibiotics is recommended. Soft tissue incision and drainage are very effective when a fluctuating abscess is present. Pain usually subsides within 24-48 hours.

LATERAL PERIODONTAL ABSCESS

Pain characteristics are similar to those of acute periapical Periodontitis. Pain is continuous, well localized, and moderate to severe in intensity; it is exacerbated by biting on the affected tooth. Examination may show swelling and redness of the gingiva, usually located more coronally than in the case of acute periapical lesion. The affected tooth is sensitive to percussion and is often mobile and slightly extruded. In more severe cases, cellulitis, fever, and malaise may occur. A deep Periodontal pocket (over 6 mm) is usually located around the tooth; probing of this pocket usually results in pus exudation. The tooth pulp, however, is usually vital, i.e., it reacts to temperature changes and electrical stimulation. Gentle irrigation and curettage of the pocket should be performed. The tooth should be ground in order to prevent contact with the opposing tooth. When cellulitis, fever, and malaise are present, systemic antibiotic administration is recommended. Pain usually subsides within 24 hours of treatment.

GINGIVAL PAIN

Gingival pain may occur as a result of mechanical irritation, acute inflammation associated with a gingival pocket or acute bacterial or viral infection[11]

Food impaction: Gingival pain caused by food impaction is characterized by localized pain between two adjacent teeth especially after meals, and particularly when food is fibrous. The pain is annoying with a feeling of pressure and discomfort. Pain gradually disappears until evoked again at the next meal and may be relieved by removing the food impacted between the teeth. Upon examination, a faulty contact between two adjacent teeth is usually noticed, where food tends to get trapped. The gingival papilla is inflamed, tender to touch and bleeds easily. The cause of the faulty contact between the teeth is often a carious lesion, and restoring the tooth will eliminate the pain.

PERICORONITIS

This severe pain is usually located at the distal end of the arch of teeth at the lower jaw. Pain is spontaneous, exacerbated by closing the mouth and aggravated by swallowing and maybe associated with trismus. Upon examination, a flap of gingiva over a partially erupted tooth is acutely inflamed, red and edematous. Occasionally, fever and malaise are associated with this infection. Treatment includes irrigation of debris between the flap and the affected tooth and eliminating contact with the opposing tooth (by grinding or extraction). Systemic antibiotic administration is commonly recommended especially when trismus occurs.

ACUTE NECROTIZING ULCERATIVE GINGIVITIS

Soreness and pain are felt at the margin of the gums. Pain is intensified by eating and brushing the teeth and is accompanied by gingival bleeding. Metallic taste is sometimes experienced, and usually there is a fetid smell from the mouth. Necrosis and ulceration are noticed upon examination of the marginal gingival, with different degrees of gingival papillary destruction and adherent grayish slough represents the pseudo membrane that is present in the acute stage of the disease. Swabbing this slough is associated with pain and bleeding. Although basically this is bacterial disease that responds to antibiotics, it is not clear whether the bacteria initiate the disease or are merely secondary to underlying local or systemic factors. Treatment includes swabbing and gently irrigating the ulcerative lesions, preferably with an oxidizing agent (Hydrogen peroxide, and scaling and cleaning the teeth). Systemic antibiotics are recommended when fever and malaise are present

REFERENCES:
1. Okeson J.P. Bell's orofacial pains. Chicago.Quintessence, 1995.
2. Grace Ly R.H. Studies of pain in normal man. In:Wall P.D, Melzack.R.(Ed). Textbook of pain Edinburgh; Churchiill Livingstone 1994; 315-336.
3. Svennsson and Graven – Nielsien T. Craniofacial muscle pain. Review of Mechanisms. J. Oroofacial pain, 2001.17:2-10.
4. Feine JS, Laigne GJ, Dao TTT et al. Memories of chronic pain and perceptions of relief. Pain 1998; 77; 137-141.
5. Melzack R. The MacGill pain Questionnaire; Measured properties and scoring methods. Pain 1975; 1; 277-300.
6. Turp JC, Kowalzki CJ, Stohler CS. Pain descriptors characteristics of persistent facial pain. J. Orofac Pain. 1997; 11: 285-290.
7. Mogini F, Italiano M. TMJ disorders in myogenic facial pain; A Discriminative analysis using MPQ. Pain 2001; 91: 323-330.
8. Sharav Y. Orofacial pain; dental, vascular and neuropathic pain. 2002- An updated review. Refresher course syllabus. Giamberardino MA, (Eds) IASP Press, Seattle, 2002.
9. Mens S, Hoheisel U Kaske et al. Muscle pain: Basic mechanisms and clinical correlate in Jenson TS, Turner JA et al. Eds, Proceedings of 8th World congress of pain, Progress in pain research and management, Vol 8 Seattle: IASP: Press, 1997, 479- 4996.
10. Sharav Y, Levine RE, Tekert A, et al. The spatial intensity and unpleasantness of acute dental pain. Pain 1984; 20:363-366.
11. Cohen S. Endodontic diagnosis In: Cohen S Burns RC (Eds). Pathways of the pulp, 7th ed. St. Louis, CV Mosby 19

Chapter 25:

Acute Dental and Temporomandibular Pain

ACUTE DENTAL PAIN

Usually, dental pain is a result of dental caries. Initially, when the carious lesion is confined to the dentine, pain is evoked due to changes in temperature or exposure to sweet substances. As the lesion penetrates deeper into the tooth, the pain produced by these stimuli becomes stronger and lasts longer (hyperalgesia). Eventually, when the carious lesion affects the tooth pulp, an inflammatory process develops (pulpitis), which is associated with acute, intermittent spontaneous pain. following pulp necrosis, microorganisms and products of tissue disintegration invade the area around the root apex (periapical periodontitis), and the tooth becomes very sensitive to chewing, touch and percussion. At that stage the explosive, intermittent pain, typical of pulpitis, acquires a continuous boring nature and the tooth is no longer sensitive to changes in temperature. In clinical practice the demarcation between these various stages is sometimes indistinct; e.g. the tooth may be sensitive simultaneously to temperature changes and to chewing.

DENTINAL PAIN:

Pain originating in dentine is a sharp, deep, sensation. It is usually evoked by an external stimulus and subsides within a few seconds. Such stimuli are normally produced by food and drinks that are hot, cold, sweet or sour and the pain evoked by such stimuli indicates a hyperalgesic state of the tooth. The pain is poorly localized, and the patient may not be able to distinguish whether it originates from the lower or upper jaw. Duplication of pain produced by control application of cold or hot stimuli to various teeth in the suspected area can aid in identifying the affected tooth.

Dentinal pain due to caries is best treated by removal of the carious lesion and restoration of the tooth. Sensitivity usually disappears within a day.

PULPAL PAIN

Pain associated with pulp pathology (pulpitis) is spontaneous, strong and often throbbing and is exacerbated by temperature changes, sweet foods and pressure on the carious lesion. When pain is evoked it outlasts the stimulus and can be excruciating for many minutes. Similar to dentine pain, localization of pulpal pain is poor and seems to be even worse when pain becomes more intense. Pain may be described by patients in different ways. It may manifest as a continuous dull ache and can be periodically exacerbated for short or long periods of minutes to hours.[2] pain may increase and throb when the patient lies down and in many instances it wakes the patient from sleep.[1] the pain of pulpitis is frequently not continuous and abates spontaneously; the precise explanation for such abatement is not clear. Localization of the affected tooth is achieved through hot and cold application and by percussion. Depending on the prognosis of the pulp (reversible or irreversible pulpitis) and that of the tooth, treatment may aim at conserving the pulp, extirpating it, or extracting the tooth. Pulpal pain usually disappears immediately after effective treatment.

PERIODONTAL PAIN:

Periodontal pain usually results from an acute inflammatory process of the gingiva, periodontal ligament, and alveolar bone due to bacterial infection. Pain is readily localized and the affected teeth are very tender to pressure. Two pathological pathways are common with pain resulting from either (1) pulp infection and pulp necrosis that results in periapical inflammation; or (2) Periodontal infection with pocket formation that results in a lateral Periodontal abscess. Although pain characteristics, ability to localize the pain, and pain producing situations are similar in both cases, treatment differs for etiological reasons and these categories are therefore discussed separately.

Acute periapical periodontitis:

Pain is spontaneous and moderate to severe in intensity for extended periods of time (hours). Pain is exacerbated by biting on the tooth and, in more advanced cases even by closing the mouth and bringing the affected tooth in contact with the opposing teeth. In these cases, the tooth feels extruded and is sensitive to touch. Frequently the patient reports that pulpal pain preceded the pain originating from the periapical area. Localization of pain originating from the periapical area is usually precise; in this respect periodontal pain differs from the poorly localized dentinal and pulpal pain. However, although the patient is able to indicate affected tooth, in approximately half the cases that pain is diffuse and spreads into the jaw on the affected side of the face.[1]

Table 1: Differential diagnosis of dental and periodontal pain

Pain origin	Localization	Character	Intensity	Intensifiers	Associated signs	Radiology
Dental						
Dentinal	poor	Evoked, does not outlast stimulus	Mild to moderate	Hot, cold, sweet or sour food	Caries, exposed dentine, defective restorations	Interproximal caries, defective restorations
Pulpal	very poor	Spontaneous, explosive, intermittent	Moderate to severe	Heat, cold, sometimes chewing	Deep caries, extensive restorations	Deep caries or restorations with pulp exposure
Periodontal						
Periapical	Good	Continues for hours: deep and boring	Moderate to severe	chewing	Periapical tenderness, redness and swelling	Usually no periapical changes at acute stage
lateral	Good	Continues for hours: deep and boring	Moderate to severe	Chewing	Periodontal tenderness, redness, swelling, tooth mobility.	Sometimes alveolar bone resorption

Table 2: Acute and chronic orofacial pain features

	Acute	Chronic
Time course	Short (hours to days)	Long (months to years)
Aetiology	Peripheral inflammatory	Central neuropathic
Response to: analgesics psychrotopics	Good poor	poor moderate to good
Behavioral response	anxiety, "guarding"	depression, "illness behavior"

During examination the affected tooth is readily located by means of tooth percussion. The periapical vestibular area may be tender to palpation. The pulp of the affected tooth is non vital, and therefore does not respond to thermal changes or to electrical pulp stimulation. In more severe, purulent cases (acute periapical abscess) there is swelling of the face associated with cellulitis, sometimes accompanied by fever and malaise. The affected tooth may be extruded and mobile.
Treatment is aimed at the source of irritation in the pulp chamber and the root canal, which are open and debrided to allow drainage. Grinding the tooth to prevent contact with the opposing teeth helps to relieve pain. If cellulitis, fever and malaise are present, systemic administration of antibiotics is recommended.

Soft tissue incision and drainage are very effective when a fluctuating abscess is present. Pain usually subsides within 24-48 hours.

Lateral Periodontal abscess

Pain characteristics are similar to those of acute periapical Periodontitis. Pain is continuous, well localized, and moderate to severe in intensity; it is exacerbated by biting on the affected tooth. Examination may show swelling and redness of the gingiva, usually located more coronally than in the case of acute periapical lesion. The affected tooth is sensitive to percussion and is often mobile and slightly extruded. In more severe cases, cellulitis, fever, and malaise may occur. A deep Periodontal pocket (over 6 mm) is usually located around the tooth; probing of this pocket usually results in pus exudation. The tooth pulp, however, is usually vital, i.e., it reacts to temperature changes and electrical stimulation. Gentle irrigation and curettage of the pocket should be performed. The tooth should be ground in order to prevent contact with the opposing tooth. When cellulitis, fever, and malaise are present, systemic antibiotic administration is recommended. Pain usually subsides within 24 hours of treatment.

GINGIVAL PAIN

Gingival pain may occur as a result of mechanical irritation, acute inflammation associated with a gingival pocket or acute bacterial or viral infection.[3]

Food impaction

Gingival pain caused by food impaction is characterized by localized pain between two adjacent teeth especially after meals, and particularly when food is fibrous. The pain is annoying with a feeling of pressure and discomfort. Pain gradually disappears until evoked again at the next meal and may be relieved by removing the food impacted between the teeth. Upon examination, a faulty contact between two adjacent teeth is usually noticed, where food tends to get trapped. The gingival papilla is inflamed, tender to touch and bleeds easily. The cause of the faulty contact between the teeth is often a carious lesion, and restoring the tooth will eliminate the pain.

Pericoronitis

This severe pain is usually located at the distal end of the arch of teeth at the lower jaw. Pain is spontaneous, exacerbated by closing the mouth and aggravated by swallowing and maybe associated with trismus. Upon examination, a flap of gingiva over a partially erupted tooth is acutely inflamed, red and edematous. Occasionally, fever and malaise are associated with this infection. Treatment includes irrigation of debris between the flap and the affected tooth and eliminating contact with the opposing tooth (by grinding or extraction). Systemic antibiotic administration is commonly recommended especially when trismus occurs.

Acute necrotizing ulcerative gingivitis

Soreness and pain are felt at the margin of the gums. Pain is intensified by eating and brushing the teeth and is accompanied by gingival bleeding. Metallic taste is sometimes experienced, and usually there is a fetid smell from the mouth. Necrosis and ulceration are noticed upon examination of the marginal gingival, with different degrees of gingival papillary destruction and adherent grayish slough represents the pseudomembrane that is present in the acute stage of the disease. Swabbing this slough is associated with pain and bleeding. Although basically this is bacterial disease that responds to antibiotics, it is not clear whether the bacteria initiate the disease or are merely secondary to underlying local or systemic factors. Treatment includes swabbing and gently irrigating the ulcerative lesions, preferably with an oxidizing agent (Hydrogen peroxide, and scaling and cleaning the teeth). Systemic antibiotics are recommended when fever and malaise are present.

TEMPOROMANDIBULAR DISORDERS

Pains in the musculoskeletal system are among the most common types of painful disorders in the body, including the orofacial region. The temporo-mandibular disorders (TMD) are currently viewed as a cluster of related pain conditions in the masticatory muscles temporo-mandibular joint (TM|J), and associated structures, i.e., they are considered a form of musculoskeletal pain.

INTENSITY OF SPONTANEOUS TMD PAIN

TMD pain can be persistent and constant, but there can also be substantial variation across time with exacerbations and spontaneous remission. Standard descriptions of persistent TMD pain usually state that the intensity ranges from mild to moderate to strong or even excruciating levels of pain and that the pain is often exacerbated by muscle function[1] of perceived pain intensity requires the use of standardized scales, such as verbal descriptor scales of visual analogue scales (VAS) [2]. A survey of recent clinical studies on persistent TMD pain indicated that the average pain level measured on a 100-mm VAS with the jaws at rest ranges between 30mm and 50mm[3]. VAS scores greater than 30mm probably represents at least moderate pain levels. The perceived pain intensity of TMD generally fluctuates with significant differences between the lowest, highest and average pain VAS scores during a week and between different facial sites. The use of diaries also can be helpful to estimate the pain because the perceived pain intensity of TMD patients can change over time simply due to regression of the mean. Furthermore the memory of pretreatment jaw-muscle pain is significantly dependent on the past and present levels of pain[4] showed that the experimental chewing increased the levels of pain in a majority of patients with persistent jaw-muscle pain.

QUALITY OF SPONTANEOUS TMD PAIN

The usual way to describe persistent TMD pain is as deep, dull ache, sometimes with a boring, pressing or tightening type of pain. The McGill Pain Questionnaires (MPQ), originally introduced as an attempt to provide a detailed description of the quality of pain[5], has become the most frequently used pain questionnaires.

In a sample of 200 patients with persistent facial pain including TMD pain, Turp et al. (1997) found that more than 30% of subjects used the words 'aching', 'tight', 'throbbing', 'tender', 'exhausting', 'nagging', 'sharp' and 'tiring'. The choice of 'radiating' (26%) and 'pressing' (22%) seems rather specific for TMD pain conditions compared to other pain conditions[6]. The quality of pain appears to be markedly different between patients with myofascial TMD pain and pain in the TMJ[7]. It is unclear whether this difference can be explained by activation of different nociceptive fibers in the muscle and joint tissue or by higher-order cognitive-emotional differences. Thus, certain words seem to be specifically related to the description of persistent TMD pain, but no word is specifically indicative of this pain condition in a similar way that 'pulsating' has been tied to migraine and 'pressing' and 'tightening' to tension-type headache.

Pain drawings made by patients are simple, but useful tools to illustrate the localization and extent of pain areas in genera. Pain drawings completed on a systematic basis by patients with pain complaints in the craniofacial region have revealed that only about 19% have pain confined to this region, whereas 66% have widespread referred pain outside the craniofacial and cervical regions[7].

The various theories on referred pain mechanisms have been reviewed recently[3]. There is a general agreement than the diffuse nature and poor localization of muscle pain is related to central convergence of afferent fibers onto common central neurons because this feature will in effect reduce the spatial resolution of somatosensory information. The nociceptive afferents from muscles, joints, skin and viscera converge onto common projection neurons. It is nevertheless unclear why muscle or joint pain can be referred to the skin, whereas the reverse is seldom encountered. Differences between cutaneous and muscular nociceptive afferents in terms of somatotopic organization, sizes of receptive fields, and laminar distribution of their terminals may explain the predominant referral of muscle pain[10]. Other mechanisms than central convergence are also likely to be involved in the expression of referred pain because there is normally a time delay between the onset of local and referred pain. One possibility is that the nociceptive barrage from muscle tissue opens up latent connections, in a form of central divergence[8]. The synaptic connections between neurons that originally had no effective drive from the myositis-induced muscle may now become effective. The neurobiology sub serving such mechanisms is probably related to central sensitization of second-order neurons and the development of hyper excitability.

MANAGEMENT OF TMD PAIN

Because the underlying mechanism of TMD pain is only partially understood, it is difficult to design therapy to cure the pain. Instead a more realistic goal will be to alleviate pain. Thus, the management strategies for TMD pain follow the same principles of management of other musculoskeletal pain conditions and may be physically, pharmacologically and psychologically oriented.

Table 3. Possible strategies for non-surgical management of teporo-mandibular disorders

Physical	Pharmacological	Psychological
Stretch therapy	Topical NSAIDs	Information
Jaw exercises	Oral NSAIDs	Counseling
Massage	Acetaminophen	Education
Ultrasound	Glucocorticosteroids	Stress management biofeedback
Heat/cold	Muscle relaxants	Relaxation
TENS	Benzodiazepines	Cognitive-behavioral therapy
Soft laser	Tricyclic anti-depressants	Psychotherapy
Acupuncture		
Oral splints	Opioids	

PHYSICAL MANAGEMENT OF TMD PAIN

There may be a significant reduction in perceived pain intensity following the intervention (e.g., acupuncture, biofeedback or splints), but that there may only be marginal or even no difference when the active treatment is compared to a placebo control. Thus, the specificity of many of the proposed treatments appears to be remarkably low. Oral splints have also been used extensively for management or even for 'curing' TMD pain.

PHARMACOLOGICAL MANAGEMENT OF TMD PAIN

Nonsteroidal anti-inflammatory drugs (NSAIDs) like ibuprofen in combination with diazepam provide significantly better pain relief compared to ibuprofen alone or placebo. A short-acting benzodiazepine, triazolam, improved sleep, but failed to provide significant pain relief in TMD patients. A combination of acetaminophen, codeine and doxylamine succinate (antihistaminic) provided significant pain relief than placebo in another study in mixed TMD patients.

PSYCHOLOGICAL MANAGEMENT OF TMD PAIN

Systematic studies on the efficacy of psychological management of TMD pain are rather scarce. A combination of biofeedback, stress management, and oral splints provides significant and long-lasting pain relief in TMD pain patients[2]. It appears to be important to tailor the treatment to each individual patient and not to consider psychological interventions on TMD pain as a treatment of last resort, but rather use it concurrently with biomedical and dental treatments.

SURGICAL MANAGEMENT OF PAIN

In some selected cases with persistent pain in the TMJ and restrictions in movement, which have not responded adequately to conservative treatment, surgical approaches may be recommended to alleviate the symptoms. The procedures range from irrigation of the upper joint space of the TMJ (arthrocentesis), direct inspection, lysis and lavage (arthroscopy), to positional changes in the condyle (modified condylotomy) or removal of the disk (diskectomy). It is clear treat that irrespective of the specific procedure, the success rate is close to 80% or more.

References

1. Sharav Y, Levine RE, Tekert A, et al. The spatial intensity and unpleasantness of acute dental pain.Pain 1984;20:363-366.
2. Grace Ly R.H. Studies of pain in normal man. In:Wall P.D, Melzack.R.(Ed). Textbook of pain Edinburgh; Churchiill Livingstone 1994; 315-336
3. Svennsson and Graven – Nielsien T. Craniofacial muscle pain. Review of Mechanisms. J. Oroofacial pain, 2001.17:2-10
4. Feine JS, Laigne GJ, Dao TTT et al. Memories of chronic pain and perceptions of relief. Pain 1998;77; 137-141
5. Melzack R. The MacGill pain Questionnaire; Measured properties and scoring methods. Pain 1975; 1;277-300
6. Turp JC, Kowalzki CJ, Stohler CS. Pain descriptors charecterists of persistent facial pain . J. Orofac Pain. 1997;11: 285-290
7. Mogini F, Italiano M. TMJ disorders in myogenic facial pain;A Discriminative analysis using MPQ. Pain 2001; 91: 323-330
8. Mens S, Hoheisel U Kaske et al. Muscle pain: Basic mechanisms and clinical correlate in Jenson TS, Turner JA et al. Eds ,Proceedings of 8th World congress of pain, Progress in pain research and management, Vol 8 Seattle : IASP: Press, 1997, 479- 4996

Chapter 26.

PAIN OF PELVIC ORIGIN

Pelvic pain is one of the most common problems affecting women of reproductive age. For clinical purposes, pelvic pain can be divided into acute and chronic presentations. Acute pelvic pain refers to pain symptoms below the umbilicus that have been present for less than six months. Chronic pelvic pain refers to menstrual or non menstrual pain of at least six months duration occurring below the umbilicus. The most common causes of acute pelvic pain include the early stages of diseases that cause chronic pelvic and problems caused by ectopic pregnancy, spontaneous abortion, ovarian cyst, endometritis, appendicitis and urinary tract calculus. The most common causes of chronic pelvic pain are endometriosis, chronic PID, adenomyosis, uterine leiomyomata, irritable bowel syndrome, interstitial cystitis, diverticulitis and fibromyalgia. Some women with chronic pelvic pain also have concomitant psychosocial problems such as depression, somatisation, narcotic dependency and history of physical and sexual abuse.

Epidemiology

Several population surveys have reported on the prevalence of chronic pelvic pain (CPP) among women of reproductive age. In one study of 2016 women responding to a written questionnaire, 24% reported that they had a history of constant or intermittent pelvic of greater than six month duration that was not exclusively associated with menstrual periods. Of the women with chronic pelvic pain, 25% reported that they also had IBS, and 9% reported that they also had genitourinary tract symptoms. In a telephone survey of 5263 women of reproductive age, 15% reported chronic pelvic pain that was active during the past three months. In this study, 61% of the women reported that a cause of their chronic pelvic pain had not been clearly identified. In a survey of the medical records of 284, 162 female patients aged 12 to 70 in the UK, the incidence of chronic pelvic pain was 38.3 per 1000 women[1].

Aetiology

Many disease processes can present as chronic pelvic pain. These conditions primarily consist of gynaecologic, gastrointestinal and urologic diseases. The relative frequency of the causes of pelvic pain is strongly influenced by the local patients, referral patterns and the specialty focus of the practice. For example in population with a low incidence of STD, endometriosis is often the most common cause of chronic pelvic pain[2,3]. Iin contrast, in populations with a high prevalence of STD, chronic PID is most common cause of chronic pelvic pain[4]. (Table)

Classification of chronic pelvic pain syndrome:-
1. Pelvic pain syndrome: (a) Urological   Bladder pain syndrome e.g interstitial cystitis
     Urethral pain syndrome
     Penile pain syndrome
     Prostate pain syndrome
     Scrotal pain syndrome e.g. testicular pain syndrome,
     post vasectomy pain syndrome
     Epididymal pain syndrome
(b) Gynecological   Endometriosis associated pain syndrome
   Vaginal pain syndrome
   General vulvar pain syndrome.
   Localized vulvar pain syndrome (vestibular pain, clitoral pain syndrome)
(c) Anorectal proctalgia Fugax
   Anorectal pain syndrome
   Anismus
  2. Others: (a) Neurological – pudendal pain syndrome
    (b) Muscular—perineal pain syndrome, pelvic floor muscle pain
     (c) Urological -Infective cystitis, prostatitis, urethritis epididymo orchitis
    (d) Gynecological—endometriosis
    (e) Anorectal—proctitis, hemorrhoids, anal fissure
    (f) Neurological—pudenal neuropathy, sacral spinal cord pathology.
    (g) Others—vascular, cutaneous and psychiatric.

The pelvic viscera receive their innervation via autonomic nervous system. The sympathetic portion originates from the thoracolumbar area of the spinal cord. The parasympathetic supply follows the distribution of the vagal nerve in combination with parasympathetic fibres from S1, S2 and S3. The autonomic nerve fibres enter the pelvis by following several routes. Most of them contribute to the formation of the superior hypogastric plexus.

Non gynaecologic causes of pelvic pain
Gastrointestinal

Irritable bowel syndrome affects an estimated 15% of adults, affecting twice as many women as men. Patients present with chronic or recurring abdominal pain associated with altered bowel habits (diarrhea, constipation or both) and bloating[5]. The pathophysiology of IBS is felt to be multifactorial, involving altered bowel motility, visceral hypersensitivity and psychosocial factors[6].

The Manning diagnostic criteria are widely used and have been validated through factor analysis. A diagnosis of IBS is likely in patients with abdominal pain with two or more associated symptoms- pain relieved by defecation, pain associated with looser or more frequent stools, abdominal distension, feeling of incomplete evacuation or mucus in stools.

Urogenital

Pain management in urological patients is a subject afflicted by failure to identify its pathophysiological origins. The problem is most commonly experienced is "interstitial cystitis" or "chronic prostates". These terms reflect the clinical interpretation of the symptoms described by the patients.

Interstitial cystitis

Interstitial cystitis is a poorly understood chronic inflammatory condition of the bladder. Altered bladder permeability from a defective gycosaminoglycan mucus layer has been proposed as the etiology of this condition. However it is not known if this is the cause or an effect of interstitial cystitis. Epidemiologic data showing an association between IC and autoimmune diseases have led to theories that IC may be immunologically mediated.

No micro organism has been found to be the cause of IC. Although cultures of urine from a minority of IC patients may contain bacteria, antibiotic treatment is ineffective in this disease.

Inflammation seems to be an essential part of the picture in classic IC. Histological examination of bladder lesions has revealed pain cystitis and perineural inflammatory infiltrates of lymphocytes and plasma cells. Inflammation is scant in non ulcer IC[7].

Mast cells are multifunctional immune cells that contain highly potent inflammatory mediators such as histamine, leukotrienes, serotonin and cytokines. Many of the symptoms and findings in classic IC such as pain, frequency, oedema, fibrosis and neovascularisation in the lamina propria may be due to the release of mast cell derived factors.[8]

Toxic constituents in the urine may cause injury to the bladder in IC. One hypothesis is that heat labile, cationic urine components of low molecular weight may exert a cytotoxic effect; defective constitutive cytokine production may decrease mucosal defences to toxic agents[13].

A decrease in the Microvascular density in the suburothelium has been observed. In a recent study, it was found that bladder perfusion decreased with bladder filling in IC patients, but that the opposite occurred in controls[14].

Clinical features and diagnosis

Patients report severe pelvic pain with bladder filled that is relieved by voiding. Pain may also be described as pelvic, vaginal or perineal, prompting evaluation for a gynaecologic etiology and delaying diagnosis. Diagnostic criteria for interstitial cystitis are symptoms of frequency, pain and urgency- findings of low bladder capacity on voiding diary or Urodynamic assessment, and the characteristic cystoscopic appearance with Hunner ulcers and granulations.

Initial evaluation

It should include a urine analysis, urine culture and cytology. A voiding diary is helpful in the initial evaluation of these patients. In women with interstitial cystitis, voiding diaries usually demonstrate 20 or more voids in 24 hours with 3 or more voids at night and average volumes of 100 ml. cystoscopy is important to exclude stone, foreign body or carcinoma and may show characteristic findings one. Sensitivity to intracellular potassium has been proposed as a diagnostic test but does not add significantly to the sensitivity or specificity of diagnosis.

Treatment approaches

These include systemic agent, instillation therapy and surgical management. Trials of systemic agents including antihistamines, azothioprine, corticosteroids, heparin, pentosanpolysulphate and tri cyclic compounds have shown inconsistent benefits. Placebo effect and intermittent remission rates of upto 50-% with an average duration of 8 months complicate the ability to assess effectiveness in small studies that are often not blinded or randomized. Dimethyl sulphoxide has been used for intra vesical therapy with response rates of 50% to 90%, although the majority of studies are uncontrolled. DMSO is teratogenic in animals and should be avoided in pregnancy.

Cystodissection

Performed at the time of diagnostic cystoscopy, may provide short term relief to 20 to 30% of patients. Surgical treatments include urinary diversion procedures, augmentation cystoplasty and denervation procedures. These are generally reserved for severe disease that is unresponsive to other therapies[15]

A frequently cited report by Bumpus claims imprecisely that hydro distension achieved symptom improvement in 100 patients over several months. Dunn claimed to have achieved complete absence of symptoms in 16 of 25 patients during a mean follow up of 14 months using the helmstein method, where an intravesical balloon is distended at the level of systolic blood pressure for three hours[16].

Acupuncture

In non curable and agonizing diseases such as IC, desperate patients frequently seek access to complimentary medicine such as acupuncture. However scientific evidence for such treatments is often poor.

Supra trigonal cystectomy with subsequent bladder augmentation represents the most favoured continence- preserving technique for the surgical management of IC. The therapeutic success of supra trigonal cystectomy has been reported in numerous studies.

Chronic prostatitis

A syndrome in men, characterized by chronic perineal and penile pain with varying degrees of urinary and sexual dysfunction, is generally recognized without difficulty by clinicians and often labeled as chronic prostatitis. As the cause of the most prevalent, non bacterial, forms of the condition remains unknown, and therefore no definitive diagnostic tests exists, diagnosis has relied on a combination of clinical features, exclusion of other diagnoses (such as bladder outlet obstruction) and the results of investigations, especially the four glass test (stamey). However there is no generally agreed clinical definition that brings together the symptomatic features and investigative findings, so it is difficult to make reliable comparisons among the many descriptive and therapeutic studies in 30 yrs of medical literature or to draw many conclusions.

Treatment

For the few patients with bacterial prostatitis, antibiotic selection should be guided by the sensitivities of the organisms cultured from urine or prostatic secretions and an agent with good prostatic penetration, usually a quinolones such as ciprofloxacin would be the agent of choice[21]. One month of initial therapy is suggested by existing studies, but upto a third of patients may relapse and need more prolonged courses or suppressive antibiotic treatment[22].

The treatment of the non infective syndrome is more problematic. Although the condition is so common, there are no published large scale randomized treatment trials. Small controlled trials and observation studies have suggested a place for selected antibiotics (which may act by non antimicrobial mechanisms such as anti inflammatory effects) including doxycycline, erythromycin and ofloxacin, (blockers such as terazosin, transurethral micro wave thermotherapy and allopurinol).[27] However no highly effective therapy has been identified. A review of the literature suggests that alpha blockers, muscle relaxants and various physical therapies improve symptoms.

Scrotal pain

Acute scrotal pain includes torsion of the testis or appendices and requires immediate diagnostic and therapeutic attention. Although it is not life threatening its manifestations affect the patient's quality of life. It can be unilateral or bilateral and continous or intermittent. It is not uncommon for examination to localize the site and distinguish between testicular and epididymal pain.

Mechanism

Afferent innervation of testis is via Genitofemoral nerve which has a femoral branch to the skin of the ventro medial region of the thigh and a genital branch to the scrotal region. The Ilioinguinal nerve conveys sensations from the groin region. The Ilioinguinal and Genitofemoral nerves are however, subject to a great deal of anatomic variability[28].

According to the traditional view the testis perceive sympathetic input from the para aortic ganglia. Studies using biochemical methods indicate that efferent fibres reaching the testis derive from major pelvic and accessory pelvic ganglia[29].

Treatment

Patients with extra genital disease are treated according to the cause. Patients without identifiable lesions must primarily be treated conservatively (adjuvant antibiotics, analgesics, TENS, nerve blocks) of Genitofemoral or Ilioinguinal nerve. If these are unsuccessful sugery can be considered. However, the results of epididectomy and orchidectomy are poor (20% and 60% success rates, respectively). Micro surgical testicular denervation represents another therapeutic option and favourable results have been reported. It has been suggested that patients with micro calcifications should be kept under surveilence because of a possible increased risk of testicular malignancy. Ganglion of Impar block with local anaesthetic has been used successfully in relieving chronic scrotal pain. If required the block is repeated and neurolysis of the ganglion of Impar is performed for chronic pain if other methods fail to provide adequate pain relief.

Urethral syndrome

Urethral syndrome represents a less well defined entity. Positive diagnostic signs are urethral tenderness or pain on palpation and slightly inflamed urethral mucosa found during endoscopy. In clinical practice, the diagnosis of urethral syndrome is commonly given to patients who present with the symptoms of dysuria (with or without frequency, nocturia, urgency and urge in continence) in the absence of evidence of urinary infection. It is the later phrase that results in difficulties because the methods typically used to identify urinary infection are extremely insensitive.

Dysuria is pain or discomfort experienced in association with micturition. The classical symptom of a burning sensation in the urethra during voiding caused by infection is well known. Less appreciated is the external dysuria experienced by women with vaginitis when urine passes over the labia.

Urethral trauma arising from intercourse may cause pain and dysuria. This used to be called as "Honeymoon cystitis", and a friction and trauma to the urethra may be the cause in the absence of infection. Women with pelvic floor dysfunction sometimes describe the symptoms, as do post menopausal women in whom the trauma is associated with estrogen deficiency, loss of lubrication and vaginal dryness.

Gynaecological causes of pelvic pain

Pelvic pain is a common complaint among women. Nearly 10% of all American women aged 18 to 50 suffer from chronic pelvic pain.

Endometriosis

It is a major cause of pelvic cause of pelvic pain characterized by the presence of functional endometrial glands and stroma outside the uterine cavity. Although many lesions have a characteristic appearance, histologic examination improves the accuracy of the diagnosis. These lesions are typically found in the pelvis but may be located on the bowel, bladder or remote locations such as lung. These lesions are hormonally responsive, typically resulting in pain that worsens just before and with menses. Approximately 40% of women with endometriosis have physical findings consistent with this disorder. Physical findings that are present in some women with endometriosis includes uterosacral ligament nodularity, tenderness or thickening; an adnexal mass, lateral displacement of the cervix and cervical stenosis.

Adenomyosis

It is characterized by the presence of endometrial glands within the myometrium, resulting most frequently in severe dysmenorrhoea and menorrhagia. Women with adenomyosis typically have a slightly enlarged, globular, tender uterus on physical examination. Adenomyosis may also be suggested by ultra sound or MRI but the diagnosis remains clinical with pathological confirmation.

Chronic pain after PID may result from persistent or recurrent infection or can be caused by scarring, tissue damage and adhesions. Chlamydial infection may be asymptomatic in women, thus no acute episode may precede the chronic sequele. Additionally with improved antibiotic treatment and radiologic and laparoscopic abscess drainage, more women with acute PID and tubo-ovarian abscess are managed conservatively.

Pelvic adhesions may result from previous infection, scarring from endometriosis and surgery. Pain is most likely to occur from adhesions when they are extensive or result in fixation of internal organs.

Evaluation of gynaecologic chronic pelvic pain
In the initial evaluation, the history helps to identify causes of pain that are hormonally responsive. For example pelvic pain that is more intense just before or during the first few days of menses is likely causes by endometriosis or adenomyosis. Woman with endometriosis report pre menstrual spotting, dyspareunia, dyschezia, poor relief of symptoms with non steroidal anti inflammatory drugs, progressively worsening symptoms, inability to attend work or school during menses, and the presence of pelvic pain unrelated to menses. Non- hormonally responsive disease should be considered for pain that is not related to menses. This category includes both gynaecologic causes of pelvic pain (e.g. chronic PID and pelvic adhesions) and non gynaecologic causes (e.g. IBS, diverticulitis, fibromyalgia or interstitial cystitis).

Laboratory and imaging test
That are useful in the evaluation of woman with chronic pelvic pain include WBC count, urinalysis, tests for Chlamydia and gonorrhoea, pregnancy test and pelvic ultrasound. Pelvic ultrasound is highly sensitive for detecting pelvic masses, including ovarian cysts and uterine leiomyomas. Endometriosis cysts of the ovary (endometriomas) often have a characteristic ultrasound appearance that allows for an ultrasound diagnosis. Sonography is very useful for identifying small pelvic masses (<4 cm in diameter) that are often not palpable on bi manual pelvic examination. For many cases of chronic pelvic pain such as endometriosis and chronic PID, a surgical procedure such as laparoscopy is required to make a definitive diagnosis.

Treatment of gynaecological chronic pelvic pain
Any authorities believe that resection/ ablation of endometriosis lesions improves pelvic pain caused by endometriosis. A non hysterectomy approach to the treatment of chronic pelvic pain is nerve transection procedures. Laparoscopic ureterosacral nerve ablation (LUNA) involves the destruction of the uterine nerve fibres that exit the uterus through the uterosacral ligament.

Pre sacral neurectomy refers to the interruption of the sympathetic innervation of the uterus at the level of superior Hypogastric plexus. Prospective and retrospective cohort studies suggest that hysterectomy is effective in relieving chronic pelvic pain from many diverse etiologies.

Danazol is a derivative of testosterone and has moderate affinity for the androgen receptor. At doses used in clinical practice (200-800mg daily) danazol suppresses endometriosis lesions by suppressing LH, FSH and the estrogen secretion and by blocking estrogen action in the lesions.

Symphysis pubis dysfunction
One problem that many pregnant women about is pubic pain which is caused by pelvic girdle area not working in the way it should, probably because of hormones, mis alignment of the pelvis, or on interaction of the two. Any activity that involves lifting one leg at a time or parting the legs tends to be particularly painful. Pregnancy hormones including progesterone tend to loosen the ligaments of the body in preparation for birth and especially woman whose joints are flexible before pregnancy are more susceptible to the effects of hormones.

Quite often it is a self limiting and pain disappears with in few weeks of delivery. Avoid the use of vaccum extractor and forceps, as these may necessitate opening the legs wider than pubic symphysis can safely tolerate. Epidural is to be avoided if at all possible as this is often associated with more severe damage. It seems logical that an elective ceaserean section might prevent damage to the pubic symphysis, but in reality the problem is caused during pregnancy and elective ceaserean won't fix it.

Levator ani syndrome
This has been described in association with a variety of organic conditions but also occurs under circumstances in which organic disorders are absent and the pathophysiology is uncertain. The pain is often described as dull aching or pressure like discomfort in the rectum, lasting several hours. Prolonged sitting and the act of defecation have been described as precipitating factors. Several studies have suggested that increased anal canal pressures and increased EMG activities often are present.

As is often the case with poorly understood entities a wide variety of treatments alone or in combination, have been reported to effective. The use of muscle relaxants such as diazepam and methocarbomol in addition to massage and sitz bath was reported to be effective, although not by all investigators. Electro galvanic stimulation through a rectal probe produced 80%-90% improvement of symptoms in unselected patients. Surgical division of puborectalis muscle showed initial optimistic results but subsequent studies reported a high incidence of incontinence for liquid or gas.

Proctalgia fugax

It is an obscure disorder that was first described more than 100 yrs ago and is characterized by sudden severe pain in the rectal area lasting several seconds or minutes, then disappearing completely, leaving the patient asymptomatic until the next episode. In contrast to levator ani syndrome patients are often asymptomatic when examined, and there are no characteristic findings to improve diagnostic certainity. In 2 uncontrolled studies of patients with proctalgia fugax who sought medical attention, a high percentage was found to have high scores for anxiety, hypochondriasis, perfectionist tendencies and somatization. There have been reports of benefits with Clonidine, nitrates, diltiazem and caudal epidural block. The presence of psychological dysfunction should lead to consideration of anti depressants anxiolysis or psychotherapy where appropriate.

Pudendal nerve entrapment

Pain caused by entrapment of pudendal nerve is confined mainly to the perineal region. It is positional in nature exacerbated by sitting and partially relieved by standing or recumbent. The diagnosis is confirmed by nerve conduction studies which show distal motor latency for the offending nerve. There was a report of surgical decompression of the pudendal nerve which was found to be flattened in the pudendal canal of Alcock and in contact with the sharp inferior border of sacrospinous ligament. After surgical decompression and rehabilitation, the patient experienced significant relief of pain and returned to normal activity.

Musculoskeletal

Fibromyalgia is a chronic condition that presents with diffuse musculoskeletal pain. There are 9 defined anatomic tender points providing 18 possible sited of excessive tenderness. Excessive tenderness in 11 or more of 18 alongwith fatigue is considered diagnostic. Fibromyalgia symptomatology has been associated with patients who suffer from chronic pelvic pain.

In myofascial pain syndromes, the tenderness is confined to one anatomic region. Palpation of trigger points produces a characteristic and reproducible pain pattern. In patients with chronic pelvic pain, trigger points are commonly found in back and abdomen. Topical medications and trigger point injections have been used to treat this disorder alongwith NSAIDs.

Role of neural blockade

Neural blockade can be used for diagnostic as well therapeutic purposes in the management of pain which originates from the pelvis. This can be used to differentiate the origin of the pain, central from peripheral and visceral from somatic. The process of therapeutic blocks should only be undertaken after evaluating the underlying pathology. Peripheral nerve blocks have a very limited application. Most of the structures are innervated by sympathetic nerves. However pudendal nerve block for entrapment of pudendal nerve is a definite option and block of this nerve with local anaesthetic alongwith steroid provides effective pain relief. Similarly Ilioinguinal nerve block in a patient following its entrapment in inguinal hernia surgery does produce good pain relief.

Sympathetic nerve blocks have been used effectively in the management of pelvic pain not responding to other means. Superior Hypogastric plexus block is an important tool in the pelvic pain management of cancer origin. This plexus is located retroperitoneally at the lower half of the fifth lumbar and the upper part of the first sacral vertebra. This is connected above with another sympathetic plexus- celiac plexus. Superior Hypogastric plexus provides sympathetic innervation to fundus of the uterus, fallopian tubes, broad ligament, part of the urinary bladder and the distal part of colon. The block of the plexuses performed either under X-ray control or this can be guided by CT. after a diagnostic block with local anaesthetic, neurolytic agent is then injected. A further confirmation of the position of the needle is achieved by using contrast media and visualizing it spread under fluoroscopy.

Ganglion of Wallther (ganglion Impar) is the termination of the sympathetic chain. It is located at the sacro coccygeal junction and a block of this ganglion is used to relieve the pain in the perineal regions and the genitals. Patients with malignancy of rectum, urinary bladder, colon and cervix have shown appreciable pain relief with blocking ganglion of Impar.

Epidural block

The role of this block lies only in terminal patients where other treatment options have failed or not possible. The other role of epidural block lies in distinguishing between central and peripheral origin of the chronic pelvic pain. Differential epidural block can be used to help clarify the segmental level of origin, after administering graded dosages through an indwelling epidural catheter. If it is decided to keep an in dwelling catheter for more than a few days, infection through the catheter should be carefully guarded against.

Intrathecal / epidural opioids

This is an option when other palliative measures of pain control have failed to produce desired pain relief. This has an inherent danger of producing respiratory depression. For long term pain relief, epidural catheter is tunneled and there is an option of implantation of injection port.

Summary

Chronic pelvic pain is difficult to diagnose and to treat because of the multiple and often overlapping causes. A systemic approach aids in the thorough evaluation and appropriate therapy. At the initial visit, a thorough history should be taken and complete physical examination performed. Screening for co-existing conditions, such as depression, narcotic abuse is crucial so these issues may be addressed immediately while additional causes for pelvic pain are evaluated.

References:-
1. Zondervan KT, Yudkin PL, Vessey MP et al. Prevalence and incidence of chronic pelvic pain in primary care: Evidence from a national general practice data base. Br J Obs Gynecol 1999:106:1149-55
2. Koninckx PR, Meuleman C, Demeyere S et al. Suggestive evidence that pelvic endometriosis is a progressive disease. Whereas deeply infiltrating endometriosis is associated with pelvic pain. Fertil Sterile 1991:55:759-65
3. Ling FW. Randomized control trial of depot leprolide in patients with chronic pelvic pain and clinically suspected endometriosis. Obs Gynecol 1999:93:51-8
4. Stacey CM, Munday PE. Abdominal pain in women attending a genitor urinary medicine clinic: who has PID? In J SID AIDS 1994:5:338-42
5. Horwitz BJ, Fisher RS. Current concepts: the irritable bowel syndrome. New Engl J Med 2001:334:1846-50
6. Manning AP, Thompson WG, and Heaton KW et al. Towards a positive diagnosis of irritable bowel. BMJ 1978:2:653-4
7. Fall M, Johansson SL, Aldenborg F. Chronic interstitial cystitis- a hetrogenous syndrome. J Uro 1987:137:35-8
8. Peeker R, Enerback L, Fall M, Alderborg F. Recruitment, distribution and phenotypes of mast cells in interstitial cystitis. J Uro 2000:163:1009-15
9. Mattila J, Linder E. Imunoglobin deposit in bladder epithelium and vessels in interstitial cystitis; possible relationship to circulating anti intermediate filament auto anti bodies. Clin Immunol Immuno Pathol 1984;32;81-9
10. Hang L, Wullt B, Shen Z, Karpman D, Svanborg C. Cytokine repertoire of epithelial cells lining the human urinary tract. J Uro 1998;159;2185-92
11. Pontari MA, Hanno PM. Reggieri. MR. Comparision of bladder blood flow in patients with/ without interstitial cystitis. J Uro 1999;162;330-4
12. Hanno PM. Diagnosis of interstitial cystitis. Uro clin north Amrc. 1994;21;63-6
13. Peters K, Diokno A, Steinert B, Yuchico M, Mitchell B, Krohta S, Gillette B, Gonzalez J. The efficacy of intravesical Tice strain bacillus Calmet Geurine in the treatment of interstitial cystitis. A double blind, prospective placebo control trial. J Uro 1997;157;2090-2094
14. Nickel JC, Prostatitis. Evolving management strategies. Uro Clin North Ame. 1999;26;737-51
15. Schaeffer AJ, Darras FS. The efficacy of norfloxacin in the treatment of chronic bacterial prostatitis refractory to cotrimoxazole and /or carbenacillin. J Uro 1990;144;690-3

16. Meares EJ, Prostatitis and related disorders in: Walsh PC, Retik AS, Stamey TA, Vaughan EDG, ad. Campbell's urology Philadelphia:WVSaunders.1992.pp807
17. Rouviere H, Delmas A: In: Anatomy human volume -2 : Parris Masson. 1985;557
18. Rab M, Ebmer and J, Dellon AL. Anatomic variability of illioinguinal and genito femoral nerve.implications for the treatment of groin pain. Plast Reconstr Surg 2001;108;1618-23
19. Gray CL, Powell CR, Amling CL. Outcomes for surgical management of orchalgia in patients with identifiable intrascrotal lesions. Eur Uro J 2001;39;455-9
20. Padmore DE, Norman RW, Millard OH. Analysis of indications for and outcomes of epididymectomy. J Uro 1996;156;95-6
21. Westrom L, Joeseof R, Reynolds G et al. Pelvic inflammatory disease and fertility. Sex Trans Dis 1992,19;185-92
22. Peters AA, Trinbos-kemper GC, Admiraal C et al. A randomized clinical trial and the benefits of adhesiolysis in patients with intraperitoneal adhesions and chronic pelvic pain. Br J Obs Gynecol. 1992;99;59-62
23. Rao SSC, Hatfield RA. Paroxysmal anal hyperkinesis; a characteristic feature of proctalgia fugax. Gut 39;609-612.1996
24. Wallace WC, Madden WM. Experience with partial resection of the puborectalis muscles. Dis Colon Rectum 12;196-200,1969
25. Barnes PRH et al. Experience of posterior division of puborectalis muscle in the management of chronic constipation. Br J Surg 72;475-477,1985
26. Thompson WG. Proctalgia Fugax. Dig Dis Sci 26;1121-1124,1981
27. Pilling LF, Swenson WM, Hill JR. The psychological aspect of proctalgia Fugax. Dis Colon Rectum 8;372-376,1972
28. Amarnath L, Welder SD. Caudal epidural block in the management of proctalgia fugax. Am J Pain Management. 4;153-155,1994
29. Ramsden CE. Pudendal nerve entrapment. Am J Phys Med Rehabl—01-JUN-2003:82(6), 479-84
30. Applegate W V. Abdominal cutaneous nerve entrapment syndrome. Surgery. 1972;71;118-24
31. Beard RW. Chronic pelvic pain. Br J Obs Gynecol 1998; 105;8-10.

Chapter 27.

ULTRASOUND

PRINCIPLES

An ultrasound probe has dual functions. It emits and receives sound waves, thus functioning both as a speaker and a microphone. As the name implies, ultrasound waves are high-frequency sound waves (20,000 cycles/s, 20 kHz) that are not audible to the human ear. Ultrasound frequencies useful in clinical medicine are in the megahertz (MHz) range. When an electrical current is applied to an array of piezoelectric crystals (quartz) within the ultrasound transducer, mechanical energy, in the form of vibration, is generated, resulting in ultrasound waves. As the ultrasound waves move through body tissues of different acoustic impedances, they are attenuated (lose amplitude with depth), reflected, and/or scattered. Waves reflected to the transducer are then transformed back into an electrical signal that is then processed by the ultrasound machine to generate an image on the screen.

Depending on the amount of wave returned, anatomic structures take on different degrees of echogenicity. Structures with high water content, such as blood vessels and cysts, appear hypoechoic (black or dark), because ultrasound waves are transmitted through the structures easily with little reflection. On the other hand, bone and tendons block ultrasound wave transmission and the strong signal returned to the transducer gives these structures a hyperechoic appearance (bright, white) on the screen. Structures of intermediate density and acoustic impedance, such as the liver parenchyma or the thyroid gland, appear gray on the screen. Knowing the speed of sound in tissue (1540 m/s on average) and the time of echo return, the distance between the probe and the target structure (depth) is calculated.

ULTRASOUND EQUIPMENT

Ulrasonography has many applications in clinical anesthesia. With appropriate probes, vascular imaging, echocardiography, and nerve imaging can be performed with the same unit. Compound imaging is an advanced feature in some of the cart-based units. The resolution of nerve images is enhanced with compound imaging when multiple lines of crystals on the transducer (as opposed to a single line) emit and receive ultrasound in multiple planes before final display of the image that is electronically reconstructed. Color Doppler is another useful feature that differentiates vascular from nonvascular structures (e.g., nerves). Compact portable units currently available with many of the sophisticated features are also suitable for peripheral nerve imaging.

Transducers (probes)

Ultrasound scanning of deep abdominal organs such as liver, gallbladder, and kidneys requires low-frequency probes (3-5 MHz). Scanning superficial structures such as the brachial plexus, on the other hand, requires high-frequency probes (10-15 MHz) that provide high axial resolution however; beam penetration is limited to 3 to 4 cm. A lower-frequency probe (4-7 MHz) is suited for scanning deeper structures, such as the brachial plexus in the infraclavicular region and the sciatic nerve in adults.

PERIPHERAL NERVE IMAGING:

Patient positioning for each block is essentially the same as is used for standard, non-image-guided peripheral nerve blocks. Sterile technique should be followed, especially when a continuous catheter technique is performed, in which case a long sterile sheath covering the probe and the cord and sterile conducting gel are recommended.

Transverse and longitudinal views are most commonly used for nerve imaging. When the probe is perpendicular to the long axis of the nerve, the transverse (short axis, cross-sectional) view shows nerves in round to oval shape with internal hypoechoic nerve fascicles surrounded by the hyperechoic epineurium. When the probe is parallel to the long axis, nerves in longitudinal view appear tubular with linear hypoechoic fascicular components mixed with hyperechoic bands corresponding to the interfascicular epineurium.[6] Nerves have different degrees of echogenicity. For example, nerve roots and trunks of the brachial plexus in the interscalene and supraclavicular regions appear mostly hypoechoic, while peripheral branches of the brachial plexus and the sciatic nerve are largely hyperechoic.

IMAGING OF THE BRACHIAL PLEXUS

High-frequency linear probes, in the range of 10 to 15 MHz, are best suited for imaging the brachial plexus in most locations, except perhaps the infraclavicular region where the cords may be more deeply located and thus probes in the 4 to 7 MHz range may be required.

The Interscalene Region

In the interscalene region, the cervical roots forming the plexus are located between the anterior and middle scalene muscles. They are best visualized when scanned in the lateral aspect of the neck in an axial oblique plane (FIG 1). In this manner, the sternocleidomastoid muscle can be identified superficially. Deep to it are the anterior and middle scalene muscles where one or more roots are visualized in the interscalene groove.[7] They appear mostly hypoechoic, with few internal punctuate echos (FIG -1). Deeper to this plane, the vertebral artery and vein are seen next to the vertebral transverse process. The carotid artery and internal jugular vein can be identified medially.

The Supraclavicular region

In the supravlavicular region, the brachial plexus is best scanned with a linear probe in a coronal oblique plane[8]. The subclavian artery is the most prominent landmark identified immediately superior to the first rib. The trunks or divisions of the plexus in this region are tightly arranged within what seems to be a single sheath, immediately lateral and cephalad to the subclavian artery. The anterior and middle scalene muscles can be identified as they insert on the first rib. The pleura can be seen immediately deep to the first rib.

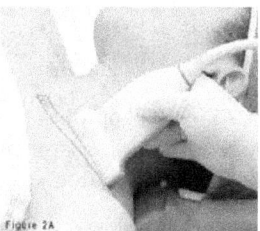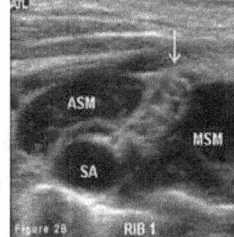

Fig 2. Ultrasound probe position for imaging the brachial plexus in the supraclavicular area.

Ultrasound image of the brachial plexus in the supraclavicular area.
ASM = Anterior Scalene Muscle
MSM = Middle Scalene Muscle
SA = Subclavian Artery
RIB 1 = First rib
The arrow signals the brachial plexus located in the most distal part of the interscalene space, just cephalad and lateral to the subclavian artery.

The Infraclavicular region

In the infraclavicular region next to the coracoid process, the cords of the plexus lie deep to the pectoralis major and pectoralis minor muscles. They can be best imaged with a linear probe in the range of 4 to 7 MHz, in a parasagittal plane, immediately medial to the coracoid process.[9] In this manner, a transverse view of the cords adjacent to the axillary vessels can be obtained. The cords appear hyperechoic, with the lateral cord commonly cephalad and the posterior cord posterior to the artery. The medial cord in this region can often be seen between the artery and vein, but is not always visible.

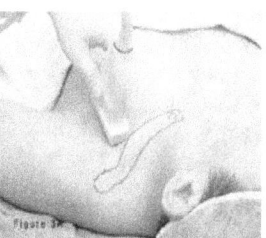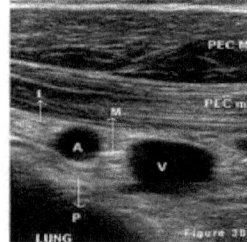

Fig 3. Ultrasound probe position for imaging the brachial plexus in the infraclavicular area.

Ultrasound image of the brachial plexus in the infraclavicular area
PEC M = Pectoralis major muscle
PEC m = Pectoralis minor muscle
A = Axillary Artery
V = Axillary Vein
L = Lateral cord
M = Medial Cord
P = Posterior Cord.

The Axillary region
In the axilla and the upper arm, the neurovascular bundle is located in the internal bicipital sulcus, which

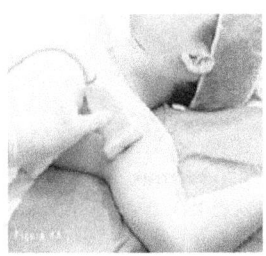

Fig 4. Ultrasound probe position for imaging the brachial plexus in the axillary area.

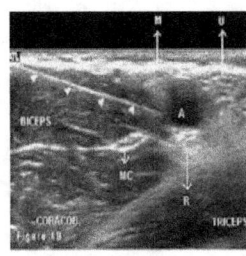

Ultrasound image of the brachial plexus in the axillary area.
A = Axillary Artery
M = Median nerve
U = Ulnar Nerve
R = Radial nerve
MC = Musculocutaneous Nerve

separates the flexor muscle compartment of the arm (biceps and coracobrachialis muscles) from the extensor compartment (triceps). At this level, terminal braches of the brachial plexus such as the musculocutaneous, median, ulnar, and radial nerves are located superficially, usually within 1 to 2 cm of the skin. A linear 10-to 15-MHz probe is therefore recommended. To obtain a transverse view of the neurovascular bundle with the arm abducted at 90 degrees and the forearm flexed, the probe is positioned perpendicular to the long axis of the arm, as close to the axilla as possible .The round pulsatile axillary artery is easily identified in the bicipital sulcus and is distinguished from the axillary veins that are readily compressed. Nerves in the axilla are round to oval shaped and hypoechoic with internal hyperechoic areas, presumably the epineurium. In the axillary region, the median and ulnar nerves are usually lateral and medial to the artery, respectively. The radial nerve is often posterior or postero-medial to the artery but nerve location is highly variable.[10] The musculocutaneous nerve often branches off more proximally, and can be seen as a hyperechoic structure. It can be found between the biceps and coracobrahialis muscles for a short distance before entering the body of the coracobrachialis muscle. When performing an axillary block, it is best to inject local anesthetic around each nerve individually to achieve consistent success. Local anesthetic spread within the sheath compartment may be restricted by presumably the septae when observed under ultrasound.[11]

LUMBOSACRAL PLEXUS
The lumbar plexus (L1 to L5) and the sacral plexus (S1 to S4) provide innervation to the lower extremity. Unlike the brachial plexus, the lumbosacral plexus and its proximal branches are quite deep. Sonographic imaging can be more challenging except for the distal peripheral branches.
Paravertebral anatomy and lumbar plexus blocks
Ultrasound imaging of the lumbar plexus in the paravertebral region in adults is technically difficult because of its deep location. Using curved 4- to 5-MHz transducers, Kirchmair and associates identified the lumbar plexus within the psoas muscle and could correlate ultrasound images with anatomic specimens. Scanning is performed with the patient prone with a pillow under the abdomen to reduce lumbar lordosis, or in the sitting position. The transducer is placed longitudinally, in a parasagital plane, approximately 3 cm from the midline to determine the location of the lumbar transverse processes. Once accomplished, the transducer is turned 90 degrees to the transverse axial plane and positioned between two transverse processes so that bony interference to ultrasound beam penetration is minimized. In the axial image, two muscles are identified deep to the subcutaneous plane, the erector spinae muscle immediately lateral to the spinous process and the smaller quadratus lumborum more laterally. The psoas muscle lies deep (anterior) to these two muscles, and is adjacent to the vertebral bodies and intervertebral discs .Previous anatomic studies demonstrate that the lumbar plexus most often lies between the posterior third and anterior two thirds of the psoas muscle; the average skin to plexus distance is 5 to 6 cm.[12] For this reason it has been recommended that local anesthetic be administered in the posterior one third of the muscle.

Ultrasound also identifies the inferior pole of the kidney (as low as the L3-4 level) and can potentially avoid renal hematoma due to inadvertent needle trauma.

Fig 5. Ultrasound probe position for imaging the paravertebral anatomy relevant to performing lumbar plexus block.

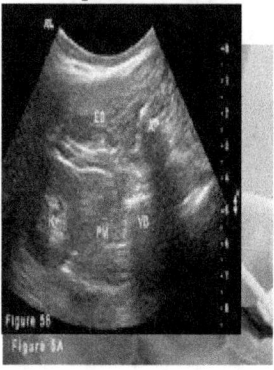

Ultrasound image of the paravertebral anatomy at the L2-3 level
AP = Articular process
VB = Vertebral Body
ES = Erector Spinae Muscle
PM = Psoas Muscle
K = Kidney
The actual lumbar plexus roots are not seen in this image. They traverse the posterior third of the psoas muscle, and are difficult to identify due to the depth and similar echogenicity to surrounding muscle tissue.

FEMORAL NERVE

The three main terminal branches of the lumbar plexus are the femoral, obturator, and lateral femoral cutaneous nerves. The femoral nerve derived from L2 to L4 is the largest branch and can be easily imaged in the inguinal region using a linear 10- to 12-MHz transducer. The probe placed over the inguinal crease in the transverse axial plane shows the femoral nerve immediately lateral to the femoral vessels, often oval or triangular in shape. It lies deep to the ileopectineal arch, and overlying the groove between the iliac and psoas muscles. The femoral nerve can be imaged further distally for a short distance until it divides into small terminal branches that become indistinguishable from the surrounding tissue. It is possible to image the saphenous nerve, which is next to the femoral vessels in the mid to distal third of the thigh.

Fig 6. Ultrasound probe position for imaging the femoral nerve in the inguinal area.

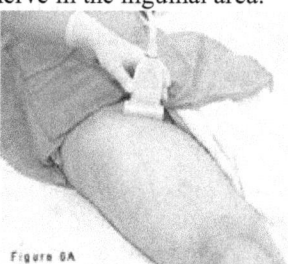 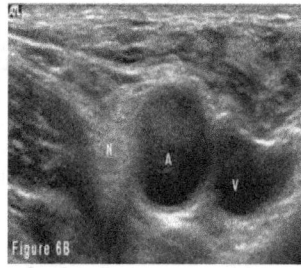

Ultrasound image of the Femoral nerve in the inguinal area.
V = Femoral Vein
A = Femoral Artery
N = Femoral Nerve

SCIATIC NERVE

The sciatic nerve also originates from the lumbosacral plexus (L4-S3) and enters the gluteal region through the greater sciatic foramen, between two muscle planes. The anterior muscle plane is formed by the obturator internus and inferior gemellus muscles, and the posterior, more superficial muscle plane by the gluteus maximus muscle. In the gluteal region the sciatic nerve is not easily identified by ultrasonography because of its depth. Lower in the subgluteal region, the sciatic nerve is more superficial, usually within 5 cm from the skin surface, and can be blocked as described by Sutherland [14] and Sukhani and associates. With a curved 5- to 7-MHz transducer, a transverse view of the sciatic nerve can be obtained showing bony landmarks, the greater trochanter of the femur laterally and the ischial tuberosity medially, when the patient is positioned semiprone with the limb to be blocked uppermost (FIG 7). The approximate location of the sciatic nerve is in the midpoint of a line uniting both landmarks. The sciatic nerve often appears hyperechoic and elliptical deep to the distal gluteus maximus muscle and lateral to the biceps femoris muscle (FIG -7). It is usually surrounded by a well-defined border, presumably the aponeurosis of the surrounding muscles.

Fig 7. Ultrasound probe position for imaging the sciatic nerve in the gluteal area.

Ultrasound image of the Sciatic nerve

IS = Ischial Tuberosity
F = Femur
Gluteus max = Gluteus Maximus muscle
SN = Sciatic Nerve

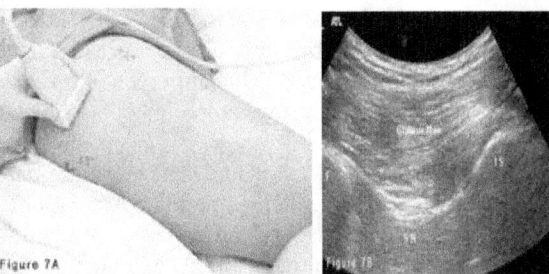

Moving caudally, the sciatic nerve can be imaged using a 7-MHz probe up to the popliteal fossa, where it divides into the peroneal and tibial nerves. Here, the sciatic nerve often appears round and hyperechoic and is located posterior to the femur, lateral to the popliteal artery, and deep (anterior) to the semitendinous and semimembranous muscles medially and the biceps femoris muscle laterally. More distally, the peroneal nerve may be followed as far laterally as the head of the fibula.

Fig 8 a,b. Ultrasound probe position for imaging the sciatic nerve in the popliteal area.

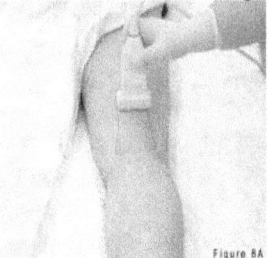 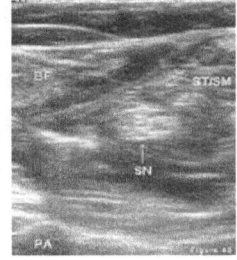

Ultrasound image of the Sciatic nerve in the popliteal area.
BF = Biceps Femoris
ST/SM = Semimembranous/ Semitendinous muscle
PA = Popliteal Artery
SN = Sciatic Nerve

Fig 8 c. Ultrasound image of the Sciatic nerve in the popliteal area after local anesthetic injection. Notice the division of the Sciatic nerve into two branches.
T = Tibial Nerve
CP = Common Peroneal.
The local anesthetic solution appears as a hypoechoic (black) space surrounding both nerve branches.

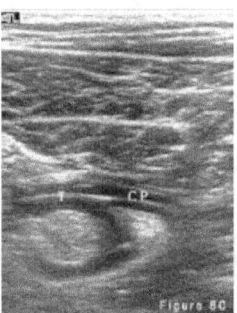

GUIDE LINES FOR ULTRASOUND-GUIDED NERVE BLOCK TECHNIQUES
1. The quality of ultrasonographic nerve images captured is dependent on the quality of the ultrasound machine and transducers, proper transducer selection (e.g., frequency) for each nerve location, the anesthesiologist's familiarity and interpretation of sonographic anatomy pertinent to the block, and good eye-hand coordination to track needle movement during advancement.
2. Optimal patient positioning and sterile technique are encouraged. This is particularly important for the continuous catheter technique, when it is necessary to use sterile conducting gel and a sterile plastic sheath to fully cover the entire transducer.
3. Nerve localization by ultrasound can be combined with nerve stimulation. Both tools are valuable and complementary, not mutually exclusive. Ultrasonography provides anatomic

information, while a motor response to nerve stimulation provides functional information about the nerve in question.
4. Observing local anesthetic spread is another valuable feature of ultrasound in addition to real-time visual guidance to navigate the needle toward the target nerve.
5. The first approach aims to align and move the block needle inline with the long axis of the ultrasound transducer, so the needle stays within the path of the ultrasound beam. In this manner, the needle shaft and tip can be clearly visualized. This approach is preferred when it is important to track the needle tip at all times (e.g., during supraclavicular block to minimize inadvertent pleural puncture).

Ultrasound-guided techniques may improve the accuracy, success, and safety of regional anesthesia. However, few prospective randomized outcome studies have been conducted and published so far. Williams and coworkers suggested that the addition of ultrasound guidance improves the quality of supraclavicular block [16] when compared to neurostimulator guidance alone. Marhofer and associates [17] also suggest that ultrasound guidance speeds the onset, improves the quality, and reduces the incidence of vascular puncture during three-in-one blocks. No study to date, however, has examined the impact of ultrasound on nerve injury. In summary, although preliminary experience has been encouraging, more outcome data are required to define the success and safety profile of ultrasound-guided peripheral nerve blocks.

ULTRASONOGRAPHY AND NEUROAXIAL BLOCKS

Neuroaxial anesthetic techniques can be challenging because of inter-individual anatomic variability and imprecise determination of the level of the vertebral interspace by physical examination alone (inaccurate 70-80% of the time).[18] Spinal needle insertion and local anesthetic injection at the wrong lumbar interspace (ie, too cephalad) may have been implicated in previously reported injuries to the conus medularis. Potentially, imaging guidance may improve accuracy and safety of needle placement during neuroaxial blocks.

Over two decades ago, attempts were made to image the ligamentum flavum using ultrasonography. Because the epidural and subarachoid spaces are surrounded by bones, anatomic assessment in this region is difficult since the majority of the ultrasound beam is reflected upon contacting the bony spinous processes. With a linear or curved 4- to 7-MHz probe, limited ultrasound beam passage is possible only through the interspinous space, especially in the paramedian region. The ligamentum flavum and the dura mater are dense tissues that appear hyperechoic on ultrasound while the low-density epidural space and the cerebrospinal fluid in the intrathecal space appear hypoechoic.

Fig 9a. Ultrasound probe position to obtain an axial view of the neuroaxial structures al the L4-L5 interspace

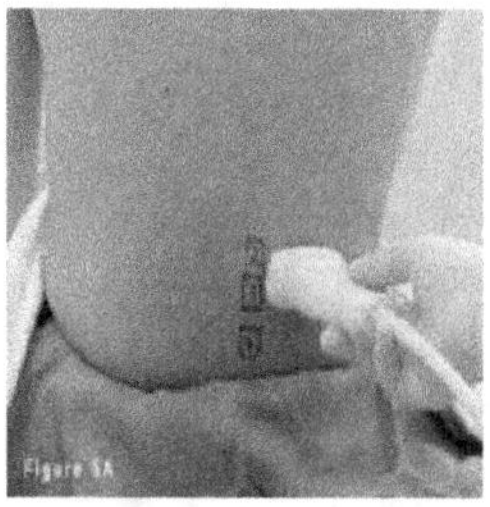

Fig 9b,c. Ultrasound image if the neuroaxial structures at the L4-L5 interspace, in an axial plane.
TP = Transverse Process
VB = Vertebral Body
IT = Intrathecal space
IL = Interspinous ligament

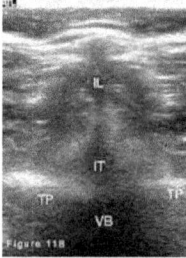

Ultrasound determination of the spinal level is more accurate than clinical examination. This has been confirmed in two recent studies showing accurate ultrasound determination in over 70 percent of patients when compared to MRI examination.[19] The markers were always placed within one interspace of the intended level. Ultrasonography can also determine the depth of needle penetration to reach the epidural space and can help reduce the number of needle puncture attempts. The paramedian region has been suggested by some to be the optimal window for ultrasound imaging, especially in the thoracic spine, because of a higher soft tissue to bone ratio.[20] In contrast to peripheral nerve blocks, real-time image-guided neuroaxial techniques have not been reported. Ultrasonography has been used primarily to help define the anatomy, depth, and angle of needle penetration immediately prior to performing the technique.

REFERENCES

1. Pavlin DJ, Rapp SE, Polissar NL, Malmgren JA, Koerschgen M, Keyes H: Factors affecting discharge time in adult outpatients. Anesth Analg 87: 816-26, 1998
2. Fortuna A, Fortuna A de O. Bupivacaine induced cardiac arrest. Anesth & Analg 71:561-2, 1990
3. Perlas A, Chan VWS, Simons M. Brachial Plexus Examination and Localization Using Ultrasound and Electrical Stimulation- A Volunteer Study. Anesthesiology 99:429-435, 2003
4. Chan VWS, Perlas A, Rawson R, and Odukoya O. Ultrasound Guided Supraclavicular Brachial Plexus Block. Anesth Analg 97:1514-17, 2003
5. Kossoff G. Basic physics and imaging characteristics of ultrasound. World J Surg 24:134-42, 2000
6. Peer S, kovacs P, Harpf C, et al. High resolution sonography of lower extremity peripheral nerves: anatomic correlation and spectrum of disease. J Ultrasound Med 21:315-22, 2002
7. Chan VWS. Applying ultrasound imaging to Interscalene Brachial Plexus Block. Reg Anesth. Pain Med 28 (4): 340-43, 2003
8. Perlas A, Chan VWS Ultrasound guided interscalene brachial plexus block.Techniques in Regional Anesthesia and Pain Management 8(4), 143-8, 2004
9. Ootaki C, Hayashi H, Amano M: Ultrasound guided infraclavicular brachial plexus block: An alternative technique to anatomical landmark-guided approaches. Reg Anesth Pain Med 25: 600-4, 2000
10. Retzl G, Kapral S, Greher M et al. Ultrsonographic findings of the axillary part of the brachial plexus. Anesth Analg 92:1271-5, 2001
11. Partridge BL, Benirschke K. Functional anatomy of the brachial plexus sheath: implications for Anesthesia. Anesthesiology 66:743, 1987
12. Farny J, Drolet P, Girard M. Anatomy of the posterior approach to the lumbar plexus block. Can J Anesth 41: 480-5, 1994
13. Gruber H, Peer S, Kovacs P et al. The ultrasonographic appearance of the femoral nerve and cases of iatrogenic impairment. J Ultrasound Med 22: 163-72, 2003
14. Raj PP, Parks RI, Watson TD et al. A new single position supine approach to the sciatic-femoral nerve block. Anesth Analg 54:489-93, 1975
15. Gray AT, Collins A, Schafhalter-Zoppoth I. Sciatic nerve block in a child: a sonographic approach. Anesth Analg 97:1300-2, 2003
16. Williams SR, Chouinard P, Arcand G, et al. Ultrasound guidance speeds the execution and improves the quality of supraclavicular block. Anesth Analg 97:1518-23, 2003
17. Marhofer P, Schrogendorfer K, Koining H, et al. Ultrasonographic guidance improves sensory block and onset time of three-in-one blocks. Anesth Analg 85:854-7, 1997
18. Broadbent CR, Maxwell WB, Ferrie R et al. Ability of Anesthetists to identify a marked lumbar interspace. Anesthesia 55:1122-6, 2000
19. Watson MJ, Evans S, Thorp JM. Could ultrasonography be used by an anesthetist to identify a specified lumbar interspace before spinal anesthesia? BJA 90 (4):509-11, 2001.
20. Grau T, Leipold R, Horter J, et al. Paramedian access to the epidural space: the optimum window for ultrasound imaging. Journal of Clinical Anesthesia 13: 213-17, 2001

Chapter 28.

Pain imaging

Spinal cord central pain:-
64-94% of patients with spinal cord injury have central pain. Aetiology includes trauma (65%), iatrogenic (12%) inflammatory neoplasm, skeletal or vascular and congenital lesions.
Brain central pain:-
98.6% incidence caused by brain lesions are more intractable than those arising from spinal cord. It is caused by vascular causes, iatrogenic trauma, infra temporal infection, syringo bulbia and degenerative diseases. Right side lesions are involved in stroke induced pain having thalamus involvement. [1]
Treatment:-
> Surgical: - The pain can disappear after removal of the tumor. Trauma pain can be relieved by exploring and excising the patient's atrophic cortex. Thalamic pain syndrome relieved by resection of post central gyrus. Cordotomy, trigeminal dorsal root entry zone, PVG stimulation relieves pain.

Features of central brain pain: - Central pain is of burning, cold, numb, tingle, sting, or itchy or aching bruise, sore, throbbing, cramping, tight or tearing.
Patho physiology is similar to peripheral neuropathic pain. The pain delays from a few weeks to months.[1]
Pattern of sensory loss:- Hemi body sensory loss- 46.5%, associated sensory-20.5%, hyperpathy, allodynia or both-6.8%, touch, position, vibration, sensory loss-5.5%.
FUNCTIONAL IMAGING IN BRAIN:-
Functional imaging is a promising tool for investigating the mechanism of central pain. Cesaro et al found that stimulating the affected half of body, so as to produce hyperpathia in patients with stroke induced hyperpathic pain, produced thalamic hyperactivity in the SPECT scans, but this was not seen after stimulation of the unaffected side.[2] Patients without hyperpathia did not show this hypersensitivity to stimulation. It was hypothesized that loss of function of inhibitory thalamic neurons after a stroke result in disinhibition of medial thalamic nucleus and possibly pain. There was a reduced perfusion in parietal lobe further reduced by induced allodynia attributed to cortical inhibition. The injection of Propofol reduced brain central pain for 5 min during which cerebral hypoperfusion improved.[3]
Flirato et al[4]- in stroke patients studied with SPECT scans, found that patients with thalamic lesions tend to have superficial pain, while those without it tend to have deep pain. In the former there was reduced back ground neural activity and reduced O_2 consumption in thalamus. The central pain resulted from a chemical imbalance between glutaminergic and GABAergic mechanisms in transmission between sensory thalamus and cortex, which opposing glutaminergic and potentiating GABAergic transmission, by administering Ketamine or Propofol respectively.
Spinal cord pain functional imaging: An associated spinal cord injury, peripheral neuropathic or cancer pain, diminished perfusion of the human contra lateral thalamus in SPECT and PET. These changes could be normalized by relief of the pain by resection of syrinx in case of spinal cord or by cordotomy in cancer pain.[2]
Imaging the Brain during Pain
The large volume of the human forebrain in relation to the spinal cord suggests that descending modulatory influences are more important in humans than in other species. In humans the forebrain occupies 85% and the spinal cord 2% of the volume of the central nervous system,1 but in rats the corresponding percentages are 44% and 35%, respectively. The human corticospinal tract contains almost a million fibers, but the spinothalamic tract contains only a few thousand. Consequently, descending forebrain influences are likely to play a uniquely important role in humans. Brain imaging depicts the activity of multiple supra spinal structures ranging from the brainstem to the forebrain. Supraspinal processing of nociceptive information activates somatic and autonomic reflexes, neuroendocrine responses, attention, arousal, evaluation of the spatiotemporal and physical features of the stimulus, hedonic experience, mnemonic functions, cognitive processes, and the ascending and descending control systems that mediate and modulate these activities and their interactions. To understand how multiple neuronal populations contribute to distinct nociceptive responses, and how they unite to produce integrated responses, requires conjoint analysis of conscious behavior and the activity of multiple synaptic populations.

Imaging Pathological Pain Most acute pain subsides with wound healing, but unfortunately, sometimes pain from injuries may persist, as in chronic complex regional pain syndromes (CRPS)[2]. In animal models, continuing afferent activity originates spontaneously from damaged nerve fibers and from their cell bodies in the dorsal root ganglion. Evidence also suggests long-term changes in the physiology of spinal and supraspinal neurons, perhaps exaggerated by abnormal inputs from damaged peripheral nerves. Functional reorganization of sensory neurons in the spinal cord, thalamus, and cerebral cortex of animals occurs after peripheral injury with or without nerve damage. It was demonstrated that the intensity of phantom limb pain experienced by amputees correlates with the extent of functional reorganization of the somatosensory cortex. Patients with central pain provide evidence that central lesions alone may produce chronic pain in the absence of any nociceptive input.3 These examples emphasize the need for information about supraspinal systems, including the forebrain, to better understand pathological pain of peripheral or central origin.

Types of Functional Imaging Functional imaging includes single photon emission computerized tomography (SPECT), positron emission tomographic (PET) studies of glucose metabolism or receptor binding, and electrophysiological methods such as magnetoencephalography (MEG) and high-density electroencephalography (EEG) with equivalent current dipole analysis (ECD). This brief review will concentrate on PET and functional magnetic resonance imaging (fMRI) methods to detect changes in regional cerebral blood flow (rCBF).

Physiological Basis for SPECT, PET, and MRI Imaged brain events correspond to activity in populations of synapses. The energy demand of synaptic activity requires rapid increases in local blood flow to deliver glucose and oxygen. Several experiments have demonstrated the close coupling of synaptic neurotransmitter release, recycling, and glucose utilization[4]. The global cerebral blood flow increased during brain activity. The, speciall optical sensors can monitor the reflectance of different wavelengths of light by synaptic populations as they respond to specific stimuli. Signals detected by this optical imaging originate within a few hundred microns of evoked synaptic activity and are thus capable of defining anatomical boundaries within the synaptic neuropil.. In PET activation, radiolabeled water or CO_2 is used, and the accumulated count of radioactivity provides an estimate of the regional cerebral perfusion during the scan (about 1 minute). This value is compared across conditions (e.g., pain or no pain) to obtain estimates of task-related or stimulus-specific changes in rCBF. When a population of active synapses uses oxygen, oxyhemoglobin is changed locally to deoxyhemoglobin. The different magnetic resonance signals of these two forms of hemoglobin make fMRI possible. The amplitude of the signal is proportional to the rCBF, which (as in PET) correlates with functional measures of neuronal activity. Among the advantages of fMRI is the lack of radiation, which offers the opportunity to repeat individual studies frequently. The fMRI provides better spatial resolution than PET or SPECT. A disadvantage of fMRI is that ferromagnetic materials, present in most electronic devices and recording instruments, cannot be brought near the scanner magnet. Subjects with implanted ferromagnetic metal prostheses or other devices thus cannot be studied with fMRI. Another disadvantage of fMRI is that the imaging of resting (unstimulated) activity and the statistical analysis of the responses of the whole brain are less well established than for PET.

What PET and fMRI reveal about Pain

Many discrete brain structures are active during pain. Although for many years multiple brain structures and pathways were known to participate in the processing of nociceptive information activity with the perception of pain which correlates specifically with synaptic activity in the primary and secondary somatosensory cortex (S1 and S2) and the anterior cingulate cortex. PET and fMRI studies have confirmed that activation of a network of interactive subsystems consistently occurs during perception of pain. Pain-related activity is found most frequently within the medial midbrain, thalamus, lentiform nucleus, cerebellum, and the insular, prefrontal, parietal (including S1 and S2), and anterior cingulate cortices. Thus, sensory, motor, association, and limbic systems combine to mediate the multiple components of the pain experience and response[6]

Normal group differences in pain perception are associated with differences in brain activation. There are differences in the spatial pattern and intensity of synaptically induced rCBF during different forms and intensities of innocuous and noxious thermal stimuli, the perceived differences between acute skin and acute muscle pain reflect differences in the intensity and spatiotemporal pattern of neuronal activity within overlapping sets of forebrain structures.

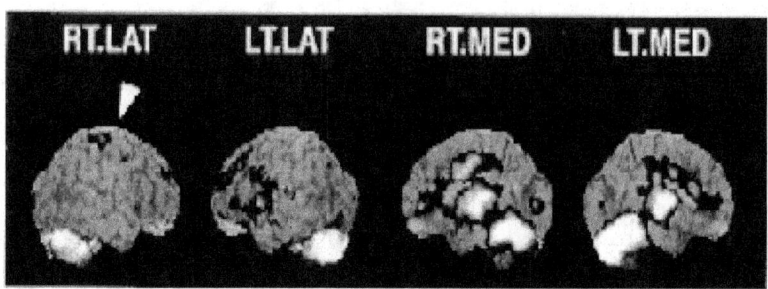

Figure - Significant pooled rCBF increases (averaged across 11 normal subjects) during immersion of the left hand in painfully cold (1°C), compared to mildly cool (29°C) water. Responses significantly (P < 0.05) above global blood flow are shown in gray scale (white corresponds to P < 0.0001). Arrow indicates a response in the right (contralateral) sensorimotor cortex. Note the strong responses in the cerebellum, bilateral thalamus, and anterior cingulate gyrus (mid-anterior and perigenual regions).7. Both male and female subjects rated 40° C contact heat stimuli as warm and 50°C stimuli as painful, and activation of the contralateral prefrontal cortex, insula, and thalamus overlapped completely in males and females. However, females rated the 50° C stimuli as more intense than did males, and showed significantly more intense activation of the responding areas, 7 perception and brain activation were similar

The functional specificity of pain-activated brain regions can be identified in imaging experiments intensity in normal subjects, pain unpleasantness correlated with the intensity of rCBF response in a far anterior (dorsal perigenual) region of the anterior cingulate cortex, but not in the S1 cortex. The information about pain intensity was widely distributed among many, but not all, pain-activated regions, including the cerebellum, these brain structures are highly heterogeneous in function. In fMRI experiments designed to separate the perception of pain from the anticipation of pain, the activation of certain regions is better correlated with anticipation of pain than with pain perception.

Unique patterns of forebrain activation occur in neuropathic pain. Imaging studies of pain caused by damage to the peripheral or central nervous system reveal that there is a thalamic hypoactivity at rest in patients with central neuropathic pain. 8Painful dysesthesiae of the left hemibody and face following a lacunar infarction at the lateral edge of the right ventral posterior lateral thalamus on sensory examination revealed deep pressure allodynia on the left and symmetrical cutaneous heat pain thresholds. At rest, rCBF was less in the right thalamus than the left. The noxious heat stimulation (55°C) is equally painful on either side. During noxious heat stimulation of the right (normal) side, there was a slight reduction in rCBF in the left thalamus compared to its value at rest. When noxious heat was applied to the patient's left (abnormal) side, there was a strong rCBF increase in the right (contralateral) thalamus compared to the left. These results suggest that pathological hypoactivity in the resting hemithalamus masks an underlying hyper-responsiveness to noxious stimulation. This pathological hyper-responsiveness may be due to a loss of resting inhibitory activity within the thalamus

Therapeutic Implications of Pain Imaging Understanding the pathophysiology of chronic, severely painful conditions could suggest preventive measures and physical or pharmacological methods targeted specifically against maladaptive central adaptations. Researchers must first distinguish between adaptive, neutral, and maladaptive reorganization. Anatomical and physiological differences among patients may require new, genetically based technology. Therapy may include local delivery of growth factors or specific suppressors, neurosurgical stimulation, or ablative procedures. Ultimately, defining each patient's pathophysiology will allow effective interventions to target specific sites and pathways based on information obtained through imaging that patient's pain.

References

1. Blinkov SM, Glezer II. The Human Brain in Figures and Tables. New York: Plenum Press, 1968.
2. Merskey H, Bogduk N. Classification of Chronic Pain: Descriptions of Chronic Pain Syndromes and Definitions of Pain Terms. Seattle: IASP Press, 1994.
3. Casey KLE. Pain and Central Nervous System Disease: The Central Pain Syndromes. New York: Raven Press, 1991.
4. Sokoloff L. In: Lassen NA., et al. (Eds). Brain Work and Mental Activity. Copenhagen: Munksgaard, 1991 52-64.
5. Casey KL, et al. In: Bromm B (Ed). From Nociception to Pain. New York: Raven Press, 1994.
6. Casey KL, Minoshima S. In: Jensen TS, et al. (Eds). Proceedings of the 8th World Congress on Pain. Seattle: IASP Press, 1997, pp 855-866.
7. Paulson PE. Pain perception and brain stimulation. Pain. 1998;76:223-229
8. Casey KL, et al. Abstracts: 9th World Congress on Pain. Seattle: IASP Press, 1999, 435.

Chapter 29.
Trauma and Pain

Depending on the site and severity of trauma- physiological change occurring can affect recovery in such patients. The goal of pain management is not only to decrease patient's pain but also to return the patient to a more normal physiologic status. Pain relief following Polytrauma is the most neglected and underestimated requirement of emergency trauma management. Most of the clinicians fail to recognize the significant detrimental impact that pain has upon the recovery of trauma patients. Many series, which followed Polytrauma patients, noted a very high incidence of residual damage, up to 30-40% in the form of pain syndromes. Rationale behind active pain relief is two folds; firstly pain relief promotes ambulation and movements which in turn help in restoring pulmonary functions, decrease venous stasis, DVT and pulmonary embolism, secondly LA and opioids used in peri dural block the nociceptive reflex are thus preventing much of the physiological derangements seen after trauma.[1]

Patho physiology of pain in Polytrauma:-
Adverse physiologic effects of pain after trauma include:
1. decreased diaphragmatic contractility
2. chest wall splinting
3. tachycardia
4. hypertension
5. increased oxygen consumption
6. hyperglycemia
7. ileus
8. splanchnic hypoperfusion
9. fluid retention
10. immobility
11. Irritation, insomnia and other psychiatric problems.

Therefore understanding of pain pathways and modalities of pain transmission from periphery towards CNS is very important. It helps in assessing the pain as well as formulating modalities of pain relief.[2]. Sports injuries can result into chronic pain in shoulder and knee joint (table 1, 2)

Methods of assessment of pain:-
Various objective and subjective methods like adjective rating scale (ARS), numerical rating scale (NRS) and visual analogue scale (VAS) can be applied for assessment of severity of pain.

Principles of management in trauma & sports injuries:-
Basic principles of active pain relief service include:
1. Decrease in the production of chemicals, which sensitize peripheral nerves.
2. Blocking nociceptive neurotransmission within peripheral nerves [3].
3. Modulating pain perception at spinal cord and CNS [4].

Factors deciding the methodology
1. Type of environment
2. Automatic location
3. Presence of complications like infection and coagulopathy
4. History of drug abuse
5. Psychological aspect – Phantom limb
6. Regional techniques.

(A) Epidural/ spinal placement of analgesic drugs has opened up new chapter in management of Polytrauma. Epidural and spinal anesthesia are not recommended as a sole anesthetic technique in acute trauma management. Low quantity of drug is used as compared to systemic route and thus avoids very many deleterious side effects. Low dose local anesthetic singly or in combination with opioids can be used in continuous infusion for to provide long duration and better quality of analgesia. These methods have additional benefits in that they help in reducing incidence of DVT as well as improve tissue perfusion by sympathetic blockade especially in vascular surgery. Most trauma textbooks have strongly recommended their use in thoracic trauma management.

Table 1: Trauma score

The trauma score

Category	Value	Points	
Respiratory rate	10-24	4	A
	25-35	3	
	>35	2	
	<10	1	
	0	0	
Respiratory effort	Normal	1	B
	Retractive	0	
Systolic blood pressure	>90	4	C
	70-89	3	
	50-69	2	
	<50	1	
	0	0	
Capillary refill	Normal	2	D
Delayed >2 sec	Delayed	1	
	None	0	
Glasgow coma score (GCS)			
Eye opening		GCS Points	
Spontaneous 4		14-15	5	E
To voice 3	1	11-13	4
To pain 2		8-10	3
None 1		5-7	2
Verbal response		3-4	1
Oriented 5			
Confused 4			
Inappropriate words 3	2		
Incomprehensible 2			
None 1			
Motor response			
Obeys commands 6			
Localizes pain 5			
Withdraw (pain) 4	3		
Flexion (pain) 3			
Extension (pain) 2			
None 1			
Total GCS Points = (1) + (2) + (3)		Total trauma score points = A + B + C + D + E	

Table 2: Principals of disaster resuscitation in 1st hour

Stage		Possible interventions
Life-supporting first aid/ Basic life support	Airway breathing	Jaw thrust, head tilt, removal of debris from pharynx, mouth-to-mouth ventilation or equivalent
	Circulation	Pulse check, closed cardiac compressions, control of external hemorrhage, leg elevation, immobilization of cervical spine
Advanced trauma life support	Airway	Intubation, surgical airway
	Circulation	Restoration of spontaneous circulation, fluid resuscitation, vasoactive agents, defibrillation, open chest compressions, treatment of pneumo/hemothorax (military antishock trousers suit)
	Other system	Cerebral preservation, degree of exposure, spinal cord injury precautions, thoracic/abdominal trauma evaluation, burn assessment, pain management, definitive studies (e.g., angiography)

(B) Regional blocks, either continuous infusion nerve blocks or infiltration anesthesia has definite role in patients with minor injuries but not in the management of acute pain inn Polytrauma where more than one area is involved. Patients who can be managed with these techniques are not subjected to unnecessary general anesthesia thus avoiding side effects.[3]

(C) Acupuncture/TENS its role in acute management is debatable but do have an appreciable role in chronic cases.

(D) Hypnosis and psychotherapy

(E) Cryo neurolysis

(F) Intrapleural medication for rib fractures and lung contusion

(G) peripheral nerve blocks- ankle/wrist

(H) intercostal nerve block
(I) subcutaneous morphine
(J) cognitive, behavioral and physical therapy.

Drugs:-

1. Opioids:- Morphine still remains the back bone as it can be given safely in many formulations. Most commonly used routes are PCA, i/v continuous infusions and epidural. Newer synthetic opioids like phentanyl, SU and al-phentanyl are short acting and with few side effects. Respiratory depression occurs rarely but can not be ignored and thus demands careful monitoring. Epidural administration can provide prolong and excellent quantity analgesia with a low dose. PCA requires sophisticated equipments and is not practiced in India.[5]
2. Local anesthetics: - lignocaine and bupivacaine are most commonly used LA drugs. Lignocaine has short duration of action and comparatively safer than bupivacaine. Continuous infusion of low dose solution through epidural catheter provides safe and excellent analgesia. Continuous axillary/femoral block gives sympathetic blockade necessary in vascular grafts.[2]
3. NSAIDs: In acute trauma NSAIDs have no role. Ketorolac and diclofenac are only i.m. preparation available at present and useful in minor injuries. In cases with circulatory compromise these i.m. preparation gives erratic results and are not recommended.[2]
4. Topical application:- refrigerant anesthetic sprays, vapocoolents, alternative delivery techniques for topical LA drugs.[2] Iontopheresis single dose injectors and tree oils have some role in such patients.
5. Other drugs: varieties of oral Adjuvants are available but useful in chronic pain. Antidepressant and other psychotic drugs are useful in chronic pain syndrome following trauma. Adrenaline, Clonidine, steroids, midazolam and neostigmine are few examples of Adjuvants, which prolong duration of/or improve quality of analgesia [6,7]
6. Physical therapy, mobilization and exercise, heat and cold care are very useful in trauma and sports injuries.

Table 3: Sports injuries causing knee pain.

Anterior pain
Patellar
    Chrondromalacia patellae, recurrent dislocation, subluxation or tracking problems, myofascial dysfunction quadriceps
Infrapatellar
    Bursitis
Tibial tubercle
    Osgood-Schlatter's disease

Anteromedial/anterolateral pain
Parapatellar
    Fat pad impingement, degenerative arthritis
Intermediate-internal derangement
    Meniscal tear, cruciate ligament tear, synovial pinching or tear, meniscal cyst, posttraumatic arthritis, osteochrondritis dissecans
Extreme lateral/medial
    Collateral ligament injury, pes anserinus bursitis or myofascial dysfunction sartorius, semimembranous, gracilis muscles, myofascial dysfunction adductor muscles, entrapment saphenous nerve in adductor canal

Posterior
Baker's cyst, myofascial dysfunction hamstring or calf musculature

Reflex sympathetic dystrophy

No single drug or method can provide complete and satisfactory pain relief. Tailor made combinations of drug and the delivery systems provide maximum benefits and have few side effects. Continuous infusions of local anesthetics and one of the opioid administrations through thoracic/lumbar epidural appears to be most effective method to provide pain relief in first few hours following trauma. For isolated limb injuries, involving vessels, continuous axillary/femoral sheath block with LA and opioid solution provide not only excellent analgesia but also help in salvaging limb. Once patient recovers after surgical intervention one can switch over to oral NSAIDs or any other method mentioned above. Prevention of post traumatic complication is prevented by early mobilization in trauma and sports injury.

Table 4: Sports injury & shoulder pain

SPORTS INJURIES RESULTING IN CHRONIC SHOULDER PAIN

Subdeltoid/subacromial pain
Tendinitis, rotator cuff, subacromial bursitis, subdeltoid bursitis, brachial plexus injury, thoracic outlet (neurovascular compression) syndromes, cervical radiculopathy

Anterior pain
Bicipital tendinitis, dislocating biceps tendon, subscapular tendinitis, impingement coracoacromial ligament on biceps tendon, rotator cuff tear, shoulder subluxation, myofascial dysfunction (infraspinatus, deltoid, scaleni, supraspinatous, pectoralis major, pectoralis minor, biceps, coracobrachialis)

Posterior/lateral pain
Hematoma deltoid muscle, myofascial dysfunction (deltoid, levator scapulae, supraspinatus, teres major, teres minor, subscapularis, serratus posterior, triceps, trapezius)

Pain at the start of throw or tennis serve
Rotator cuff tendinitis, subdeltoid bursitis, subacromial bursitis

Pain at the end of throw or tennis serve
Insertional tear long head triceps, tear posterior capsule, posterior osteophytes

Pain with movement/restricted movement
Posttraumatic arthritis, recurrent dislocation

Reflex sympathetic dystrophy
Shoulder-hand syndrome

Table 5: Phases of burn management

Phase	Management issues
Resuscitation (First 24 hours)	Airway assessment, carboxyhemoglobin level, 100% oxygen, pulmonary toilet, blood gases, chest x-ray management, of adult respiratory distress syndrome
	Hemodynamic assessment, large-bore IVs, Blood pressure above 90 systolic, Urine output above 0.5 cc/kg/hr, Pulse under 130, Colloid for shock
	Wound care
Postresuscitation (2 to 6 days)	Airway maintenance, pulmonary toilet, adequate gas exchange, infection control
	Hemodynamic maintenance, fluid for hypovolemia, inotropes for ↓ cardiac output, acid-base and electrolyte regulation
	Nutritional support, wound care
Inflammation (7 days to wound closure)	Prevention of nosocomial pneumonia, pulmonary toilet, infection control measures, appropriate antibiotics, prevention of adult respiratory distress syndrome
	Adequate nutrition, parenteral if needed
	Maintenance of adequate oxygen delivery, blood transfusions as needed
	Prevention of pain, stress, sepsis
Rehabilitation/wound remodeling	Restoration of function to affected area
	Control of scarring/contractures
	Restoration of whole patient to functional activity
	Pain control
	Psychological support

References

1. Rybrol, Schurizer BA, Peters et all. Post operative analgesia and lung functions: a comparison of intramuscular with epidural Ketamine. Acta. Anesthesio scand 198,26;514-518
2. Raj PP; Practical management of pain 3rd edi. St Louis, Mosby year book; 1998.
3. Kehleth. The endocrine metabolic response to post operative pain. Acta. Anesthesio Scand(suppl) 1982;74:173-175
4. Lund C, Selmar P , Hensen OB et al . Effect of epidural bupivacaine on somatosensory evoke potential after dermatomal stimulation.Anesth. Analg. 1987,66:34-38
5. Mathor LE, Parentral opioids for post operative analgesia. Res, anaesthe. 1982,7:144
6. Islas JA, Astorgc J, Laredo M. Epidural Ketamine for control of post operative pain, Anaesth. Analg. 1985;64:1161-1162
7. Kinahata LM. Spinal analgesia with morphine and Clonidine. (Editorial). Anesth. Analg. 1989; 65:194
8. Maron RR. Orthopedic aspects of sports medicine. In Appenseller O(Ed): Sports medicine, Ed, Baltimore, Urban and Schwarzenberg 1988.
9. Callilet R. Soft tissue pain and disability. Philadelphia, F A Davis, 1983.

Chapter 30.
Palliative Care: Magnitude of cancer pain and related symptoms

The World Health Organisation estimates that, worldwide, there were 14 million new cancer cases and 8.2 million cancer-related deaths in 2012.Of these half of them occur in developing countries. As majority of these present in advanced stage, the only realistic options are pain and palliative care.
The cancer patient faces a wide range of psychological and physical problems. There is a fear of death, physical disability and dependence on others. But the most feared consequence of cancer however is pain. Moderate to severe pain is experienced by 30 to 60 % of cancer patients during active therapy and in 90% of patient with advanced disease. Pain is often a remainder of an impending death and has profound impact on the patient's emotions, mood and distress. Thus the cancer patients with pain are more likely to develop psychological disorders than those without pain[1].

Pain also heightens the burden on the patient's family, in terms of financial difficulty due to the cost of patients care and treatment. There are associated emotional burden and physical strain on the attending relatives. Similar problems are faced by staff nurses and physicians who face complex diagnostic and therapeutic challenges, inability to cope with treatment failures. Cancer patients need more nursing care with the aim of improving the quality of life of the patients[2].

The management of associated problems like poor nutrition, problems related to urogenital, renal and CNS & CVS also need a multidisciplinary approach by a specialized team consisting of an oncologist, surgeons, psychiatrist, anesthesiologist, radiotherapist and trained nurses. This has lead to specialized cancer wards in major hospitals. The challenges posed during terminal stage of cancer needs special care homes called hospices where care, rehabilitation and treatment are provided by a dedicated team. In spite of technological advances, made in last 50 years, the physicians' attitude towards the cancer patient is of resignation, relegating him to doom. Most of the terminal patients are sent back home to die. The physicians & care givers lack knowledge of the pain & other related symptoms. The attitude of care givers should be changed from treatment of malignancy only to specialized care, rehabilitation and quality of life especially in the end stage. The no availability of morphine which is due to government restrictions is another hurdle in our country which incidentally is the highest producer of opium in the world. There is a baseless fear of addiction in the cancer patients which is basically a drug dependence and not drug abuse. The WHO and Indian Society for Study of Pain have been guiding the physicians and technological know how with a little success. It is heartening to note that there are opening more and more pain clinic services at district level every year. Amen.

World Health Organization has documented following reasons for inadequate cancer pain control[2].
1. Absence of national policies on cancer pain relief and palliative care.
2. Lack of awareness on the part of health care provide4rs, policy makers, administrators and the public that most cancer pain can be relieved.
3. Shortage of finances, limitation of health delivery systems and personal.
4. Concern that medical use of opioids will produce psychological dependence and drug abuse.
5. Legal restrictions on the use and availability of opioids.

Following factors contribute to under treatment of cancer pain
  A) Patient related-pain under reporting.
   1. Fear of disease progression.
   2. Perceived lack of time or inadequate time spent with physician
   3. Poor compliance with prescribed medications.
  B) Physician related-
   1. Legal issues – opioid prescriptions
   2. difficulty assessing pain complaints
   3. lack of information, expertise on cancer pain management
   4. Desire to provide untried, latest pain management techniques.

This can be dealt with by: 1) Education of patients and health care providers
2) Establishment of pain management practice/programmes
3) State cancer pain initiative parallel to advanced cardiac life support and advanced trauma life support programmes.

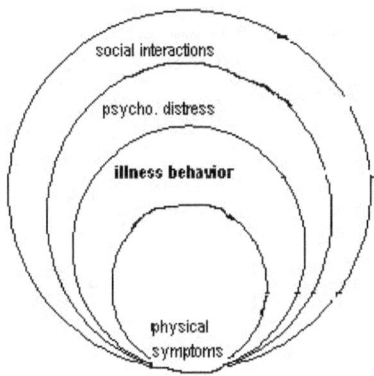   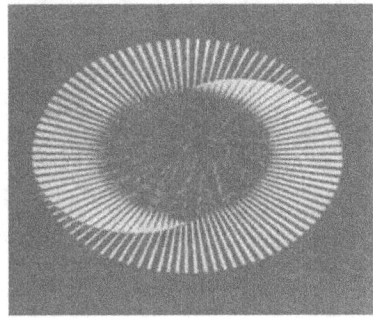

Fig 1. Biopsychosocial phenomenon   Fig 2. Whirlpool of pain

Paradigm of pain: A joint report of the than College of Anaesthetist and The Royal College of Surgeons highlighted the need to treat acute pain. The acute pain later becomes chronic following tissue damage and becomes a complex biopsychosocial phenomenon. The figure 1 shows an illustration of pain in cancer management[3].

The figure shows the author's conception of the patients' suffering from pain. The center of the diagram shows electric shock like sensation represented by electric ray fish sending electrical shocks which in turn leads to somatic and psychological changes in the body and its surroundings as well thus causing a whirlpool in the surrounding waters. [5]

Every year, about 800,000 new cancer patients get registered with the National Cancer Registry Programme in India. This shows that cancer is one of the major health problems in India at present. Lung and oral cancer are the most common types of cancers among men, where as cervical and breast cancer among women in India. There were 5,56,400 cancer-related deaths in India in the year 2010. Out of which, 71% of cancer patients (3,95,400) were of the age group between 30-69 years.

Prevalence and magnitude of cancer pain in India [3]

At any given time there are about 1.5 million people suffering from cancer in India. As cancer detection facilities are poor, most of the patients are already in an advanced stage of the disease and need palliation for cancer-related and other symptoms.

As accurate statistics are not available, it is difficult to say how many of these patients are having pain and the degree of severity of their pain. Based on figures from some more affluent developed nations it may be estimated that about 70% (1.05 million) of the victims of cancer are in pain at some stage or the other of their disease and require relief by effective intervention by pain clinicians.

Of the various possible interventions, neurolytic nerve blocks, continuous patient-controlled analgesic administering devices and use of skin patches of narcotic and other analgesic are beyond the reach of a majority of these patients either because of the non-availability of experts or because of high costs.

Oral morphine and adjuvants, therefore, remains the only universally applicable intervention for relief of pain in these patients. All palliative care centres should ensure continued availability of oral morphine and adjuvant drugs.

There is almost a total lack of awareness amongst our people on how cancer presents and progresses. The facilities for early detection and so-called early curative interventions are also few and far between. As a matter of fact, medical facilities in general are still beyond the reach of the common man, both logistically and financially.

As a result of this, patients with cancer when they present for medical consultation have already reached a stage when their disease is beyond any curative intervention. Palliative care remains the only choice in these circumstances.

Pain – the most important symptom in cancer, requiring relief

As conscientious members of the Indian Society for Study of Pain (ISSP), we have to endeavour to chalk out plans for relief of pain in not only in cancer patients but also in patients with pain of other categories, whose number may run into millions at any given time.

Patients are suffering unnecessary pain, according to a survey in USA. More than three-quarters of patients questioned say they had experienced pain as a result of drugs or surgery either for cancer or for other diseases.

However, fewer than half had been told to expect this by a care-giver, and only one in ten had been given any written material on techniques for pain control. Adequate pain relief is generally thought to be possible in nine out of 10 cancer cases, but most patients were unaware of any methods of doing this including - pain relieving skin patches, and suppositories containing pain-relieving drugs, which could be within the reach of some of such patients.

The suffering resulting from pain

Pain is subjective and unpleasant feeling and results in psychological, behavioural, and even physical changes. Pain can be a destructive disease as well. Persistent pain, when the threat of injury has past and the wound has healed, no longer serves its useful protective purpose. Persistent chronic pain can be as disruptive as the original injury with far reaching consequences that impact on every aspect of human existence. These physiological and psychosocial consequences result in decreased mobility, anger, depression (incidence 30 - 100%) disrupted family life, loss of earning power and significant cost to society.

This multidimensional nature of chronic pain entitles it to be considered a disease entity in and of itself. Pain is a universal experience that a staggering number of people live with every day. Estimates of the number of chronic pain sufferers vary and have grown significantly in the last ten years. In 1983, it was estimated that more than 75-80 million people in America alone suffered chronic pain. In 1996 more than 120 million Americans suffered from chronic pain. A few other current estimates from varying sources include arthritis pain - 16 million, low back pain - 19 million of which 11.7 million are impaired and 2.6 million are permanently disabled, headache - over three million, chronic neuralgia - eight million, cancer pain - 2.5 to 3 million, and post-herpetic neuralgia 28,000. Although estimates vary, it is obvious that pain is a very prevalent health problem in India also; in fact, it may be the greatest healthcare problem in India. A study in 1999 for the American Pain Society estimated that nine percent of U.S. adult population are suffering from moderate to severe non-cancer related chronic pain. 2.

Categories of pain

The three major categories of pain are:
1. Cancer pain,
2. Non-malignant pain,
3. and, Psychogenic pain.

Cancer patients may be classified into five groups:
1. Patients with acute cancer related pain (Table 1)
2. Patients with chronic cancer-related pain due to either progression or therapy
3. Patients with pre-existing chronic benign non-malignant pain and cancer-related pain
4. Patients with chemical dependency history and cancer-related pain
5. Dying patient who must be provided comfort m

Problems of Management

Management to be effective has to be preceded by an accurate assessment of the type and severity of pain and the impact of pain on the life of the pain sufferer. When the assessment is complete, ancillary testing performed, and a diagnosis is reached, a plan for managing the pain must be formed.

The treatment will depend on the aetiology of the pain. However, there are some basic principles for managing pain. The most important principle is that pain is a multidimensional problem that impacts all aspects of the patient. All of the

Table 1. Characteristics of pain[6]

1. Number of pains
   - (a) Single site of pain - 46
   - (b) Multiple sites of pain - 68
2. Duration of worst pain
   - (a) 1 Month - 46
   - (b) 1 – 3 Months - 31
   - (c) > 3 Months - 37
3. Intensity of pain
   - (a) No pain - 0
   - (b) Mild pain - 4
   - (c) Moderate pain - 38
   - (d) Severe pain - 62
   - (e) Excruciating pain - 10
4. Temporal pattern
   - (a) Continuous - 64
   - (b) Intermittent - 48
5. Radiation of pain
   - (a) Present - 67
   - (b) Absent - 47
6. Palliative factors
   - (a) Lying down - 2
   - (b) Rest - 10
   - (c) Fomentation - 8
   - (d) Others- Massage, Rubifacient - 1 each
7. Provoking factors
   - (a) Eating food - 48
   - (b) Coughing - 25
   - (c) Ambulation - 23
   - (d) Change of position - 8

Table 2. Distressing and annoying symptoms other than pain[6]

1. General symptoms
   - (a) Fatigue - 86
   - (b) Fever - 20
   - (c) Breathlessness - 22
   - (d) Sleep disturbance - 94
     - Due to pain - 84
     - Due to anxiety - 3
     - Due to both - 9
2. GI symptoms
   - (a) Hiccups - 3
   - (b) Fullness after meals - 10
   - (c) Anorexia - 35
   - (d) Nausea - 16
   - (e) Vomiting - 9
   - (f) Constipation - 37

Table 3. Number of patients with various mechanisms and various causes of pain[5]

1. Mechanism of pain
   - (a) Somatic nocciceptive - 23
   - (b) Visceral nociceptive - 0
   - (c) Neuropathic - 19
   - (d) Somatic & neuropathic - 62
   - (e) Somatic and visceral - 4
   - (f) Visceral and Neuropathic - 3
   - (g) Somatic, visceral and neuropathic - 3
2. Cause of Pain
   - (a) Tumour related - 97
   - (b) Treatment related - 1
   - (c) Related to both - 14

physiologic effects of pain must be treated but equally important are the psychological, social, spiritual, and economic components. No one practitioner is adequately prepared to manage all of these aspects. A multidisciplinary approach draws together specialists from many specialties to work collaboratively to develop and implement a treatment plan. An interdisciplinary team composed of pain practitioners, medical, nursing, rehabilitation, and psychosocial specialists and clergy coordinated by a case manager has the best chance of improving the quality of the chronic pain sufferer's life. Not all patients will need all specialties but the program can be tailored to meet each patient's needs. The goals are to identify and treat aetiologies that can be managed medically or surgically, provide physical, occupational and recreational rehabilitation to maximize the level of activity, identify and treat psychosocial problems and maladaptive behaviours, and give the patient the necessary education and tools to take control of the pain and his life.

Medical, surgical, and anaesthetic treatment will be diagnosis-specific. Pain can be managed medically with both non-opiate and opiate analgesics. Specific pain syndromes or aspects of pain may respond to antidepressants, anxiolytics, anticonvulsants, hormones, psychoactive agents, cardiovascular agents, and radiopharmaceuticals to name a few. Transcutaneous electrical stimulation may provide non-pharmacological pain control. Surgical procedures may correct a pain producing aetiology, correct a complication of chronic pain, or may be aimed at interrupting a nerve pathway. Anaesthetic blocks can help diagnose or treat pain. Implantation of catheters along nerves or in the spinal canal can be used for long-term administration of local anaesthetics or opiates. Spinal cord stimulators that can control pain without drugs may be appropriate for some patients.

Rehabilitation is aimed at improving the patient's overall level of function. Physical Medicine may be specifically indicated for some pain syndromes but all chronic pain patients can benefit. Chronic pain patients tend to be deconditioned from restricted activity. Physical Medicine (physiotherapy) can improve strength, flexibility, and cardiovascular condition. Occupational therapy can help get the patient back to work, either in the home or in a paying job, improving the sense of self-esteem and easing financial strain.

Recreational therapy improves physical and mental well-being and helps the patient develop activities that divert attention away from pain. The psychosocial team is a very important component of pain management. Psychological testing can help diagnose pain and its effects. It can then help the patient deal with anxiety, anger, depression, and stress associated with chronic pain. Behaviour modification techniques are crucial to gaining control and keeping control of chronic pain. Patients can be taught relaxation, guided imagery, distraction, and biofeedback to gain control of pain. Since chronic pain impacts the family as well as the patient, attention to family can be provided. Social services can help the patient take full advantage of resources available in the community.

Nurses are often the health care professionals that spend the most time with the patient. They are an invaluable resource for assessing pain and implementing therapy. **Nurses may act as case managers or patient advocates.** Clinical specialists and nurse practitioners may provide services in many disciplines.

Poor diet and weight gain or loss may often be side effects of chronic pain or its treatment. Opiates may suppress appetite and cause constipation. The inactivity resulting from pain contributes to obesity. A dietician can work with patients to correct these problems.

Alternative therapies can be useful for some patients. Yoga acupuncture, massage therapy, chiropractic treatment, therapeutic touch, and meditation, to name a few, have all been found to help some patients and should be utilized. [2]

Team leadership
With multiple disciplines involved, good communication, integration, and coordination are of paramount importance to good management. One person, usually the pain specialist, should act as the team leader. The leader brings the specialties together to formulate a management plan and then on a regular basis as indicated to evaluate and reformulate the management plan. The leader facilitates communication between specialties and assures that treatment progresses according to the plan. The leader is the patient's primary contact for questions, concerns, and problems.

Conclusion
Cancer pain is an unsolved problem in India. The number of patients is overwhelming. The available resources are limited and there is hardly any awareness on the part of patients of their right to seek and obtain relief from pain. The ISSP owes it to the millions of victims of pain to evolve ways and means for an effective pain relief in the cancer patients.

Reference:
1. Firzgbbon DR & Chapman. Cancer pain In: Bonica's Management of Pain, Loeser J.D (Ed), Lippincott Williams & Wilkins, Philadelphia, 2001; 623-703.
2. World Health Organization. Cancer pain relief and palliative care. Technical report series, 804, Geneva, Switzerland, 1990.
3. Aitkenhead AR, Rowtham DJ & Smith G. Textbook of Anaesthesia. 5th Ed. Churchil-Livingstone, Edinburgh. 2000
4. Kumar P. Souveneir (cover page) Proceedings of XVII National ISSPCON, ISSP, Jamnagar.2002.
5. K.Pandey. Prevalence and magnitude of cancer pain.Proceedings of XVII ISSPCON, Jamnagar .2002.
6. Joad A.K. Gupta P. Pain profile in patients of advanced Head and neck cancer seen at a pain a clinic at Jaipur. INDPAIN, 2001;15(2)- 18-27.

Chapter 31.
CANCER PAIN

Pain is not a simple sensation, but a complex physiological and emotional experience. The many reasons for a failure to relieve pain have been well described.

Causes of failure to relieve pain	Consequences
Belief that pain is inevitable	Failure to treat
Inaccurate diagnosis of the cause	Inappropriate treatment
Lack of understanding of analgesics	Prescribing of inappropriate, insufficient or infrequent analgesics
Unrealistic objectives	Dissatisfaction with treatment
Infrequent review	Rejection of treatment by patient
Insufficient attention to mood and morale	Lowered pain threshold

Table 1. ACUTE AND CHRONIC PAIN

Acute pain (e.g. fracture)	Chronic pain (e.g. cancer)
Patient : obviously in pain	May only seem depressed
Complains loudly of pain	May only complain of discomfort
Understands pain	Sees pain as unending and meaning less
Primarily affects the patients	Pain overflows to affect family
Doctor : treatment straight forward Parenteral analgesics acceptable	Treatment may be complex Oral analgesics preferable
Analgesic side Effects acceptable	Side effects unacceptable

CAUSES OF PAIN:

Table 2 Treatment of pain depending on cause.

Cause of pain	First line treatment	Second line	To consider
Visceral from involvement of abdominal, pelvic or intrathoracic organs	Analgesics	Steroids may help if compression by tumor is implicated	Nerve blocks-celiac axis for retroperitoneal pain, spinal for pelvic pain
Bone pain Direct spread or distant metastases	1. palliative radiotherapy 2. analgesics 3. NSAIDS	Immobilization (eg. orthopedic pinning long bone) (NSAID)	Nerve blocks
Colic -constipation -obstruction	Clear lower bowel Fecal softeners Antispasmodics	Laxatives Analgesics	Enema Celiac nerve blocks
Soft tissue infiltration	1. analgesics 2. NSAIDS	Steroids may be helpful	Nerve block

Nerve pain -compression -dysaesthetic -stabbing	Analgesics Amitriptyline Valproate Carbamazepine	Radiotherapy Steroids Nerve block Nerve block	Nerve block Transcutaneous nerve stimulation
Infection- deep -Superficial without cellulitis	Systemic antibiotics Local disinfectants with debridement	Analgesics analgesics	Nerve block local surgery topical local anesthetics
Pleural pain	Antibiotics	Intercostal block if localized, analgesic if extensive	NSAIDs
Lymph edema	1.gentle massage 2.exercises 3.compression hosiery 4.elevation	1.intermittent positive pressure bandaging 2.analgesics	Steroids if due to recurrence Diuretics don't help
Headaches from raised intracranial pressure	Steroids	Analgesics	
Gastric -irritation -distension	Stop irritants Antacids Asilon	H2 blockers Metocloparamide,domperidone	
Rectal -tenesemoid	Chlorpromazine	Diazepam	Nerve block
Pain in paralyzed limbs	Physiotherapy, passive movements	NSAIDs	Muscle relaxants, NB

1. Visceral pain may result from hepatic metastasis, lung tumors, pancreatic carcinoma with retroperitoneal involvement and peritoneal involvement by tumor. Pain is often a continuous dull ache but may be interrupted by sharp pains if an organ moves when the patient changes the position.
2. Bone pain may cause local tenderness, or dull ache worsened by movement. Increasing pain on movement with time suggests an impending fracture.
3. Nerve pain will usually be with in the distribution of one or more nerves. Compression produced by variable qualities of pain, with or with out motor and sensory changes. Nerves destruction may produce dysaesthetic (hypersensitivity, pins and needles, burning pain) or a stabbing pain.

PRINCIPLES OF PAIN CONTROL
1. DO NOT WAIT FOR A PATIENT TO COMPLAIN –ASK AND OBSERVE.   Patients with chronic pain do not always look in pain. Clues lie in what drugs have failed. Whether sleep is disturbed and if the activity is limited. Some patients prefer to be asked about "discomfort" rather than "pain". The family's comments are often helpful.
2. ACURATELY DIAGNOSE THE CAUSE OF PAIN .80%of the patients have more than one site of pain, 34%have more than four separate pain.
3. USE REGULAR ANAESTHESIA, IN DOSES TITRATED TO EACH INDIVIDUAL SUCH THAT PAIN IS PREVENTED FROM RETURNING. if a drug is known to give effective relief for 4 hours ,then it needs to be prescribed 4 hourly .CONTINOUS PAIN WILL NOT BE CONTROLLED BY "AS REQUIRED "OR "PRN"PRESCRIBING .

4. SET REALISTIC GOALS. Initially a pain free. Full –night's sleep should be the aim, followed by relief during the day, freedom from pain on movement is more difficult to achieve in nerve compression and bone pain.
5. REASSESS REPEATEDLY AND REGULARLY. Accurate analgesic titration demands reassessment. This is an essential requirement for effective care.
6. EMPATHY, UNDERSTANDING, DIVERSION AND ELEVATION OF MOOD ARE ESSENTIAL ADJUNCTS TO ANALGESICS. Drugs are only part of overall management.

Table 3. ANALGESIC CLASSIFICATION

> **NON OPIOIDS**   aspirin and others non –steroidal anti-
> Inflammatory drugs
> Paracetamol

Opioids | **opioids**
Opioids agonist's | **Agonist/antagonists**
Weak | Weak
Codeine | (pentazocine)
Dihydrocodeine |
Dextropropoxyphene |
Strong | Strong
Morphine dextromoramide | buprenorphine
Diamorphine (Pethidine) | (meptazinol)
Phenazocine (dipipanone) | (nalbuphine)
Oxycodone |

Comparison of analgesics

Mild analgesics | opiates
1. Less effective in large doses-ceiling | 1. dose related analgesia
2. Used orally- less effective, no dependence | 2. i.v., i.m, s.c., Epidural, intrathecal
3. Used in chronic low grade pain in OPD | 3. used in acute pain
4. Diverse mechanism of action, treats cause | 4. opiate receptor, nonspecific
5. Fewer side effects – gastric | 5. more side effects- n/v
6. Used in combination | 6. administered individually
7. Aspirin, NSAIDs, paracetamol | 7. morphine, buprenorphine, Fentanyl

OPIOIDS = any chemical capable of stimulating opioid receptor.
1. Opiates = Analgesics derived from opium (e.g. morphine)
2. Agonists = Analgesics with morphine like effects only
3. Agonist/antagonists = Analgesics with effects similar to morphine but which may antagonize the effects of an agonist analgesic; if both are given together.
4. Narcotics = Now obsolete as a term to describe strong opioids.
5. Analgesics in (brackets) in this classification are not recommended for routine use in cancer pain.

The analgesic staircase

Choosing an analgesic solely on the basis of pain severity often fails since clinical estimates of pain severity are highly subjective. A choice based on analgesic response tailors the analgesic to the patient .if pain fails to respond to a non opioid, then a weak opioid is the next step. If a weak opioid fails then a strong opioid is the next logical step

-Strong opioids
E.g. morphine
Diamorphine

-Weak opioids
E.g. codeine
Dihydrocodeine

Non opioids
E.g. aspirin
   Paracetamol
Fig 2: The analgesic staircase

1. CHANGING FROM ONE WEAK OPIOID TO ANOTHER WILL NOT ACHIEVE BETTER PAIN CONTROL.
2. THE DECISION TO START A STRONG OPIOD IS MADE BY A LOGICAL SERIES OF DECISIONS. NOT AS A LAST RESORT.
3. PATIENTS WITH CANCER DO NOT AUTOMATICALLY NEED STRONG OPIOIDS.

Table4. First step: The Non Opioid

NON OPIOID ANALGESICS			
Drugs	strength	dose	comments
Aspirin Dispersible BP	300 mg	300-600mg 4-6 hourly	useful adjuncts in bone pain. gastric irritant
Paracetamol	500mg	0.5-1g 4hrly	lack of gastrointestinal effects
Ibuprofen	400mg	400mg 4 hrly	gastritis
Diclofenac	50 mg	50-75 mg 8 hly	gastritis, renal dysfunctions
Naproxen	250 mg	250-500 mg 8 hrly	gastritis, renal dysfunctions

Table5. Second step: THE WEAK OPIOIDS.

Weak opioids			
Codeine phosphate Tablets BP Syrup BP	15/30/60mg 25 mg/ml	15-60mg 4 hourly	Approximately 1/12th as patent as morphine
Dihydrocodiene tablets elixir	30mg 10mg/ml	30-60mg 4 hourly	Approximately 1/10th as patent as morphine
Dextropropoxyphene Capsules **BP**	Equivalent of 65mg HCL salt	One capsule 4-8 hourly	Accumulation occurs, especially with poor renal function
Dextropropoxyphene And **paracetamol** (co-proxamol)	32.5mg)each 325mg)tablet	2 tablets 4-8 hourly	Dose interval may have to be increased in the elderly

Third step: THE STRONG OPIOIDS
The strong opioids are often necessary to treat cancer pain adequately. They are not euphoriants or sedatives.
Mechanism of pain – pain impulses travel from the site of injury because of receptors. 5 HT Bradykinins release locally. The impulse ascends in the dorsal horns crosses to other side in spinothalamic tract reaching thalamus and internal capsule & terminating in cortex.
The aspirin and NSAIDs act through prostaglandin / COX inhibition etc.

Mechanism of action of opiates – the opiate drugs act on opiate receptors present on brainstem, spinal cord dorsal horn, amygdala, limbic system, thalamus, and substanitia gelatinosa

Types of opiate receptors - μ receptors – supraspinal analgesia, γ- dysphoria produced by opiates & k-receptors produce spinal analgesia & sedation. δ- act selectively on leu encephalin. There are further subdivisions of above receptors depending upon the ligand blocking their action. This has lead to cloning of various receptor types with the aim to produce an ideal opiate without any side effects.

Endogenous opioids – body produces endogenous opioids like substance which control the nociception most of the times. This works in the pain relief due to various non-conventional methods. They can be released by stimulating the sites given below.

1) Endorphins – in hypothalamus, III rd ventricle
2) Leu –enkephalin – brain stem and spinal cord
3) Met enkephalin – dorsal horn, morphine like

The actions of all these can be reversed by naloxone.

Patient Controlled Analgesia (PCA)

It involves the self administration of a small dose of analgesic drug according to patient's own experience of pain. PCA is available for i.v., epidural, or subcutaneous route. PCA is better liked by patients providing better satisfaction, relieving coughing, and overall morbidity, as compared to i.m. routes. A watch on instrument malfunction, careful planning of doses by physicians, loading a requisite dose of analgesic with a periodic review of pain, lock out interval & costs, are to be effectively worked out.

Opioids like morphine, fentanyl, and butorphanol alone or with additives like Ketamine, ketorolac, droperidol can be used in PCA.

Advantages – patient less apprehensive about demanding analgesic, non addiction, round the clock pain relief, available with fewer burdens on nursing staff.

Neurosurgical ablation:
1. Dorsal rhizotomy by interrupting spinothalamic tract
2. Dorsal route entry zone lesioning for refractory de afferentation pains in plexus avulsions
3. Deep brain stimulation through implants in peri aqueductal, peiventricular gray matter
4. Cryo or thermal lesioning of Gasserian ganglion & pituitary (75% success)

Dependence

Psychological Dependence is not observed in advanced cancer on opioids[1]

Patients treated with infrequent or insufficient analgesics will ask for more, but this is not dependence, simply an appropriate demand for adequate pain relief. Physical dependence does occur, but clinical experience shows that when pain is relieved by other means such as nerve blocks, opioid dose can be reduced without precipitating withdrawal symptoms.

Tolerance

TOLERANCE TO OPIOD ANALGESIA IS SLOW TO DEVELOP. Tolerance to analgesia is easily matcher by small dose increases. After three months a plateau is reached whereby effective analgesia can be maintained for long periods at fixed doses[2]. Respiratory tolerance is very rapid and respiratory depression is not a problem in patients on long time oral morphine.[3] The only exception is when pain (a stimulus to respiration) is suddenly relieved by other means (e.g. a nerve block), when respiratory depression can occur if the dose has not been reduced beforehand. Most patient on a fixed dose of opioids can be reassured that any residual drowsiness will disappear within 3-5 days. Tolerance to nausea and vomiting takes longer, but prophylactic anti emetics such as haloperidol can usually be stopped after 10 days. In contrast there is no observable tolerance to constipation and regular laxatives must be prescribed with opioids.

If the initial dose of opioid is low enough not to cause side effects the dose can be increased until pain control is achieved, knowing that the patient is becoming tolerant to most of the side effects, but not to the analgesia.

Choice of opioid
Oral morphine or diamorphine are the strong opioids of choice. They are of equal efficacy and there is no evidence that regular oral medication with one has any advantages over the other. This is not surprising since diamorphone as rapidly metabolized to 6-mono acetyl morphine and morphine[4]. Their differing rates of absorption result in different potencies, but a higher potency does not implicate increased efficacy, simply less drug can be given to have the same effect.

$$\begin{array}{cc} \textbf{3 mg} & \textbf{2 mg} \\ \text{ORAL MORPHINE} = & \text{ORAL DIAMORPHINE} \end{array}$$

Morphine sulfate is chemically stable in water and its shelf life is determined by microbial contamination. The addition of 0.25% v/v chloroform prevents microbial contamination upto 3 weeks. Sodium metabisulphate 200 ppm may be a more effective anti microbial for al long time [5].

Initial dose
Opioid requirements depend on previous analgesic requirements and age, weight, height and surface area correlate poorly with the amount of opioid needed. Patients with poor hepatic function appear to metabolize morphine normally and there is now some evidence that the kidney has an important role in eliminating opioids such as morphine [6].
The initial dose should be chosen as follows:
1. Previously on non-opioid: Dihydrocodiene 30mg 4 hourly.
2. Previously on weak opioid: 10mg oral morphine 4 hourly.
3. Previously on strong opioids: equivalent dose of morphine. Calculate the 4 hourly doses and increase this by 50% if the patient was not pain controlled.

These rules can be safely followed for those with poor hepatic function. For the elderly, frail or those with poor renal function these rules still apply but the doses may have to be increased more slowly.

Conversion to controlled –release morphine 60 mg diamorphine or morphine solution per 24 hours (i.e. 10 mg 4 hourly) is approximately equivalent to 60 mg controlled –release morphine per 24 hours (i.e. 30 mg -12 hours).
The last dose of morphine or diamorphine solution and the first dose of controlled release morphine should be given together.
Controlled trials have been shown formulation to be equivalent, mg for mg with oral morphine sulphate solution. However two observational studies suggest it was also equivalent, mg for mg, with diamorphine. This disparity may be due to the 22% greater bioavailability of controlled –release morphine compared with morphine sulphate solution. This would suggest that in practice patients can be transferred from either morphine or diamorphine solution with little or no adjustment of the controlled release morphine needed.

Night time doses
On a four–hourly regimen for oral morphine it is possible to avoid giving in the middle of the night by increasing the bedtime dose by 50-100%. This gives sufficient analgesia over the following 8 hours; possibly reduced renal function overnight keeps plasma morphine levels elevated. There is no evidence that higher bedtime doses increase night-time mortality in advanced cancer patients, even when these patients are receiving a hypnotic. Patients on more than 100 mg oral morphine for hourly are likely to need a 2 am dose, although the reason for this is not clear. An alternative is then to transfer the patient completely too controlled release morphine. There is no logic in using controlled release morphine at night and four hourly morphine solution at daytime.

Dose increases
Doses should be titrated to the Patient's pain. Effective dose ranges from 5mg or less of oral morphine, 4-hourly to more than 500 mg 4-hourly. Recommended maximum dose has no relevance to the control of cancer pain.
Doses are increased in 30-50% steps. A typical sequence of increases of 4th hourly morphine sulphate solution would be 5mg/10mg/15mg/20mg/45mg/60mg/90mg.for pain that needs rapid control two or more steps can be taken each day. Elderly patients or those with poor renal function may only need increases every 3-5 days because of morphine accumulation.

Table 6. Oral strong opioids of choice.

Drug	Typical starting dose	Equivalent doses of oral morphine	Dose interval	Comments
Morphine hydrochloride Or sulphate solution	10mg	10mg	4 hourly	Titrate dose of the individual patient
Diamorphine hydrochloride -solution -tabs(10mg)	7.5mg	10mg	4 hourly	Interchangeable with morphine as long as potency difference taken into account
Controlled – released morphine sulphate(MST continuous)tabs	30mg	See notes below	12 hourly	Effective over 12 hour's .Unnecessary to prescribe more often than 8 hourly. Do not use for breakthrough pain since it takes 4 hours before effective blood levels are reached. Do not crush or cut the tablets

Table7: Approximate oral opioid equivalents

Opioid	Conversion factor to oral morphine	Opioid	Conversion factor to oral morphine
dextropropoxyphene	X 1/10	diamorphine	X1.5
dihydrocodeine	X1/10	dextromoramide morphine Parenteral	X2 X2
pethidine oral	X1/8	diamorphine Parenteral	X3
dipipanone	X1/2	phenazocine	X3
papaveratum	X2/3	levorphanol	X5
oxycodone	X1	hydromorphone	X6
methadone	X1	buprenorphine	X50

Other strong opioids
The following strong opioids have few or no advantages over those already described. They are discussed in alphabetical order.

Buprenorphine: Side effects are similar to morphine and although it is said to have little action on bowel cancer patients. Buprenorphine require laxatives.[7]. It is a partial agonist and shows a ceiling effect to analgesia. It has a high affinity for morphine receptors.

Table 8. Alternative opioids to morphine and diamorphine

Opioid	Typical starting dose	Equivalent dose of morphine	Route	Dose interval	comments
Phenazocine 5mg tablets	2.5mg	7.5mg	Oral sublingual	6-8 hourly	Possibly causes less nausea when given sublingually
Levorphanol 1.5mg tablets	1.5mg	7.5mg	Oral	6-8 hourly	May be less well tolerated at higher doses
Dextromoramide 5/10mg tablets 10mg suppos.	5mg	10mg (po) 5mg (pr)	Oral /sublingual/ PR	3hrly	Little evidence that it is effective for more than three hours in cancer pain
Pentazocine Butorphanol Buprenorphine	20 mg 2mg, 0.5mg 0.3mg, 0.1 mg	10mg 15 mg 10 mg	i.m. /i.v. i.m Epidural i.m. epidural	4-6 hrly 6 hrly 6 hrly 6-20 hrly	Limited use in cancer Psychomimetic sedation Withdrawal symptoms

Dipipanone with cyclizine dos increases are limited due to sedation caused by the 30 mg cyclizine in each tablet.

Nefopam: A non opioid analgesic that can be given orally or sublingually. It appears to be approximately 1/3 as potent as oral morphine. There is a ceiling effect to analgesia. It may induce convulsions and should be avoided in the presence of cerebral metastases. It has no place in advanced cancer pain.

Pethidine: Its short duration of action of 2-3 hrs makes it impractical for use in cancer pain.

Phenazocine: It commonly causes dysphoria and hallucinations.

ALTERNATIVE ROUTES OF ADMINISTRATION
THE ORAL ROUTE IS ALWAYS PREFERABLE AND USUALLY POSSIBLE.

Sublingual or buccal route:
This route may be useful in patient with vomiting or dyspghagia.the following analgesics can be used in this way.

Sublingual only: Buprenorphine.

Sublingual buccal or oral: dextromoramide, diamorphine, morphine nefopam, phenazocine.
The sublingual route is usually unacceptable in very ill patient with little saliva.

Rectal route:

This route may be the route of choice when the oral route is no longer practical. Injections however can be easier to give, cause no great discomfort and may be better tolerated

Table 9: **Rectal analgesics.**

Suppository and strength	Typical starting dose	Equivalent dose of morphine	Route	Dose interval	Comments
Oxycodone pectinate Suppose:10mg	30mg	30mg	PR	6-8th hourly	Sedative and long acting, useful overnight.
Morphine(as hcl or sulphate) Suppose.10/15/30 60mg	10mg	10mg	PR	4th hourly	Can be made up to any dose upto 150mg
Dextromoramide Suppos.10mg	10mg	10mg	PR	3 hourly.	Short duration limits its use

Spinal routes
Extradural or intrathecal routes may have a place in treating some patients but these routes are not free of side effects, including delayed respiratory depression and itching[8] the method needs practitioners skilled in this technique.

Intrathecal injections – opioids neurolytics used for accurate placement of neurolytic agents in indoor patients
Indications – carcinoma of cervix, rectum, pelvis
Agents used – absolute alcohol (95%) hypobaric, diffuses fast, relief shorter, inflammation, burning at site
Phenol – 5% hyperbaric, local analgesic. Used aqueous or in glycerol, effective diffusion
Chloro eresol – 5% in glycerol, hyperbaric, effective diffusion
Complications – patchy degeneration, arachnoiditis, retention of urine, paresis headache, nausea & vomitin

Table 10.Drug delivery implants by spinal routes.

Type I - simple epidural, intrathecal catheter. Analgesia for few days provided
Type II - tuned catheters, for pain relief for a few weeks
Type III-reservoir port, provides analgesia for a few months
Type IV-continuous infusion; provide analgesia for more than six months
Type V -programmed infusion, analgesia for more than a year
Drug delivery systems:

Type I	Type II	Type III	Type IV	Type V	Type VI
Simple Epi, S.A.Catheter	Tunneled Catheter	Reservoir port	Manually activated	Continuous infusion	Programmed infusion
Days	Weeks	Months	Years	Years	

Epidural - opioids, neurolytics
Indications – same as intrathecal catheter & infusion pumps
Diagnosis and therapy – vascular phenomenon, visceral pain
Agents – 3-5 ml of 3-10% phenol

Advantage – easy injection, no complication due to dural puncture, position
Disadvantages – less precise, dural puncture, neurological complications

Parenteral route

THERE ARE FEW INDICATIONS FOR PARENTERAL ANALGESICS IN CANCER PATIENTS.
1. In the last few hours, or occasionally days of life.
2. Vomiting while anti emetic treatment is thing effect
3. Acute pain for rapid effect (although rectal or sublingual route can be almost as rapid)
4. Dysphagia

Small volume injections are kinder in thin patients and the high solubility of diamorphine hydrochloride is a useful advantage. Morphine sulphate is less soluble but suitable alternatives are morphine acetate and hydromorphine .subcutaneous injections through 25G needles is kinder and as effective as intramuscular injections.Continous subcutaneous infusions can be given by using small battery driven pumps. When changing from the oral to parenteral routes the following dose equivalents apply.

3mg oral morphine	=	**2mg** oral diamorphine	=	**1mg** inj.diamorphine SC/IM
	=	**1.5mg** inj.morphine SC/IM		

CONTINOUS INTRAVENOUS OPIOIDS ARE UNNECESSARY. There is no evidence in chronics cancer pain the intravenous route provided more analgesia than regular subcutaneous, sublingual or rectal administration. Few very ill patients with cancer either need or want an intravenous infusion.continous subcutaneous administration is an alternative.

PAINFUL PROCEDURES

There are occasion when procedures such as dressing changes or manual evacuation of faecal impaction produce pain which is not covered by regular prophylactic analgesia. **Nitrous oxide and oxygen**: In equal parts (Entonox) inhaled from premixed cylinders is useful when a rapid onset of analgesia is needed, but the effect only lasts a few minutes. Ideally the patients should self administer the gases under supervision, in this way titrating the correct dose for themselves.
Diazepam: It is rapidly effective given intravenously (absorption from the intramuscular route is unreliable). It must be given in a titrated dose no faster than 2.5mg /minute, until the patients eyes droop and speech becomes slurred. The aim is to stop short of patient losing consciousness .the patient, may still feel some pain during the procedure but will have no memory of the event later. Diazepam emulsion (diazemules) is expensive but causes less local pain and thrombosis. The rectal route can be used but titration is more difficult and less accurate.
Extra dose of morphine: can be given by repeating the normal; oral 4 hrly dose 1 hour before the procedure, or giving the equivalent dose of diamorphine parenterally. The effect will last upto 4 hours. The next 4 hourly doses should be given on time.
Coanalgesics: These are drugs other than analgesics which indirectly relieve pain; they include corticosteroids antibiotics, and antispasmodics. They may be effective without concurrent analgesics.
NSAIDs: These are mild analgesics but their ability to inhibit prostaglandin synthesis makes them of particular value in bone pain when prescribed with a strong opioid.
The logic is that prostaglandins may contribute to the osteolysis in bone metastases and to the resulting pain. Radiotherapy is the treatment of choice in the pain of bone metastases but NSAIDs can be used while the effect of radiotherapy is developing or if it is impractical such as with multiple rib metastases. The combination of cutaneous pain pruritis and erythema in breast carcinoma ('Cupitch' syndrome) may also be caused by local prostaglandin production and response to NSAIDs[9]. The choice of NSAID depends mainly on cost and patient acceptability.
ASPIRIN: is cheap and often effective in a dose of 3g daily.

Side effects are less common at this dose, but the full anti inflammatory action doses of 4g or more are needed which may not be tolerated. Patients who are hypoproteinemic may not tolerate even the lower doses. Flurbiprofen is a potent inhibitor of PGE_2 synthesis and clinically effective at doses of 50-100mg 12 hourly. An alternative is the salicylates diflunisal in doses of 250-500 mg 12 hourly.

Corticosteroids

Corticosteroids have wide application in advanced cancer. They can reduce the edema and inflammation that surrounds the tumour and therefore ease the pressure on surrounding structures. Although they have anti inflammatory action, they have a less specific effect on synthesis of prostaglandins and less effective than NSAIDs in bone pain. They can improve appetite and occasionally produce a useful sense of well being. Side effects are not often troublesome:

Table 11: Side effects of corticosteroids

Side effects	Incidence	Comments
Oral candidiasis	31%	Treatment is simple and effective
Peripheral edema	20%	Usually mild
Moon face	18%	An advantage in thin patients
Dyspepsia	7%	Usually mild
Hyperactivity	4%	Do not prescribe corticosteroids later than 6pm

Approximately 2% of patients on corticosteroids develop peptic ulcer disease while upto 5% of patients with advanced cancer may develop complicated ulcer disease. In view of the benefits they bring such risks are accepted by most physicians.

Table 12: Corticosteroids in advanced cancer.

Low dose (eg.2-4mg dexamethasone daily)	
Nonspecific uses	Specific uses
Improved appetite	Haemoptysis
Advanced wellbeing	
Improve strength	
High dose (e.g. 16-24mg dexamethasone daily)	
Co analgesic	Specific uses
Raised intracranial pressure	Cold compression
Nerve compression	Superior vena caval compression
Head and neck tumour	Air ways obstruction
Pelvic tumour	Carcinomatous lymphangitis
Metastatic joint involvement	Leucoerythroblastic anaemia
Malignant pleural pain	Cough due to malignancy

Dexamethasone is the corticosteroid of choice. It is more potent than prednisolone (2mg dexamethasone =approx.15mg prednisolone), resulting in fewer tablets for the patients. Low doses should be taken once in the morning, higher doses can be taken in divided doses but no later than 6 pm to avoid insomnia. High doses should be reduced gradually over 10days to the lowest dose that controls symptoms. For those unable to swallow tablets dexamethasone suspension (4mg/5ml) is easily made up by pharmacists and is significantly cheaper than soluble prednisolone or betamethasone.

Muscle relaxants

Skeletal muscles spasm may be due to nerve involvement or direct irritation by tumour. Local heat, massage and relaxation techniques may help. The following drugs may be useful [10].

Diazepam: tablets 2/5/10mg, syrup 2mg /5ml, suppositories 5/10mg. Effective, but at the expense of drowsiness. It has a prolonged half life so that a single bedtime dose of 5-20 mg is usually sufficient.

Baclofen: tablets 10mg. The dose needs to be gradually increased from 5mg 8hourly to a maximum of 30mg 8hourly. It should be taken with food. Nausea, vomiting, drowsiness and confusion limit its use.

Dantrolene: capsules 25/100mg. The dose is slowly increased over several weeks from 25mg daily up to 100mg 6 hourly. Drowsiness and weakness are problems, especially in the first weeks of treatment. The therapeutic effect may take several weeks to develop.

Psychotropic drugs

Phenothiazines: There is no clear evidence that drugs such as chlorpromazine or methotrimeprazine potentiates morphine or diamorphine. There is no place for routinely combining an opioid and phenothiazines.

Butyrophenones and **benzodiazepines**: Pain in an anxious or agitated patient is likely to improve with counseling and the judicious use of psycho tropics such as haloperidol or diazepam.

Antidepressants can be effective in nerve destruction pain which is characterized by a burning sensation and local hypersensitivity. Amitriptyline or dothiepine can be used at a dose of 25mg increasing every few days until the pain eases or side effects arise.

Anticonvulsants

These can be useful in stabbing pain that can accompany nerve compression. Sodium Valproate starting at 200mg 12 hourly upto 400mg 6 hourly can be used.

COANALGESIC THERAPY

These modes of therapy are adequately covered elsewhere and include radiotherapy, nerve blocks, neurosurgical procedures including pituitary alcohol block transcutaneous nerve stimulation hypnosis and acupuncture.

Persistent pain.

If after multiple increases of a strong opioid the pain is still not adequately controlled, a complete reassessment is necessary.

- Has the cause of pain is correctly diagnosed?
- Are analgesics appropriate? Has a new pain developed that needs different treatment?
- Has basic principles followed?
- Has the analgesic staircase been followed?
- Have appropriate strong opioids used?
- Have co analgesic drugs been considered?
- Is the patient lonely, frightened anxious or depressed?

Communication Skills in Patient Treatment:

Consultation skills:

Consultation skills of doctors: Patients preferred those who introduced themselves, were sympathetic, appeared self-confident, listened to them, responded to verbal cues, asked precise and simple questions, did not repeat themselves[13].

Patients want eye contact, partnership, communication, time, appointments within a reasonable time, listening and good communication skills[14].

Benefits

- Patients problems are identified more accurately
- Adherence to treatment instructions is improved
- May improve health outcomes – better emotional health, symptom resolution and pain control
- Likely to reduce the incidence of clinical error
- May relieve pressure in an emotionally demanding profession
- Job satisfaction may be enhanced
- Patients are less likely to complain
- Reduced likelihood of being sued

Barriers for physician

- Lack of skills

- Inadequate knowledge & training
- Undervaluing the importance of communicating
- Lack of time
- Uncomfortable topics (e.g. child protection)
- Lack of confidence

Barriers for patients
- Tiredness/ Stress
- Language barriers (e.g. overseas doctors/patients)
- Personality and class differences between doctors and patients
- Concerns regarding confidentiality
- Lack of knowledge of illness/condition

Components of a consultation
- Building the doctor–patient relationship
- Opening the discussion and gathering information eg what can I do for you, what are your concerns?
- Understanding the patient's perspective.
- Listening skills show you are listening, nonverbal behavior, clarifying, summarizing.
- Sharing information by checking understanding, eye contact, asking questions
  Offer other sources of information, letters, leaflets, and internet.
- Reaching agreement on treatment reduces anxiety and distress, improves, willingness to engage, break the ice
- Offer choice to see them alone first
- Involve children by eye contact, patience, using name, open posture.
- Rapport building
- Closure by summarizing an action plan, safety netting, telling them what happens next.

Sharing bad news
Preparation
- Are you the right person to give the news?
- Environment--ideally a quiet, comfortable, private room
- Minimize interruptions
- Do not appear rushed
- Know as much about the case as you can start.
- Consider who should be there. Consider an interpreter.
- Consider whether there may be cultural attitudes
- Introduce any members of the team or students
- Brace yourself for an emotional task!

Sharing the news
- Try to know what is known by the patient/family already.
- Give information in a simple language with honesty but sensitivity, taking care with prognostication.
- Do not take all hope away--find some reason to be optimistic.
- Allow time for questions; listen to what the relatives say, let them be able to make any decisions.
- Don't be worried by periods of silence, cope with family denial, recognize and acknowledge their feelings of anger or sorrow .
- Do not impose the truth but if the patient asks, do not lie, avoid false reassurances and uncertainty.
- Show empathy but do not lose control, acknowledge that dealing with is often harder than knowing the diagnosis.

- Try not to let your own opinions interfere even if parents push you to make a decision for them
- Don't stay too long. Closure can be difficult--make sure you have arranged follow-up---then leave the room, leaving a nurse with the parents for a period of time,

Follow up
- Arrange a review appointment relatively soon
- Provide written information if available (patient-information leaflets, support-group literature).
- Suggest writing down any questions they think of
- Document in the notes what information the parents have been given and who was present.
- At review appointments, update the news, for instance if further test results are available.
- There may be ongoing bad news to communicate..
- Liaise with the primary healthcare team (GP, health visitor) and any other relevant professionals.
- Consider debriefing for the staff involved.
- Bereavement counseling

References:
1. Twycross RG. Principles and practice of pain relief in terminal cancer. Update 1972 5(2/115-121).
2. Twycross RG. Clinical experience with diamorphine in advanced malignant disease. International journal of paharmocology.1974: 9(3)184-198.
3. Walsh TD. Opioids and respiratory functions in advanced cancer. Recent results in cancer research 1984; 89:115-117.
4. Locktidge. Hydrolysis of diacetylmorphine by cholinesterase. Journal of pharmacology 1980; 21(1)1-8.
5. Regnard CFB, Edward S. Chloroform in morphine soln. Pharmaceutical journal 1984; 233:745-746.
6. Mcquay AJ. High systemic relative bio availability of oral morphine, Royal society of medicine. Int. Cong.series. 1984; 64:149-154.
7. Twycross RJ. Narcotic agonist antagonism symptom control in advanced cancer pain relief.1983; 253-269.
8. Yaksh TL. Spinal opioid analgesia. 1981; 293-346.
9. Twycross RJ. Pruritis and pain in encuirass breast cancer. Lancet. 1981; 696.
10. Consumers association. Drugs to relieve plasticity. Drugs and therapeutic bulletin. 1983; 21(1:1-3).
11. Doyle D. Nerve blocks in advanced cancer. Practitioner. 1982; 226:539-544.
12. Myles J. Chemical hyphophysectomy. Advances in pain research, 1979; 373-400.
13. Dr Sanjay Suri. Communication skills in medicine. Where art meets science. Rotherham NHS Foundation Trust. 2014.
14. Langewitz, W. et al. Spontaneous talking time BMJ 2002; 325:682-683.

CHAPTER 32.

Neuro-psychological symptoms

Cerebral tumours
Features vary from subtle mood changes to Confusional states, with focal signs such as dysphasia, ataxia, or hemi paresis. As intracranial pressure rises there may be headache, nausea and vomiting. Dexamethasone in high doses reduces oedema around a primary or secondary tumour. The daily dose is reduced over 2-3 weeks to the lowest dose that will control symptoms. This dose should continue until there are clear signs that symptoms are progressing. It is then sometimes possible to increase the dose again with good effect, but it is often necessary to remain at this dose to control symptoms. If it is clear that the patient is deteriorating rapidly despite dexamethasone, the dose can be reduced and stopped. Focal neurological signs may respond to radiotherapy. Side effects of whole brain irradiation are alopecia and occasionally nausea. Increased survival is not claimed when treating metastases. It is less effective than corticosteroids in reducing oedema and these should be given concurrently. Cyclizine is the antiemetic of choice for nausea and vomiting due to raised intracranial pressure. Opioids may be required to control headache. Since respiratory depression is rare with oral oplolds there is little risk of carbon dioxide retention raising intracranial pressure still further.

Spinal cord compression
This neurological emergency requires an early diagnosis. Pain with local spinal tenderness is early signs, and subsequent leg weakness or sensory changes strongly suggest compression. Sensory changes can be varied and non-specific. Altered reflexes are useful localizing signs. Sphincter disturbance is a late sign. Metastases from primaries of breast, lung or prostate are the commonest malignant cause.

On suspicion of cord compression dexamethasone should be started, 8mg IV stat, followed by 24 mg daily in divided doses. This should be followed immediately by radiotherapy. Laminectomy alone appears to be less effective with more complications[1]. The best results are obtained in slowly developing lesions - acute compression is usually the consequence of local cord ischemia and therefore irreversible.

Lumbo-sacral plexopethy
Pelvic tumours may involve the lumbo-sacral plexus on the posterior wall of the pelvis. Features of a pelvic tumour include leg or perineal pain, leg weakness and sensory loss, sphincter disturbance, tenesmus or bladder irritability and leg oedema. These symptoms may respond to high dose dexamethasone. Symptoms of nerve destruction (stabbing or burning pains, hypersensitivity) may respond to antidepressants or anticonvulsants. Tenesmus may respond to chlorpromazine 25-50mg 8 hrly.

Anxiety
DRUGS CAN NEVER BE A SUBSTITUTE FOR EMPATHY. True Anxiolytics that are capable of 'Iysing' anxiety do not exist - at best such drugs suppress anxiety. But this can be very helpful in allowing patients to express their fears, an essential first step in treatment.

Haloperidol is relatively non-sedating and can be given in doses of 5-10mg nocte or 12 hrly. Extrapyramidal symptoms occasionally occur at higher doses (restlessness, dystonia, parkinsonian features).

Diazepam can be effective in a single night-time dose of 2-1O mg at the expense of some daytime sedation. A half-life of up to a week makes divided doses unnecessary but accumulation can occur which may be mistaken for deterioration due to the cancer. A short course (4-6 weeks) should be planned. Longer courses can result in rebound anxiety starting within 2 weeks of stopping diazepam[2] and this withdrawal syndrome can last several weeks. Doses should be reduced gradually. Midazolam provides better and reliable anxiolysis.

Hypnotics e.g. nitrazepam (half-life 30 hrs), temazepam (half-life 8 hrs) can be useful in elderly patients to reduce the risk of accumulation. Treatment should be short and the dosage reduced gradually.

Agitation
An agitated patient is frightened and treatment needs to be rapid. Agitation may stem from anxiety alone, or be the result of an acute confusional state. Pain, constipation or urinary retention can also be precipitating factors and must be excluded.

Haloperidol 10mg patient is given hourly until the patient settles. It can be given intravenously. Diazepam is useful it a greater sedative effect is required in a dose of 10mg po or PR repeated hourly until the patient settles. Up to 50mg may be required. Rectally, the injection solution is absorbed faster than the suppository form. Repeated use of the injection solution may cause local irritation. Diazepam can be given intravenously. If a patient becomes increasingly agitated on diazepam, this is an indication to change to chlorpromazine. Initially give 50mg po or 100mg PR, repeating hourly until the patient settles. Titrate the dose to an 8-hourly regimen. Midazolam 1-2 mg. IV can be better than diazepam.

Depression

DEPRESSION CAN BE MISTAKEN FOR SADNESS, which is a natural emotion felt by most patients. Indicators of depression are early morning wakening and feelings of guilt or worthlessness. Suicidal ideas may reflect a wish to retain control over life or a wish to be less of a burden, and are not always a consequence of depression.[3] Somatic symptoms (e.g. weight loss, anorexia, insomnia) cannot be used as markers of depression. A skilled counselor is invaluable for depressed patients, in addition to a course of antidepressant. Amitriptyline is the first choice, starting at 25mg and increasing every few days up to 150mg

Anticholinergic side effects occur (dry mouth, constipation, blurred vision, difficulty micturition) Dothiepine can be tried in the same doses, or Mianserin 30-90mg. In general agitated and anxious patients respond to sedative drugs such as amitriptyline and dothiepine, where as withdrawn and apathetic patients will require less sedative drugs such as Imipramine 25-150mg. It may take a month or more to see a response, after which the doses can be reduced gradually to half of the highest daily dose.

Confusional states

CONFUSION IN CANCER IS NOT INEVITABLE AND CAN OFTEN BE TREATED OR MADE TOLERABLE. It may present as disorientation, misinterpretation, short term memory loss include drugs (sedative, opioids, corticosteroids) infection, metabolic disturbances, cardiac or respiratory failure, and in susceptible patients, a full bladder or bowel.

When trying to understand confused patient a useful concept is that confusion reduces the number of messages from the environment and increases those from the body and memory stores, while making it difficult to differentiate the source of the messages[4].

The implication is that self awareness is at least partly intact. while this may cause some patient to be very frieghtened by the confusion it does provide a means of managing confusion. A further implication is that sedatives drugs should not be used routinely in order to preserve awareness.

Guidelines for managing confusion

Table 1..Hallucinations arise without an outside stimulus and may need treatment (h

Diagnose cause :(always suspect drugs)	Treat if possible
Provide	A company (family or friends) A constant routine Light, quite environment
Listen for clues	To understand confusion (ask the attendant)
Explain the cause	It may make the confusion less frightening
Reassure	The patient is still sane
Reorientate	Provide hooks on to which they can hang their reality

Differentiate between misinterpretation and hallucinations.

Psychotropic drugs may be required if a patient is too agitated to be helped.

HALOPERIDOL 10mg po/sc should be given hourly until the agitation settles. if more sedation is required use a short acting sedative such as chlorpromazine 50mg po/im or 100mg pr, repeated hourly until the agitation settles.

Refusal of medication should be respected unless a patient is likely to injure him or others.

Listening for clues may uncover a fear of dying, guilt or anger which at least will allow an understanding of the patient's behavior.

Misinterpretation results from garbled environmental messages poorly interpreted. they can be made worse by droperidol 5-10mg nocte).

References:
1. Gilbert RW. Epidural spinal cord compression from metastatic tumor.
2. Annals of neurology, 1978; 3(1): 40-51.
3. Power KG. Controlled study of withdrawal symptom and rebound anxiety after diazepam, BMJ, 1985; 290: 1246-1248.
4. Stedford A. In: Facing death patient's family and professionals, 1984; 109-121.

Chapter 33.
Psychological aspects of cancer pain patients.

Caner patient faces various stresses like fear of death, physical disability, disfigurement and growing dependency on others. These fears may vary between individuals depending upon patient personality, coping abilities, social support and medical factors. Pain has a profound impact on mood, anxiety, along with complex diagnostic and therapeutic challenges. A multidisciplinary approach, recognizing the importance of psychological symptoms and psychiatric complications (anxiety , depression, delirium) 1

Psychological impact of cancer

After an initial period of shock, denial and disbelief, follows a period of anxiety and depression leading to disturbed sleep, diminished appetite, irritability and pervasive thoughts about cancer. These stress responses generally occur temporarily for a few weeks at specific points in the course of cancer eg. After diagnosis, with relapse, prior to diagnostic tests, surgery, radio and chemotherapy. Psychiatric intervention is not necessary, although anxiolytic, sedation and relaxation techniques along with support of family, social workers and hospital staff helps the patient. 1

Pain is the most feared consequence of cancer. Pain is a psychological process involving nociception, perception and expression and requires addressing both physical and psychological issues, requires services of neurology, neurosurgery, anaesthesiology, rehabilitation medicine, inaddition to psychiatrists. Unfortunately psychological variables which are consequences of pain often propose to be the sole cause of pain without addressing to medical factors.

Psychiatric disorders in cancer

After an adequate control of pain, it is imperative to reassess the patients mental state for psychiatric disorders which may increase mood disturbances and thus morbidity and mortality. After a thorough assessment and accurate diagnosis, the treatment of depression , delirium and anxiety can be done with psychotherapy, behavioral and psychopharmacology.

Depression :

Depression occurs roughly in 20-25% of all cancer patients and prevalence increases with higher levels of disability, advanced illness and pain. (2)

the somatic symptoms of depression(eg. Anorexia, insomnia, fatigue, weight loss) are unreliable and lack specificity. Thus psychological symptoms of depression eg. Hopelessness, guilt, suicidal tendency are of greater diagnostic value (3). A family history, h/o past episodes and organic causes like corticosteroids, chemotherapy, amphotericin, whole brain radiation, etc. further supports the diagnosis of depression. Carcinoma of pancreas patients are associated with higher rate of depression than that of other intra-abdominal malignancies.

Treatment – depressed cancer pain patients are treated with a combination of antidepressant medication, psychotherapy and cognitive, behavioral techniques(2). Psychopharmacological treatment is the mainstay of symptom management.

Table 2. Tricyclic antidepressants

Drugs	Doses (mg/day)
Amitriptyline	25-125
Doxepin	25-125
Imipramine	25-125
Decipramine	25-125
Nortryptiline	25-125
Clomipramine	25-125
Second generation	
Bupreprion	200-450
Trazodone	150-300
Serotonin specific reuptake inhibitors	
Fluoxetine	20-60

Sertraline	50-200
Heterocyclic antidepressants	
Maprotiline	50-75
Amoxapine	100-150
MAO inhibitors	
Isocarboxazid	20-40
Phenalazine	30-60
Tranylcypromine	20-40
Psychostimulants	
Dexamphetamine	5-30
Methylphenidate	5-30
Pemoline	37.5-150
Neuroleptics	
Haloperidol	20-100
Benzodiazepines	
Alprazolam	0.75-6
Others	
Lithium carbonate	600-1200
Buspirone	15-60

ECT for severely depressed patients, or when antidepressants pose unacceptable side effects.

Anxiety in cancer pain patients

Anxiety syndromes in cancer patients are due to
1) reactive anxiety related to the stresses of cancer an its treatment
2) manifestation of a medical or physiological problem eg. uncontrolled pain (organic anxiety disorder) and
3) phobias, panic and chronic anxiety disorders

Reactive anxiety
Anxiety at critical moments (i.e. waiting for diagnosis, surgery, procedures) can isrupt ability to function normally, interfere with relationships and ability to understand/comply cancer treatments. Benzodiazepines, behavioral techniques, relaxation can reduce the distress.

Organic anxiety
Uncontrolled pain, infection, metabolic derangements can be treated with analgesics, oxygen, antibiotics and antihistamines, steroids related anxiety can be treated with benzodiazepines or low dose antipsychotics.(4). Encephalopathy, hyperthyroidism, carcinoid, primary and metastatic brain tumour also leads to anxiety.

Phobias and panic
Panic attacks, needle phobia or claustrophobia follow a critical moment and can complicate treatment of cancer. Relaxation training, systematic desensitization and antipsychotic drugs often help control the patients fear.

Organic disorders- delirium and dementia incidence may vary from 15-75% depending upon the progress of disease. Other organic disorders are dementia, amnesia, delusion, hallucinations, intoxications, personality and withdrawal disorders.

Delirium is a global cerebral dysfunction characterized by concurrent disturbance of consciousness level, attention, thinking, perception, emotion, memory and sleep awake cycle. Aetiology of delirium is unknown and there is a waxing and waning of above symptoms. Often reversible except in terminal multiple organ failure. Haloperidol cn control delirium but produces extrapyramidal symptoms, dystonia, hyperthermia, confusion and high CPK levell. Later can be treated by dantrolene sodium. In the last days of patient, methrimepraazine, or Midazolam can be used as an alternative to neuroleptics.

Confusional states[6] in cancer is not inevitable and can often be treated or made tolerable. It may present as disorientation, misinterpretation, short term memory loss include drugs (sedative, opioids, steroids), infection metabolic disturbances, cardiac or respiratory failure and susceptible patients- a full bladder or bowel.

When trying to understand a confused patient a usefull concept is that confusion reduces the number of messages from the environment and increases those from the body and memory stores, while making difficult to diffentiate tahe source of the messages. The implication is that self awareness is at least partly intact. While this may cause some patients to be very frieghtened by the confusion, it does provide a means of managing confusion. A further implication is that sedative drugs should not be used routinely in order to preserve awareness. Haloperidol 10mg per hour until agitation settles.

Table 3.Guidelines for managing confusion (6)

Diagnose cause: drugs ?	treat if possible
Provide	accompany, constant routine
Listen for clues	to understand confusion (ask relatives)
Explain the cause	makes confusion less frightening
Reassure	the patient is still sane
Reorientate	provide ooks on to which they can hang their reality

Cancer pain and suicide - inadequately controlled pain or poorly tolerated pain can cause suicidal tendency. N addition mood disturbances, hopelessness, depression, delirium in advanced stage of cancer, pre-existing psycopathology, suicide history and inadequate social support

Euthanasia- persistent pain and terminal illness are the primary reasons for those who request for physician-assisted suicide. From a medical perspective, uses of suicide as manifestation of psychiatric disturbance to be prevented. However philosophically, many in our society view suicide in those who face the distress of a fatal and painful disease like cancer as 'rational' and a means to regain control and maintain a 'dignified' death. This subject is often debatable by physicians (active euthanasia) and public (passive euthanasia).

Active euthanasia is often tolerated under condition that- i) the patients consent is free, conscious explicit and persistent. ii) The patient and physician agree that suffering is intolerable. iii) Other measures of relief have been exhausted. iv) Second physician must concur v) these facts must be documented. Incidence is 1.8% of deaths in Netherlands. Common reasons for requesting euthanasia (vandermass 1999) loss of dignity-57%, pain-46%, unworthy dying 46%, dependence on others 33%, tired of life 23%.

Cancer Pain and family (Second order patients)

Family members are called upon to provide emotional support, basic care taking, share responsibility for medical decision making, weathering financial and social cost. A programme for family members should include in pain management issues like assessment, administration of medicines, addict emotional support and stress management. In addition to family the staff nurses are also intensively involved in the palliative care and face treatment failures & psychological burnouts.

Cognitive- Behavioural Interventions in Cancer Pain –

Hypnosis, biofeed face and multifunctional behavioural interventions are used as adjuncts in cancer pain management. Behavioural includes self monitoring, anticipating anxiety & avoiding it.

Relaxation Technique:-

Achieve a physical and mental state of relaxation. This includes (1) Passive relaxation (2) Progressive muscle relaxation (3) Medication (4) Focused breathing. Once relaxed patient can use imaginationto manipulate or distract pain.Patient imagery includes (1) Pleasant distraction (2) transformational (3) Dissociative imagery. The patient can imagine pleasant pain free experience, a pain free walk & breaking pain cycle.

Hypnosis-

A stage of heightened focus concentration can manipulate pain perception. Three principles of hypnosis are self hypnosis, relax, not fighting the pain & use a mental filter to ease the hurt in pain.

Biofeedback –
Includes electromyographic & electroencephalographic assisted relaxation. However analgesia is not maintained after treatment stops.

Music Therapy:-
Can capture focus of attention away from pain while aroma therapy can have relaxaing & stimulating qualities.

In the end it can be concluded that cancer pain patients are most vulnerable to psychiatric complications needing proper management with antipsychotic dugs along with psychotherapy & cognitive behavioural therapy.

References:-
1. Massive M J, Holland J. C.The Cancer patients with pain; Psychiatric complications and their management; Medical Clinics of North America 1987 ,71:243-258
2. Massive M J, Holland J C. Depression and the cancer patient, Jour Clin. Psychiatry, 1990, 51:12-17.
3. Plumb M M, Holland J C. Comparative studies of psychological function in patients with advanced cancer, Psychosomatic Medicine, 1977, 39:264-276.
4. Stiefel F C, Breitbart W, Holland J C. Corticosteroids in cancer: Neuropsychiatric complications. Cancer Investigation, 1984, 7:479-491.
5. Helig S. The San Francisco Medical Society euthanasia survey, Results and Analysis, San Fransisco Medicine, 1988, 61: 24-34.
6. Kumar P. A Hand book of Management of pain & related symptoms. Samvedna, New Delhi, 2003,29.

CHAPTER 34.
Gastro intestinal symptoms

Constipation

CONSTIPATION CAN MIMIC SOME FEATURES OF CANCER, particularly abdominal masses, nausea vomiting, pain confusion and diarrhea. Colic combined with fixed abdominal masses can be easily mistaken for tumour, resulting in inappropriate use of analgesics. If the facility is readily available suppository can be invaluable in this situation. Constipation should be anticipated in all patients on opioids or drugs with anticholinergic actions and in patients who are immobile and with reduced fluid intake or on low fiber diet.

Table 1. **The treatment of constipation.**

Clear lower bowel.	Start laxative
High arachis oil retention enema overnight.	Contact laxative:
In the morning:	With danthron: Co danthramer
If rectum full-glycerol suppository	Co danthrusate.
If rectum empty-high phosphate enema	With sennoside:senna
If no success:	
Repeat enema after 24 hrs if faeces are palpable in descending colon. Start laxative.	Upto 20 mls bd Co danthromer forte.
If rectum is impacted:	If colic precipitated
Soft faeces: biscodyl suppository or tablet.	-reduce dose of contact laxative
Hard faeces: manual evacuation.	-add osmotic agent e.g. lactulose.

Table 2. **Contact laxative equivalents**

6 Co danthromer capsules =30 ml of co danthromer syrup =3 co danthrusate capsules =10 ml Co danthromer syrup.	=10 ml senna syrup =2 senna tablets

Nausea and vomiting

ANTIEMETIC CHOICE DEPENDS UPON CAUSE.

Commonly overlooked causes of nausea and vomiting in advanced cancer are constipation, hypercalcemia, pharyngeal stimulation by copious sputum, gastric stasis and drugs such as metronidazole.Tolerance to opioid induced nausea and vomiting occurs in 7-10 days. Patients transferred from strong opioids to weak opioids are already tolerant so that an antiemetic is not needed. A single anti emetic is usually sufficient[1.]

In some situations such as bowel obstruction, second antiemetics may be needed but should have a different but appropriate site of action. During the initial period of control of nausea and vomiting the oral route may not be practical. All the anti emetics given below are available in injectable form but only cyclizine, prochlorperazine domperidone and chlorpromazine are available in suppository form. In the subcutaneous infusion pump only haloperidol, cyclizine, metoclopramide should be used.

Table 3. The treatment of nausea and vomiting.

Stimulation of vomiting centre	First line treatment	Second line treatment
Higher centers -Anxiety, fear	Counseling	Add diazepam 5-10 mg or chlorpromazine 25-100mg 8th hrly
Directly -DXT to head and neck? -raised ICP	Cyclizine 50mg 8th hrly Corticosteroids +/- Cyclizine 50mg 8th hrly.	Chlorpromazine 25-100mg 8th hrly

Via vagal and sympathetic afferents. -cough	Simple linctus PRN	Add morphine soln 5-10 mg 4t hourly
-bronchial secretions	Hyoscine hydro bromide 0.3-0.8 mg 6-8 hourly	Add gentle chest physiotherapy.
-stretched liver capsule	Corticosteroids	Add Cyclizine 50mg 8 th hrly
-gastric stasis	Metoclopramide 10mg 8t hourly Or domperidone 10mg 8th hourly.	Add dimethicone 10ml 4th hourly
-constipation	Clear constipation	Add Cyclizine 50mg 8th hrly
- bowel obstruction	Cyclizine 50mg 8 th hrly	Add haloperidol 3-5mg
Via Chemoreceptor trigger zone - drugs inc.opioids, hypercalcemia,uremia	Haloperidol 1.5-3mg	Chlorpromazine 25-100mg 8th hourly
Via vestibular nerve	Add Cyclizine 50mg 8 th hrly	Chlorpromazine 25-100mg 8th hourly

Anti emetic

Haloperidol preparations: tabs 0.5, 1.5,5,10, 20 mg.inj:5/10 mg/ml. routes: PO/IM/SC. antiemetic of choice on CTZ. Reduced risk of extra pyramidal effects at low doses.

Cyclizine preparations: tabs 50 mg suppose 50mg in 50mg/ml dose: 50-100 mg 4 – 8th hrly. Routes: PO/PR/SC/IM. Antiemetic of choice acting directly in vomiting center, anticholinergic side effects at higher doses. Occasionally local irritation when injected subcutaneously.

Metoclopramide preparations tabs 10 mg, elixir 5mg/ml Inj 5mg/ml dose: 10-20mg 8th hrly.dose 10-20mg 8th hrly. Routes PO/SC/IM. Antiemetics of choice to speed gastric emptying.may cause extra pyramidal effects at large doses. Can be given subcutaneously.

Alternatives to the above anti emetics

Prochlorperazine preparations tabs 5, 25 mg.syrup 5mg/ml, and suppose.5, 25 mg.
Inj12.5 mg/ml.dose:5-10 mg 8th hourly .routes: PO/IM/PR. More sedative and likely to cause dry mouth than haloperidol .shorter half life than haloperidol. Too irritant to use subcutaneously. Suppository can be useful.

Domperidone.preparations.tabs 10mg.susp 5mg/ml suppose 30 mg. doses: oral 10 mg 8 hourly. Alternative to metoclopramide especially if extra pyramidal reactions are a risk and rectal route is required.

Chlorpromazine preparations tabs 10, 25, 50,100 mg.elixir 25mg/ml, suppose 100 mg.inj 25 mg/ml.dose:10 – 100 mg 8th hrly. Routes: PO/IM/PR. Comments: Too sedative for routine use. Too irritant for subcutaneous use.

Anorexia.

IT IS NORMAL FOR LESS ACTIVITY TO REDUCE ENERGY INTAKE and this should be explained to the patient. It need not be treated, underlying causes which can be treated include pain, constipation, nausea and vomiting, gastric distension, oral problems, body odours, anxiety and depression, drugs, unappetizing food and food odours.patients may develop taste abnormalities and may prefer sweeter, colder and spicier foods. While others cannot tolerate the bitterness of urea in red meats.[2] So all, attractively presented meals are more likely to be eaten.

If the cause of anorexia is unclear, or difficult to treat, corticosteroids can be effective.dexamethsone 4mg mane reducing to 2mg after one week can improve appetite and taste. Side effects are unlikely at this dose, but dexamethasone should be stopped if there is no improvement after two weeks

Intestinal obstruction.

OBSTRUCTION CAN BE MANAGED AT HOME. The traditional pre operative "drip and suck" is successful in controlling the symptoms of obstruction in less than 15% of patients unfit for surgery.[3] These patients can be managed medically without "drip and suck"; free of nausea and pain. An outline of management is given below.

Patients are little troubled by short episodes of vomiting provided that the most distressing symptom, nausea, is controlled by anti emetics. Obstructions distal to the upper small bowel will allow sufficient fluid to be absorbed to prevent significant dehydration. Patients with complete small bowel obstruction have been managed in this way for several weeks before succumbing to the cancer. It is possible to achieve a peaceful phase without the need for nasogastric suction or intravenous hydration which is rarely justified in the last days or weeks of life.

Table 4. The medical management of bowel obstruction.

Explanation	Eliminate nausea and reduce vomiting
Dietary advice	AVOID Metoclopramide or domperidone
No fluid/food restriction	START Cyclizine 50mg 6-8 hrly (PO/SC/PR/IM)
- Small meals earlier in the day.	-if no success
Reduce colic	ADD haloperidol 3-5mg nocte.
Stop osmotic or contact laxatives.	- if no success
Hyoscine hydro bromide 0.3 mg sublingually 4-8 hrly.	REPLACE Cyclizine and haloperidol with Hyoscine hydro bromide. 0.4 mg sc. 8th hrly.
- if no success increase Hyoscine to 0.8mg subcutaneously 4-8hrly	
Reduce background pain.	**Soften bowel contents**
Opioids (oral route often possible)	Docussate tabs or syrup
- Codeine phosphate 30-60 mg 4 hrly.	100-200 mg 8th hrly
- morphine sulphate (titrate dose)	
	Reverse obstruction.
	Clear constipation.
	Consider dexamethasone 12 mg daily for 1 week.(only occasionally successful)

1. Contact laxatives are withheld to avoid colic, osmotic laxatives to avoid bowel distension and Metoclopramide or domperidone to avoid the upper gut trying to contract against high obstruction.
2. Hyoscine butyl bromide (buscopan) is an alternative to Hyoscine hydro bromides and may have less peripheral anti cholinergic effects such as dry mouth. The dose is 10-20 mg 4-6 hrly PO/SC.

Causes of obstruction.

Recurrent abdominal pelvic cancer can often cause multiple malignant blockages; usually in the small bowel. **metastatic obstruction** from outside the abdomen is most commonly due to melanoma or due to primaries of breasts or lung. **constipation** can cause distension, nausea. Vomiting and abdominal masses that may not change position far a week or more. A supine abdominal x ray will differentiate constipation from other causes of obstruction. **Benign adhesions** may occur in upto 20% of patients with recurrent abdominal; cancer. Adhesions are more likely if the ileum is obstructed and if the abdomen is previously irradiated[4].

Surgery: The possibility if benign adhesions or a single site of obstruction means that surgery can be considered, relative simple surgery is often all that is required, such as forming a loop colostomy or dividing adhesions. An understanding surgical opinion can be helpful; lthough radiology may be needed to show a single level obstruction that is amenable to surgery.

There will be many patients, however, whose tumour is too extensive, who have had previous surgery for obstruction, who are too ill or frail, or who have no wish for further intervention. These should be managed medically as described before.

Proximal obstructions: duodenal or **pyloric** obstructions are more likely to cause vomiting, but less likely to cause distension. They cause gastric stasis with features of the "squashed stomach syndrome" and must be differentiated from other causes of this syndrome which may respond to Metoclopramide or domperidone.use of these drugs in intraluminal obstructions are likely to cause increase discomfort and colic the nausea can be treated with Cyclizine but vomiting may still occur several times. These patients may need gastric aspiration to reduce vomiting and IV hydration to prevent thirst.

Esophageal obstructions present special problems with regurgitation of swallowed saliva, painful dysphagia and epigastric pain. Gastric acid causes precipitation of protein from the tumour producing tenacious material which is difficult to bring up, antacids or H_2 receptor blockers can help. Hyoscine hydro bromide 0.3-0.6 mg sc 8t hrly will reduce saliva production at the expense of the dry mouth which can be treated with local measures. Painful dysphagia can be helped with mucaine and tumour pain with opioids.consideration should always be given to insertation of an esophageal tube or to radiotherapy.

Feeding and hydration: Some patients will absorb sufficient fluids from their upper gut to prevent significant dehydration. As patient deteriorate and eventually become comatose their fluid intake reduces, but contrary to common belief, the resultant dehydration need not be distressing.

Ascites.

The commonest causes for malignant Ascites are primary tumour of the breast, ovary, colon, stomach, pancreas and bronchus. Nearly one third of the primary tumors lie outside the abdomen. Symptoms include abdominal distension or pain, a squashed stomach syndrome, leg lymph edema and dyspnoea due to diaphragmatic splinting.treatement plan is outlined below.

Diuretics: the finding of increased Renin and sodium retention in malignant Ascites has prompted the successful use of spironolactone.the addition of a oral loop diuretic increases the diuresis,although the reduction of the Ascites is as much due to redistribution of fluids as by diuresis[5].

Paracentesis this is best carried out using a peritoneal dialysis catheter connected to a urinary drainage bag via a urinary catheter with the balloon and tip cut off. The use of 0.5% bupivacaine as local anesthetic for the puncture site allows pain free drainage for upto 8 hours if necessary. Puncture sites should be away from scars and the inferior epigastric artery which runs 3-5 cm from the midline in the abdominal wall.ideal sites are in the left iliac Fossa (atleast 10 cm from the midline) and in the midline suprapubically (the bladder should be empty). A lateral approach is advisable in patients with distended bowel-marked distension is a contraindication to paracentesis.if diuretics have been unsuccessful, or the prognosis is short, the slow drainage of 5litres or more of fluid may be indicated. Contrary to popular belief, there is no evidence that the patient deteriorate rapidly after such a large Paracentesis as long as it is done slowly over 8-12 hours.

Peritoneo venous shunt. Insertion of a shunt can be done under a short general anesthetic and causes fewer problems than for Ascites due to benign liver disease. There is no evidence that increased metastatic disease occurs after such a procedure, a tense ascites is preferred prior to insertion since this encourages drainage. Thereafter inspiratory exercises are used to further encourage drainage.

Diarrhea

Table 5.Treatment of diarrhea in advanced cancer.

Cause	1st line treatment	2nd line treatment
Infection **Drugs**(e.g. antibiotics, laxatives)	Loperamide-4mg tabs/syp with each loose stool.	
Constipation	Clear rectal impaction	Treat constipation
Obstruction	Manage obstruction	
Pancreatic steatorrhoea(reduced lipases and bicarbonates)	Pancreatic enzymes	Cimetidine 400mg at least 30 min before a meal (a night time dose is not necessary) pancrex gelatin capsules (5-10) or granules 93-6 5ml tspns should be used if cimetidine is prescribed.
Post gastrectomy	Loperamide 2-4mg tabs /syrup with each loose stool then 12 hrly.if bacterial overgrowth suspected :oxytetracycline 250 mg 6th hrly for 2-4 weeks	Pancreatic enzymes
Post radiotherapy	Low residue diet loperamide-4mg tabs/syp with each loose stool then	NSAIDs consider cholestyramine 4g in water 6 hrly

	12 hrly	
Bile salt irritation(e.g. ileal resection)	loperamide-4mg tabs/syp with each loose stool then 12 hrly	cholestyramine 4g in water 6hrly
Rectal discharge	Predsol enema Metronidazole 400 mg 8 hrly if anaerobic infection present	Local Cryotherapy or diathermy Radiotherapy

Table 6. Other problems and management

Problem	Causes	Features	Treatment
Dry mouth	Dehydration, Phenothiazines, Tricyclic, Hyoscine.	Dry tongue thick saliva, difficulty in speaking	Oral hydration if possible, sucking: crushed ice, butter, frozen tonic water. Chewing: pineapple chunks Change drugs e.g. Amitriptyline to mianserin,prochlorperazine to haloperidol
Coated tongue	Debility, poor oral hygiene, dehydration, Candida	White/brown or black tongue, reduced taste, halitosis	Cleansing:2%soda bicarb or 6% h2o2 Dissolving:1g effervescent ascorbic acid on tongue Brushing:gently with tooth brush Chewing: pineapple chunks
Candidiasis (thrush)	Debility, cross infection, poor oral hygiene	White adherent patches, coated tongue, dryness redness, soreness or dryness cheilitis only ulceration only	Ketoconazole 200 mg mane for 1 week Soak dentures in week Milton-do not use denture solution Mouthwash: betadiene
Ulceration	Apthous ulcers Radiotherapy Chemotherapy Dentures Poor oral hygiene	White depressions in mucosa with surrounding inflammation Painful	Tetracycline syrup 10 ml(250 mg mouth wash for 2 min then swallowed) Triamcinolone in oro base Betamethasone 1mg dissolved in water as a mouth wash
	Herpes simplex. zoster	Pale vesicles with surrounding redness Painful, unilateral in zoster,	Treat as for painful mouth Consider: acyclovir 200 mg po 4 hrly for 5 days
Painful mouth	Ulceration, candidiasis, poor oral hygiene, oral cancer oral sepsis	Soreness talking, eating and swallowing	Benzydamine as mouth wash 1-2 hrly Choline salicylates to local lesions Consider: local anesthetic prior to cleansing mouth

Candida: normally inhabitant of mouths of many patients with cancer, especially of irradiation of head and neck. Most overt candidiasis is the result of over growth of Candida following reduction of host immunity. Fungicidal disinfectants such as betadiene should be used for hand washing in units treating patients with candidiasis[6].

Ketoconazole vs. nystatin. Ketoconazole 200mg once daily for one week is at least as effective, more convenient and its cost is similar to one week's treatment with 2ml nystatin 4 hrly.gynecomastia and hepatic toxicity have been reported with Ketoconazole. The incidence of serious hepatic injury is very low and should not preclude its use in advanced cancer[7].

Oral analgesia Benzydamine hcl mouth wash provides local anti inflammatory action and analgesia for 1-2 hours with minimal numbness. choline salicylates is also effective but can cause pain on application.

Table 7. Dysphagia

Cause	Features	Treatment
Obstruction Esophageal tumors	Painful dysphagia with patient describing level of obstruction	Celestin tube Bouginage Radiotherapy Corticosteroids And lasers
Extrinsic compression	As above	Radiotherapy corticosteroids
Neurological Neuromuscular	e.g. brain stem tumor MS &MND disorganized swallowing	Hyoscine hydro bromide 0.3-0.8mg 8th hrly to reduce chocking Physical help with swallowing
Perineural spread of tumor(5th,9th and 10th)	Disorganized swallowing Altered sensation in throat and face	Corticosteroids
Mucosal Candidiasis	Painful swallowing, back or retrosternal pain	Ketoconazole 200 mg maine for 1 week
Radiotherapy	As above	Mucaine 10ml 2-4 hrly Diflunisal 250 mg bd

Esophageal tube (Celestin tube) it can be inserted using an endoscope under light anesthesia.
Hydration and feeding. There are special situations in which it is worth considering hydration and feeding Esophageal gastric and intestinal candidiasis[8]. Radiological appearance in a barium swallow is characteristic in case of esophageal candidiasis. gastric and intestinal candidiasis may present with abdominal pain and watery diarrhea. Treatment of both is Ketoconazole.

Table 8. Squashed stomach syndrome

Cause	Features	Treatment
Drugs (opioids, anti depressants), Ascites, hepatomegaly.	Nausea vomiting, epigastric pain, regurgitation, hiccups, early satiation, heart burn	Metoclopramide 10-20 mg 8th hrly po/sc/im.
Obstruction	As above	Treat as per obstruction

References

1. Hanks G.W. Antiemetics for terminal cancer patients. Lancet. 1982; 1410.
2. Dew Y. S. Changes in taste sensation and feeding behavior in cancer patients. Journal of human nutrition, 1978, 32:447-453.
3. Glass RL, Le Duc R.J. Small intestinal obstruction from peritoneal carcinamatosis. The American journal of surgery, 1973; 125:316.
4. Walsh H.P.J. Is laparatomy for small bowel obstruction justified in patients previously treated malignancy? British journal of surgery,1984; 71:933-935
5. Amiel SA, Blackbuin AM and Rubers RD. Intravenous infusion of furosemide as treatment of ascites in malignant disease. Brit. Medical journal, 1984; 288:1041
6. Burnie JP., Lee W, Williams JD et al. Control of an outbreak of systemic Candida albicans. British Medical journal 1985; 291:1092-1093
7. Lewis JH, Zimmerman HJ, Benson GD. et al. Hepatic injury associated with ketaconazole: injury analysis of 33 cases. Gastroenterology.1984 503-513.
8. Trier JS & Bjorkman DJ. Esophageal, gastric candidiasis. American journal of medicine, 1984; 77(4d): 39-43.

CHAPTER 35.

Urinary symptoms

Hematuria

It is unusual for blood loss to be severe so that iron supplementation may be sufficient to prevent anemia. Infections should always be excluded both by clinical and urine culture.

Palliative radiotherapy may cause trouble some hematuria arising from bleeding from a malignant lesion in urinary tract.

Bleeding can be minimized by 1%alum irrigation solution. It acts by precipitating proteins in mucosal surface. It is given by continuous bladder irrigation; it is not absorbed, and has no systemic toxicity.

Table 1.Urinary retention

Cause	First line	Consider
Constipation	Laxatives	……………..
Drugs(anti cholinergic)	Reduce dose	Change drug
Tumor obstruction	Phenoxybenzamine or dexamethasone	Catheterization or suprapubic catheter
Naturopathic bladder Spastic	Phenoxybenzamine	Intermittent self Catheterization
Flaccid	Phenoxybenzamine	Distigmine 5mg on alternate days; Intermittent self Catheterization

Urinary incontinence

Investigation of incontinence is rarely appropriate in patients with advanced cancer, and a clinical diagnosis must be made .although surgical repair is also inappropriate, the advice of an urologist can be invaluable .drugs are often the first line of treatment.[1]

Table 2. Urinary incontinence

Cause	First line	Second line	Consider
Post prostatectomy	Propanthiline,15mg before meal +30mg nocte(upto 90mg daily)	Imipramine 50-100mg nocte	Comdom,urethral catheter or bag decompression nasally may help
Stress continence	Ring pessary	Ephedrine 30mgBD,last dose no later than 6 pm	Absorbant pads, tampons ,surgery
Urge incontinence	Propantheline 15mg before meal=30mg nocte(upto 90 mg daily	Imipramine 50-100mg nocte	NSAID (flurbiprofen),pads,condom,urethral catheter or bag
Neuropathic Bladder -spastic -flaccid	Large capacity: manual stimulation to void , small capacity : intermittent catheterization regular voiding	Permanent condom.urethral catheter or bag Intermittent catheterisation	Desmopressin nocte may help

Bypassing catheter	Exclude infection or bladder spasm	Have balloon volume	Change to smaller size catheter
Vesico-vaginal fistula	Absorbant pads or tampons	Desmopressin nocte may help	
Over flow	Catheter	Phenoxybenzamine	Distigmine

1. Desmopressin: this synthetic analogue of vasopressin (anti-diuretic hormone) will reduce urinary output overnight and is occasionally helpful in otherwise intractable nocturnal incontinence .A fluid intake /output chart should be started, and no fluids given after 6 pm .20microgram of desmopressin is given nasally at 10pm. It is important the patient produces a daytime output of at least 500mls .otherwise water intoxication can occur.
2. Intermittent self catheterization is an alternative at home to a permanent catheter .The technique is usually only suitable for women. Catheterization is done at least four times a day. The catheters can be washed after use then boiled or kept in sodium hypochlorite solution.
3. Condom catheters for men are an alternative to a permanent indwelling catheter but have the disadvantage of leaking if not carefully fitted. An alternative is a urostomy bag fitted over the penis and adherent to the pubic skin.
4. Sex and the catheter : Some patients and their partners are still able and willing to consider intercourse ,but frightened to the catheter .many women are able to have satisfactory intercourse with an indwelling catheter ,although intermittent self catheterization is a better alternative .Men who are able to achieve an erection can do so with a catheter present .Gentle intercourse is possible with a disconnected catheter (after draining the bladder), and placing a condom over penis and catheter. If the ejaculatory mechanism has not been damaged this can still occur with a catheter, but may be painful. Self re-catheterization or a condom catheter is better alternative.

Table 3 **Bladder pain or spasm**

Cause	First line	Second line	Consider
Infection	Appropriate antibiotic	Bladder washout if catheter present	Phenazopyridine 100-200mg 8 hourly
Irritation –catheter -tumour	Remove half water from balloon radiotherapy	Phenazopyridine Phenazopyridine	Exclusion of bladder calculus Analgesics
Neuropathic bladder spasm	Propantheline 15mg before meal+30mg nocte(upto 90 mg daily)	Hyoscine hydrobromide 0.3-o.6mg SL/sc pm	
Anxiety	Empathetic listening	Propantheline 15mg before meals+30 mg nocte(upto 90 mg daily)	Diazepam 5-10 mg

Note: Radiotherapy can occasionally cause bladder pain and spasm. Try phenazopyridine which is a topical analgesic .It colours the urine orange /red.

Cardiovascular symptoms
Vena caval obstruction
This needs urgent treatment .Superior vena caval obstruction may cause distressing and painful swelling of the head, neck and arms .inferior vena caval obstruction has a similar effect on the lower half of the body.
Initial treatment consists of high doses dexamethasone 8mg IV stat, followed by 24mg daily in divided doses (the last dose no later than dose required to control symptoms .If possible the patient should be urgently referred for radiotherapy.
Anaemia

ANAEMIA IN ADVANCED CANCER DOES NOT ALWAYS REQUIRE TREATMENT .It is usually an anaemia of chronic diseases and does not respond to iron or other supplements .consequently transfusion is often considered if the anaemia is profound .This needs careful consideration .If the anaemia is causing postural dizziness or weakness, and the patients is likely to remain active then a transfusion may help. Transfusions are not helpful in controlling drowsiness or dyspnoea and are contraindicated when the prognosis is a few weeks or less. Transfusions are not without risk and repeated transfusions do little to improve a patients comfort and quality of life.

Leucoerythroblastic anaemia due to marrow infiltration may respond to hormone therapy (e.g. Tamoxifen in breast cancer) or appropriate chemotherapy .If these have been tried consider high dose dexamethasone.

Respiratory symptoms

Dyspnoea is subjective and unrelated to the severity of the pathology. The fear of suffocation and anxiety from any cause will make the situation worse. Consequently simple measure such as cooling fan, opening a window and the security of someone's presence will do much to ease the sensation of dyspnoea. Causes of dyspnoea such as bronchospasm or pulmonary edema are treated conventionally.

Pleural effusion if symptomatic this should be drained almost to dryness, not taking more than 1-1.5 liters at a time. It is a common fallacy that fluid will reccumulate within days of tapping several weeks is more usual and this may be sufficient in an ill patient. Occasionally more rapid accumulation occur, or the patients prognosis such that a regular tapping is impractical. In these cases it is worth instilling a fibrotic agent to prevent re accumulation. Tetracycline 500mg is the choice, and is dissolved in 20 ml 0.25%bupivacaine just before use. It is instilled after tapping and the patient asked to lie on each side, front and back for two to three minutes each way. Mild, temporary, pleuritic pain is usually the only problem.

Lobar collapse which is recent and due to bronchial carcinoma may respond to radiotherapy.

Lymphangitis Carcinomatosa may br helped by dexamethasone, 16 mg daily in divided dose (the last dose no later that 6 pm) reducing to 2-6 mg once daily over the following week. Inhalation of bupivacaine 0.25 % nebulae using ultrasound produces 2 A size particles which will reach the alveoli and may ease dyspnoea, but the inhalation are not always tolerated[2].

Opioids are effective at reducing the demand for ventilation with out causing clinically significant respiratory depression. Even in the presence of chronic bronchitis or bronchial carcinoma, carbon di oxide retention is unusual. Patient not previously on opioid should be started on 5 mg oral morphine 4 hourly, titrating the dose upward to the response.

Midazolam (1-2mg) & diazepam has a place in a very anxious, dyspnoeic patient, 5-10 mg stat (po or pr) followed by 5-10 mg nocte.

Respiratory infection

Whether or not to treat a chest infection in a patient with advanced cancer often cause great concern. First it must be remembered that cancer will progress despite antibiotic .second what matter is whether the patient is distressed by infection (e.g. fever, purulent sputum, pruritis chest pain). In such situation there is a duty to treat in order to preserve right to comfort. Whether to control symptoms with antibiotic or other methods (e.g. cooling for fever, Hyoscine for secretion, analgesic for pain) must depend on the prognosis. If this is likely to be weeks or months then antibiotics should be considered. If the prognosis is likely to be hour or days, however, there is no time to wait for antibiotic to work and the other treatment should be used for the patients comfort.

Cough

Cough may be dry (e.g. mechanical irritation of the pharynx, trachea, bronchial tree, pleura, pericardium or diaphragm) or moist (e.g. infection, chronic obstructive disease, asthma or heart failure). It is not always possible to treat the cause.

Peripheral suppression: Simple linctus or humidified air are soothing preparation which can be repeated as often as required.bupivacaine0.25%(maximum 30 ml per day) in 2 –10 A size particles (via a bird nebulae) is helpful to suppress cough arising anywhere down to the larger bronchi. It is not always tolerated and the larger particles may cause numbness of mouth and throat, preventing safe eating and drinking for several hours. High dose dexamethasone may reduce pleural, pericardial or diaphragmatic irritation by tumour.

Central suppression: oral morphine sulphate 3-10 mg 4 hourly in a dose that is titrated to the cough. Methadone should not be used since its long half life results in sedation.

Haemoptysis

MAJOR HAEMOPTYSIS IS A RARE EVENT. Slight blood stained sputum in bronchial carcinoma is a normal part of the disease. Infection can be simply treated with appropriate antibiotics. Hemoptysis from a pulmonary infarct will settle and needs no treatment.

Frequent hemoptysis due to bronchial carcinoma can be treated with radiotherapy to the mediastinum or low dose dexamethasone. In the rare event of a major hemorrhage and if the patient remains conscious then diamorphine 5-10mg stat IV and diazepam 5-10mg iv will easy the fear and distress.

Noisy breathing

Bronchial secretion can produce a "death rattle "which is distressing to relatives and staff, although rarely to the patient who is usually comatose. A few very debilitated but conscious patient s are troubled with secretion but are too weak to cough. Treatment is with Hyoscine hydro bromide 300-800micrograms 2-4 hourly. It is sedative but preferable to atropine which can cause CNS stimulation. If high dose are used repeatedly paradoxical agitation can occasionally occurs.frusemide 40 mg im/iv has been used in resistant cases.

Grunting respiration is occasionally seen in comatose patient. Repositioning often helps. If the patient is breathing rapidly, diamorphine 5-10 mg sc 2-4 hourly will reduce the respiratory rate to normal level and ease the grunting. High dose of diamorphine may be needed if the patient is already receiving an opioid for pain relief. If the respiratory rate is normal them diazepam 5-10mg rectally 2-4 hourly can help.

Hiccups

Exclude a squashed stomach syndrome. Diaphragmatic or phrenic nerve irritation from tumour may respond to high dose dexamethasone. If simple remedies fail (e.g. swallowing granulated sugar) and the hiccups are persistent, try chlorpromazine 25-50 mg as a slow IV injection, oral or in routes being less effective[3].

DERMATOLOGICAL SYMPTOMS

Ulcers

Many unrelated treatments have been proposed for the management of decubitus and malignant ulcers, which reflects the low success rate of any one method. The simplest methods are the best.

1. Debridement to remove slough requires the active removal of all dead tissue with forceps and curette. In some areas of established pressure damage access to the underlying dead tissue may be prevented by a hard, dark eschar of dead skin. Wet dressings (gauze with normal saline) will soften the eschar sufficiently to allow debridement.

2. Cleansing does not imply sterilization since ulcers are invariably colonized by bacteria. Antiseptics such as povidone-iodine (Betadine solution) will control overt infection and allow healing to take place. Topical antibiotics in powders, sprays or tulles should not be used since they result in the selection of resistant organisms and can cause local sensitivity which may lead to systemic hypersensitivity. Systemic antibiotics will not reach dead tissue which must be removed by debridement. They should dead tissue which must be removed by debridement. They should only be used if cellulites is present (after sensitivity tests), or in controlling odors. Chlorine releasing solutions may damage viable tissue and are best avoided.

Radiotherapy should be considered for all fungating tumours.Bleeding can be a problem from superficial vessels that are damaged during debridement or dressing changes. Gauze soaked in 1 in 1000 adrenaline solution usually stops oozing after a few minutes application. More persistently bleeding vessels can be sealed by applying absorbable gelatin sponge

Dressing: Dressings should provide a moist environment and the simplest and cheapest is gauze soaked in normal saline or Ringer's solution. Granuflex is suitable after debridement and can be left for one week between dressing changes. Op-site can protect superficial ulcers in areas subject to repeated trauma (e.g. sacrum). It is semi-permeable and should be left in place until it peels away naturally. Exudate accumulation can be removed with needle and syringe, the puncture hole being sealed with a small square of Op-site. Silastic foam[4] can be useful in deep ulcers where a comfortable dressing is needed, or in facial ulcers.

Generalized pruritis

An attempt to diagnose the cause should always be made since specific treatments may then be indicated. In particular drugs, eczema, infestations, contact dermatitis, iron deficiency and uraemia should be excluded. In advanced cancer, however, diagnosis is often difficult and treatments have to be non-specific.

General measures: Patients should avoid heat, hot baths, rough underclothing and rough drying after bath. Preventing a dry skin is essential and measures include; adding oil to the bath, aqueous creams or crotamiton. Calamine is too drying and should be avoided.

Cupitch syndrome (cutaneous pain and itch): This is occasionally seen in patients with en cuirass breast cancer. The skin surrounding the tumour is often red, painful and itchy and may be due to local prostaglandin production. Both pain an itch may respond to an anti-prostaglandin e.g. flurbiprofen or diflunisal.

Jaundice: Pruritis is not always to the severity of the jaundice, probably because the balance of dihydroxy salts seems more important than the total amount of bile salts present. Cholestyramine 4G 6 hrly preferentially binds dihydroxy salts in the bowel, but the granules are unpleasant to take. Cholestyramine will be ineffective in total biliary obstruction since there are no bile salts in the bowel to be absorbed. Methyltestosterone 10-25 mg 8 hrly has been used successfully in ill patients with severe pruritis, despite occasionally increasing the jaundice due to cholestasis"'.

Topical drugs: Corticosteroids can be effective when appropriately applied to inflammatory skin disorders. They tend to be ineffective if applied to itchy skin without lesions. Topical anaesthetics and antihistamines are best avoided.

Systemic drugs: Antihistamines are often used with no evidence of histamine release and any positive effect is probably due to a central sedative effect. Morphine is a rare cause of histamine release, but should be considered with itching starting soon after commencing an opioid. Cimetidine has occasionally been used in itching due to various causes and specifically in Hodgkin's disease[5].

Sweating

Some patients suffer from profuse sweating, particularly at night. It is difficult to treat. It may be due to fear or anxiety. Occasionally the malignancy itself will produce a fever with sweating. Simple measures such as cooling with a fan or sponge are effective. Naproxen has been shown to relieve the fever due to cancers of the breast, lung, and bowel and to Hodgkin's The usual dose is 250-500 mg bd.

ODOURS AND DISCHARGES

Odours

Most odours are the result of infection and foul-smelling odours are associated with anaerobic bacteria. ATTEMPTS TO MASK A SMELL WITH OTHER ODOURS WILL FAIL (e.g. air fresheners, perfumes). The patient comes to associate the new odour with the unpleasant one and soon it too becomes intolerable.

1. Reducing Infection. For anaerobic Infections Metronidazole (Flagyl) 200-400mg 8 hrly is the drug of choice. Suppositories (500mg or 1G) and a suspension (200mg/Smi) are available. There is little evidence that topical Metronidazole is effective[4]. Other methods aimed directly at the tumour should be considered such as radiotherapy or Cryotherapy with liquid nitrogen since these may reduce tumour bulk and so reduce the amount of dying tumour tissue that predisposes to infection and odour.

2. Isolating the odour may be possible using adsorbants such as charcoal dressings. (Actisorb, Bandor, Denidor), or appliances such as colostomy bags for fistulae. Oxychlorodene (Ostebon) has no inherent odour and is effective in removing unpleasant odours. It cannot be applied directly to tissues but can be sprinkled between dressings or into colostomy bags. Granuflex (hydrocolloid) and Sorbsen (calcium alginate) are expensive dressings which can slightly reduce odour.

Discharges

Discharges may occur from fistulae, colostomies and the vagina or rectum. Impacted faeces should always be excluded in rectal discharges.

Fistulae: It maybe possible to fit colostomy bags over the fistula - the Paediatric types are easier to fit because of a softer flange. Odour can still pass through "odour-proof" bags and oxychlorodene (Ostobon) can then be used (see above). Silastic foam can be used when it is desirable to reduce the amount of discharge as in external fistulae connecting with the oral cavity. The dressing forms a close fitting, comfortable and washable dressing which reduces fluid loss. The foam dressing formed can be washed and re-used frequently

Vaginal and rectal discharges due to local carcinomas can be helped with antiseptic douches/lavage e.g. povidone-iodine (Betadine vaginal gel or douche). Corticosteroids (given rectally or vaginally) can help. A recto-vaginal fistula may cause stool to be passed vaginally which can be reduced by allowing the stool to become firmer (reduce the laxative or give a low dose of Loperamide). Vaginal discharges from a recto-vaginal fistula can also be reduced with regularly changed tampons. Perineal and perianal skin often need protection from the continual moisture with barrier creams e.g. zinc oxide paste. Referral for radiotherapy, diathermy, and cryotherapy or laser treatment should be considered.

HYPERCALCAEMIA

Malignancy is the most common cause of Hypercalcemia, occurring in nearly 10% of patients with advanced cancer. Primaries of the breast and bronchus are the commonest causes. THERE IS NO CLEAR

RELATIONSHIP WITH BONE METASTASES and their absence should never preclude a search for Hypercalcemia. The mechanism appears to be Increased bone and renal. Resorption of calcium due to a parathyroid-like hormone produced by the tumour.

Drowsiness occurs in over half of patients[2] other symptoms include thirst, polyuria, nausea, vomiting, anorexia, constipation and a confusional state. It is all too easy to attribute many of these to the cancer or the analgesia, although a combination of drowsiness, thirst and polyurla should always lead to a check of serum calcium. The calcium level should be corrected according to me albumin (true calcium approx. equals measured calcium + 0.02 x 140 - albumin).

The intensity of treatment will depend on the severity of symptoms and the advanced stage of the cancer.

Severe symptoms require intravenous rehydration with 0.9% saline (4-6 litres in 24 hours may be required), together with Parenteral Frusemide to promote calcium excretion. Mithramycin is a cytotoxic agent which in single doses of 25 micrograms/kg has a delayed but sustained effect which may last several weeks.

Repeated doses increase the risk of side effects, particularly bone-marrow depression.

Moderate symptoms will respond to intravenous hydration and parenteral Frusemide.

Mild symptoms may respond to oral rehydration and maintenance therapy alone.

Maintenance therapy: Keeping the calcium within normal limits can be achieved with oral phosphate. Diarrhea is a common side effect, which may be minimized by Loperamide 2-4 mg daily and by increasing the phosphate dose gradually. Reduced renal function due to renal calcification is a long term risk. Patients not tolerating or responding to phosphate may be controlled on the expensive etidronate, a diphosphonate which has a slow onset of action, but a more sustained effect than mithramycin. Corticosteroids are not helpful in Hypercalcemia due to solid tumours (breast, bronchus) but can be useful in myeloma. Hormones should always be considered in primaries of breast (tamoxifen, medroxyprogesterone, aminoglutethemide) and prostate (stilboestrol)

References:
1. West Moore. Urinary incontinence drugs.1979; 17:418-422.
2. Heyse Moore. Respiratory symptoms in the management of terminals diseases,
3. 1984; 113-119.
4. Williamson BWA. Management of intractable hiccup. British Medical journal, 1977; 2; 501- 503
5. Warrender TS. Op-site and the dhss. British Medical journal., 1982; 285:378-9.
6. Imard JOP. Cimetidine for pruritis. British Medical Journal., 1980;280:151-2.
7. Stevenson JC. Malignant hypocalcaemia. British Medical journal, 1985; 291: 421-2.

Chapter 36.
Management of Cancer Pain

10 lakh new cancer patients are diagnosed every year in India. 60% are diagnosed in advanced stage, so require only pain management and palliative care. 30%-50% have pain at the time of diagnosis. 70% to 90% have severe pain when the disease is advanced. 40% die with severe pain. 60%-80% complains of inadequate pain relief by their physician. 30% are not relieved by drug treatment alone, so require interventional pain management. More than 90% cancer pain can be adequately controlled.

THREE DIMENTIONS OF CANCER PAIN:

Pain is an unpleasant sensory and emotional experience associated with actual or potential tissue damage, or described in terms of such damage[1]. There are three components or dimentions of pain on the basis of physiology.

1. **Sensory** – tumour associated pain including a nociceptive, somatic or visceral or neuropathic.
   Somatic pain is further subdivided into a) well localized cutaneous, diffused dull deep tissue pain and b) a sickening visceral pain c) The neuropathic component arises due to tumour compression and invasion of nerves. This pain is associated with loss of motor and sensory functions and is characterized as a burning pain e.g. brachial & Lumbosacral plexus.

   The somatic pain can be treated by analgesics & neurosurgical techniques while neuropathic pain responds to these partly, making pain management in some patients very difficult.

2. **Emotional and suffering** – A sustained nociception and other problems lead to suffering due to negative emotional arousal and elicit associated stress responses.

   There is a perceived threat to the self leading to perceived helplessness in the face of threat and exhaustion of psychological & personal resources for coping with that threat[2]. This suffering is different from pain by affecting ability to cope, depletion of physical, psychological & social resources.

3. **Psychological factors** – Psychological factors enhance pain severity. Thus the relation between pain severity and disease pathology is not in a linear fashion. The cancer related pain has higher level of perceived disability & fear responses, reducing their activity and leading to hopelessness & depression Consequences of Pain and depression in Cancer Patients.
   1. Suffering – significant contribution in major organic disease
   2. Medical evaluation and disease can be complicated
   3. Outcome & severity are adversely affected.
   4. Recovery and compliance is delayed
   5. Suicidal tendency due to undetected depression
   6. Pain when poorly managed leads to reactive depression in life threatening disease.

APPROACH TO THE PATIENT
1. Knowledge of the temporal aspects of pain – acute, chronic or incidental
2. Understanding of the physiological mechanism – Somatic, Visceral & Neuropathic.
3. Identifying the types of patients with pain.
4. Diagnosis of cancer pain syndrome.

ASSESSMENT APPROACH [1]
1. Believe the patients complaint of pain.
2. Take a careful history of pain complaint.
3. Assess the characteristics, site, pattern, aggravating & relieving factors of pain.
4. Clarify the temporal aspects of pain, acute, sub acute, chronic, and intermittent.
5. Assess type of patient – psychological state & degree of suffering.
6. Careful medical & neurological examination and monitoring.
7. Performing & reviewing the diagnostic procedures, knowledge of their limitations.
8. Evaluation of extent of disease – site, metastasis, stages periodically
9. Defining & treating specific pain syndromes.
10. Treat the pain to facilitate necessary work up.
11. Provide continuity of care from evaluation to treatment to ensure patient's compliance & to reduce anxiety, using single prescribers.
12. Individualize the management approach to the needs of the patient.

13. Informed consent explaining the risks of treatment including opioids, neurolysis, etc.

PAIN MANAGEMENT

1. WHO 3 – step ladder for pain relief is the most commonly used method of starting simple analgesics at first, than switching over to opioids & adjuvant in moderate pain.
2. The severe pain needs neurosurgical interventions e.g. patient controlled analgesia (PCA). The PCA offers patients a sense of control over their pain and is preferred over by most patients to intermittent injections.
3. Spinal analgesia using epidural opioid or analgesic adjuvant injected intermittently or infused continuous through a catheter of implantable infusion pump device.
4. Intermittent continuous local neural blockade e.g. intercostal, deep cervical, stellate, intra pleural, brachial & peripheral nerve blocks using analgesic ajuvants or neurolytics.
5. Physical agents e.g. massage application of hot or cold, TENS & others.
6. Cognitive behavioral interventions e.g. relaxation, distraction bio feedback pain imagery. These methods reduce pain and anxiety but do not substitute pharmacological management.

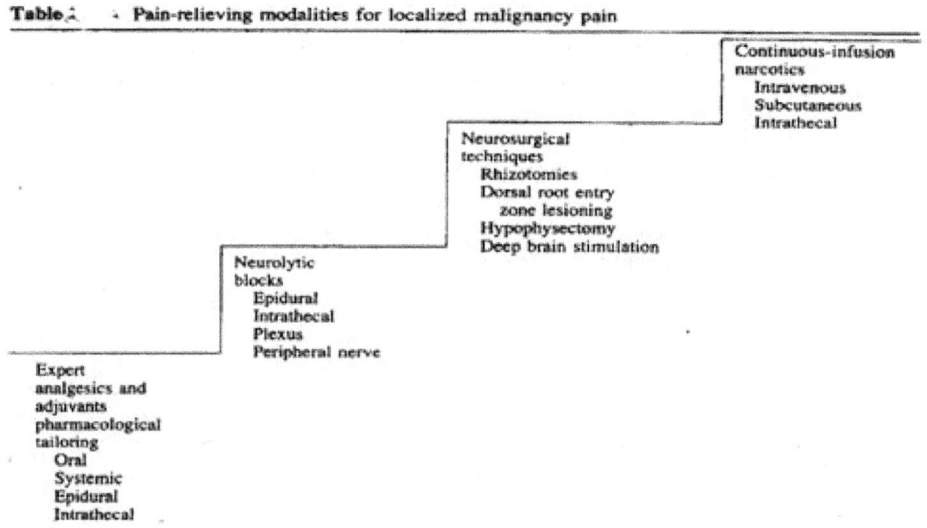

Table : - Pain-relieving modalities for localized malignancy pain

Pain syndromes in cancer- Acute pain is related to diagnostic and therapeutic interventions, while chronic pain is caused by direct tumour infiltration[2].

1) Acute pain associated with diagnostic interventions.
   Lumbar puncture headache
   Transthorasic needle biopsy
   Arterial & venous blood sampling
   Bone marrow biopsy, percutaneous biopsy
   Colonoscopy
   Myelography
   Thoracocentesis
   1. Acute post operative pain after
   Pleurodesis
   Tumour embolisation
   Suprapubic catheterization
   Inter costal catheter
   Nephrostomy insertion
2) Acute pain associated with analgesic technique
   Local anaesthetic infiltration
   Opioid injections
   Opioid headache
   Spinal opioid hyperalgesia syndrome
   Strontium – 89 induced pain flare
3) Pain associated with chemotherapy

Intravenous infusion pain due to venospasm, phlebitis
Hepatic artery infusion, intrathecal methotrexate meningitis
Intra peritoneal chemotherapy pain
Bone pain, colony induced chest, palmer, gynecomastia, digital ischemia pain, mucositis, perineal discomfort, peripheral neuropathy, joint pain.
4) Corticosteroid induced pain
5) Pain associated with hormonal therapy
   Leutinising hormone releasing factor tumour flares in prostate cancer
   Hormone induced pain flare in breast cancer
6) Immunotherapy- Interferon-induced acute pain
7) Radiotherapy induced pain
   Incident pains associated with positioning
   Esophageal mucositis
   Acute radiation enteritis and proctocolitis
   Early onset brachial plexopathy
   Radiation myelopathy
   Strontium-89 induced pain flare
8) Infection associated herpetic neuralgia
9) Pain associated with vascular events- thrombosis in limbs, superior vena caval obstruction.

Tumour related chronic pain

Bone pain – metastasis, marrow expansion, vertebrae C_7-T_1, T_{12}-L_1, sacrum, joints
Muscle cramps and skeletal muscle tumours
Headache and facial pain-intracerebral, base of skull metastasis, IX N.neuralgia
Ear & Eye syndromes- otalgia, eye pain.
Peripheral nervous system- radioculopathy, herpes, plexopathy
Visceral pain – hepatic, retroperitoneal, intestinal obstruction, peritoneal, Perineal Pelvic floor neuralgia – adrenal, ureteric, ovarian & lung cancer pain
Tumour related gynecomastia

CANCER THERAPY ASSOCIATED CHRONIC PAIN

Post chemotherapy- peripheral neuropathy, avascular necrosis of femur & humerus
Post surgical- after mastectomy, radical neck dissection, thoracotomy, phantom stump pain, pelvic floor myalgia & frozen shoulder.

CHRONIC POST RADIATION PAIN

Plexopathy – brachial, Lumbosacral, peripheral nerve tumour induced by radiation
Chronic radiation myelopathies.
Chronic radiation induced enteritis & proctitis
Burning perineum, bone necrosis

Pain intensity scores[1]
1. Patient self reports continuously in adults should take precedence
2. Simple descriptive pain intensity scale of no pain, mild, moderate & severe, worst possible (verbal descriptor scale)
3. Visual analogue scale- A graphic rating scale using a ten centimeter baseline with no pain at one end (0) to worst possible pain. The frequency and evaluation of self report with VAS should be done in any new pain or changes in pattern.

```
0_____10
No pain                                worst possible pain
```

MULTIDIMENSIONAL PAIN SCORES

Numeric rating scale – A number is assigned to intensity of pain on a scale of 0 to 10; with 0 reflecting no pain and 10 reflecting the worst possible pain. This score is easy to work with in clinical settings

0   1   2   3   4   5   6   7   8   9   10

RADIOLOGICAL INVESTIGATIONS
1. Plain film radiography e.g. for breast cancer and skeletal metastasis, in later Scintigraphy, bone scan with tracer isotope may be better with SPECT.
2. CT scan- more sensitive for detection of destructive bone lesions.
3. M.R.I. - is highly sensitive to skeletal metastasis especially in bone marrow, M.R.I. differentiates between traumatic and pathological compressions and delineates the whole spine.
4. F DG- PET scanning is an area of current research.

HOSPICE CARE IN CANCER PATIENTS
In medieval period Hospices were shelters for the pilgrims. Hospice programs take bedside care of the dying by ensuring continuity of care across home and inpatient settings. The programmes address needs of patient's pain which left unattended can lead to hopelessness and disability along with patient's family who are emotionally and physically depleted.

AIMS OF INTRACTABLE CANCER PAIN IN HOSPICE[1]
1. Identify cause to better treat.
2. Prevent pain- anticipate and prevent rather than treat.
3. Erase pain memory – thus decrease the dosage.
4. An unclouded sensorium.
5. Normal effect relate to environment.
6. Decrease of suffering, increase function & setting therapeutic goals with the help of family.

The hospice model of pain management is as per WHO three step ladders using following methods by a physician, nurse, family and social workers.
1) Drugs 2) Neural blockade 3) Neuroaugmentive- TENS 4) Physical/occupational therapy- exercise, hot/cold applications. 5) Behavioral: Hypnosis, imagery, relaxation, prayer. 6) Symptom treatment – constipation, vomiting, diarrhea, bedsores.

Central place of family- In 80% of patient days of care, family members are involved. The family members are helped by nurses, counselors, social workers. There should be one or more people on call for emergencies 24 hours a day.

The terminally ill patient relies heavily on family members for toilet, bath, medications & the fear of being alone. Adult sons, daughters, relatives, neighbors all are expected to play particular roles depending on their jobs & personal ties to the family.

Psychological & spiritual support: The social workers, priests can listen to fears, worries, help clear planning and control the fear, anger, forgiveness to the patient & the family members. They provide bereavement services & transport, cremation for the dead patient.

The palliative care in the hospice enhances comfort & improves the quality of the patients' life. The disease has taken over and the goal of controlling its spread is no longer realistic.

PROTOCOL OF HOSPICE PROGRAMME
1. Support staff members of the team meet the patients & family.
2. Proper authorization by physicians for treatment of pain and related symptoms.
3. Informed consent about protocols of hospice management.
4. Radiotherapy- No active treatment, only conservative radiotherapy on an as needed basis for pain & disease control.
5. Chemotherapy, IV antibiotics, blood transfusions, hyper alimentation.
6. Intravenous hydration if tube feeding fails.
7. Minor colostomy can be performed for relief of symptoms.
8. Oxygen- can be used as a comfort measure.

REASONS FOR HOSPICE CARE
1. A perception of physicians & patients that technology would overcome disease and death always leads to disappointments in terminally ill.
2. Health profession not geared to deal with treatment failure.
3. Obligation to dying patient and family not fulfilled by therapy.
4. Care during active treatment re-emphasized

Hospice ownership-
Hospital owned-46%,
Independent-35%,
Community-25%.

Types of Hospice care-
Home care, 56%
Inpatient + home care- 31%

REFERENCES:
1. American society of anesthesiologist's Task force on pain management. Cancer pain section. Anesthesiology. 1996; 84: 1243-1257.
2. Wall PD & Melzack R. Textbook of pain. 4th edition. Churchil-Livingstone, Edinburgh, 2001; 1018-1019.

CHAPTER 37.
PALLIATIVE CARE: SPECIAL PROBLEMS

Hydration and feeding

There is sometimes an overwhelming need for relative and staff to give patient water and food .this natural feeling should not be allowed to override the patients need for comfort. There is no evidence that symptoms of experimental water deprivation or hyponatremia are seen in patients with advanced cancer.[1] Indeed, intravenous hydration can be distressing and in a very ill patient some dehydration can actually improve comfort. Urinary output drops so reducing the need for catheterization, and troublesome bronchial secretion lessen. In bowel obstruction gastric secretions are less , so reducing both vomiting frequency and the need for nasogastric suction .energy requirement are usually so low and anorexia so complete that feeding is unnecessary .

There are special circumstances, however, when hydration and feeding is both possible and reasonable .these are usually patients with the neurological problems with swallowing. Some of these patients may still have many months of life that they wish to live to the full. In contrast, by the time patients with oesophageal or gastric tumours have completely obstructed they are usually far too ill for feeding or hydration to be justified.

Assistance with feeding

In patients with neuromuscular dysphagia it is possible with practice and patience to help some patients to swallow by positioning, manual pressure at specific points and the gentle use of droppers to deliver fluids.

Clinifeed tube

This is a fine bore; soft and self lubricating nasogastric tube which is usually well tolerated by patient's .the tube is too soft to allow aspiration of the gastric contents and needs a wire introducer to stiffen it sufficiently to allow easy passage. It can pass into the trachea during insertion and gastric placement should be confirmed by:
1. A chest X ray (when the tip should be below the diaphragm),
2. Injecting 20 ml air into the tube (when bubbling should be heard over the stomach with a stethoscope).
Of the two methods chest x ray is preferable.

Pharyngostomy may be useful in the very few patients requiring lengthy nasogastric feeding because of swallowing or feeding difficulties. It can be performed under a short GA and results in a small permanent fistula below the jaw angle into which a fine bore feeding tube can be easily inserted.

Diabetes in advanced cancer
Drug requirements

The need for hypoglycemic agents usually reduces as the disease progresses. Reduced food intake and weight loss are major factor. The aim of treatment changed from preventing future complication to preventing symptomatic hypoglycemia or hyperglycemia. Acceptable blood glucose ranges are wider, 6-12 millimole /litre fasting and 8-20mmol/l none fasting.

Noninsulin dependent diabetics can usually reduce and even stop their oral hypoglycemic drugs without symptomatic hyperglycemia occurring.
Insulin dependent diabetics may wish to simplify bd or tds regimens to long acting once daily insulin such as ultratard. Postprandial blood glucose peaks of upto 20mmol/l may be well tolerated. This is preferable to distressing symptoms of repeated hypoglycemia and insulin requirement can often be halved. As the disease progresses insulin requirement will drop further. It is not necessary to continue insulin in patient comatose because of their cancer.

Diabetes and corticosteroids

Corticosteroids induced diabetes: latent diabetes may become hyperglycemic on corticosteroid but are usually asymptomatic. Thrust and Polyurea can be treated with diet if the patient still has an adequate intake. A short acting oral hypoglycemic such as tolbutamide bd may be needed.

Non-insulin dependent diabetics already on an oral hypoglycemic may do better once daily insulin if the hyperglycemia is symptomatic. The simplest regimen is as follows:

Day 1	Insulin 20 units
Day 2	Insulin +stop oral hypoglycemic
Day3	Insulin +check fasting glucose

Thereafter: adjust insulin dose according to the fasting glucose (6-12 mmol/l)

Insulin dependant diabetics may need more insulin but at the same time insulin requirements are reducing because of reduced intake and weight loss. Consequently it is often possible to leave insulin dose unchanged.

HEAD AND NECK CANCER

Pain is the commonest complaint, followed by dysphagia (38%), airway obstruction (28%), fungating ulcer (14%) and mucosal dryness with major bleeding occurring in less than 1 %[2].

Pain

Co-analgesics are often required. Tumour expansion with small fascial compartment and nerve compression by perineural spread of tumour will respond to high dose dexamethasone.pain from local bone invasion is treated in the same way as bone metastasis with a combination of analgesic and NSAIDs.infection is often present and the resulting pain may respond to antibiotic. Nerve destruction is likely in locally invasive lesions and may respond to amitriptyline. Nerve blocks can be of help, especially in brachial plexus involvement. Radiotherapy should always be considered.

Dysphagia

This may be due to tumour obstruction, neuromuscular incardination due to Perineural spread of tumour, or splinting of the pharynx by fibrosis and local tumour. Short term relief can be achieved from high dose dexamethasone and radiotherapy. Dysphagia due to esophageal candidiasis is easily treated. It is now always helpful to feed or hydrate very ill patient but when this is appropriate fine bore tube feeding system or even a pharyngostomy are well tolerated.

Airway obstruction

Strider due to tracheal obstruction by tumour is frightening to the patient and needs urgent treatment. High dose dexamethasone starting with 8 mg IV stat, followed by radiotherapy is the treatment of choice. Fortunately obstruction usually develops over several days, making urgent tracheostomy unnecessary .referral for excision /vaporizations by carbon di oxide laser should be considered if this is available.

Fungating ulcers

Once the area is cleaner and has less odour there may be a large fascial defect or an orocutaneous fistula which leaks saliva, water and food needing frequent dressing changes. Silastic foam comes as a liquid which is mixed with a catalyst (0.2ml catalyst to every 10ml silastic foam) and poured into cavity. a soft , well fitted sponges formed which is comfortable , cosmetically preferable to bulky dressings , and easily washed .to prevent the liquid from the pharynx before it has set , "cling film " can be fitted in and around the fistula , allowing the foam to be poured in with complete safety. The film peels easily away from the set sponge.

Mucosal dryness

Excessive crusting with in the nose following radiotherapy can be softening with 25% glucose in glycerol drop 8 hourly. Secretion and crust can then be loosened with steam inhalation and removed by regular normal saline douches.

Lymphoedema

Oedema due to fluid retention or a low albumin will usually respond to simple measures such as elevation and mild compression (eg shaped tubugrip) .In cancer patient's lymphoedema is due to blockade of lymphatics by malignancy or fibrosis consequent on previous radiotherapy or surgery. It can cause severe swelling, pain and loss of mobility and often needs more intensive treatment. It is a condition that can be treated.

Initial treatment consists of doing the following daily elevation of the arm or leg when sitting or resting. Gentle exercises morning and evening, elastic sleeves and stocking to be worn all day, but which can be taken off at night, and massage. More intensive treatment consists of a compression pump which gently squeezes fluid out of the arm with an inflatable sleeve or, in some centers, a combination of bandaging and massage.

The swelling may resolve in days. However it can take a year to reduce swelling especially if the lymphoedema has been present for many years. Even if the swelling has not gone down by much, the limb is often more comfortable and easier to move. Most people find they have to continue indefinitely with some treatment such as gentle exercise or wearing a sleeve or stockings. The fluid removed finds its way into general circulation and excreted by kidneys.

Swollen arms and legs are more likely to become infected and dry, cracked skin provides an entry for infection. Careful and thorough skin care is therefore essential to keep the skin supple.

Elevation

Arms: when resting in chair or bed during the day arm should be raised to shoulder height by using pillows on the arm rest or small table next to the chair. A sling can worsen the lymphoedema.

Legs: the leg should be up when sitting, at least level with the hips. The foot of the bed can be raised at night by 2-3 inches.

Exercise

This should be gentle, each being done 5-10 times twice a day.

Compression stocking and sleeves

Stocking and sleeves prevent fluid accumulating and give firm support; they must provide enough pressure which should be graduated, being highest at the hand or foot. Some sleeves are made to measure by fitter(in the hospital or shock). "Of the self" sleeves are usually cheaper and as effective. Some firms make half and full gloves for those patient with finger or hand swelling. Most leg stocking will take care of foot swelling.

When fitting ensures that there are no crease or wrinkles, and never roll the tops over since this area will act like elastic bands. Initially it is best to wear the stocking / sleeves all days, but taking it off at night. After a few months it may be possible to leave them off for a few hours. If a separate mitten is used it should never be taken off while the sleeve is still on.

Massage

Massage stimulates the lymphatics near the skin to drain fluid more efficiently and helps to relieve discomfort. The simplest method is to use a hand held electric body massager, the massager comes with an assortment of detachable heads, but the smooth, rounded head need to be used. No lubricant should be applied. Switch to the lowest setting the massager is rested on the skin with gentle pressure and moved in a circular motion. Massage should start on the unaffected side, front and back, moving across to affected side and down the affected to the fingers or toes, concentrating on the root of a limb.

Compression pumps

These are only needed for swelling that is resolving slowly. They are powered from the mains and intermittently pump up an inflatable sleeve into which the limb has been placed. In the first week the pressure is gradually built up from 30mm of hg for 30 minutes once daily to 60 mm hg 60 minutes twice daily. When using pump keep the limb elevated and support it on pillow. It is best to remove a compression sleeve or stocking when using a pump, but if they are left the pump pressure should be reduced to 40mm hg. Larger pumps with sequentially inflated sleeves can be used in resistant cases.

Cellulitis
This should be suspected in a limb which is red, feels hotter or if the patients complain of acute pain, a burning sensation and feels unwell. Phenoxymethyl penicillin (penicillin V) 500 mg 6 hourly (or erythromycin500mg 6 hourly) should be started immediately, continuing on half this dose after one week for at least 6 weeks.

Skin care and general advise
The patient should be advised that careful skin care is essential to prevent an entry of an infection, with consequent risk of cellulites .care includes protection in gloved in garden or kitchen, prompt antiseptic care of cuts and scratches, avoiding direct sun light or heat, care when manicuring nails, using moisturizing cream at night, avoid shaving with wet razors, and wearing a thimble when sewing. The limb should be used as normally as possible but the patient should not carry heavy shopping with an affected arm or do any exercise actively that makes the limb tired or uncomfortable. Restrictive clothing is best avoided. Finally injections, blood pressure reading or blood samples should not be taken from the affected limb,

References:

1. Billings JA. Comfort measures for the terminally ill. Is hydration painful? American Geriatrics Journal, 1985; 33(11): 808-810.
2. Aird DW. Clinical care in head and neck cancer patients, ENT Journal 1983; 62: 10-30.

CHAPTER 38.
Children and elderly patients

SYMPTOM CONTROL IN CHILDREN WITH CANCER

As with the adults, a trusting relationship, together with the maintenance of a reassuring environment is the keystone to effective symptom control in children. This section, however, deals only with the physical control of the commoner symptoms.

Pain

An understanding of child development is essential, particularly when confirming the presence of pain in the pre-school child. It is necessary to look for secondary effects such as the different quality of a cry, irritability, anorexia, insomnia or anxiety. Patients are usually the best judges. Diagnosing the cause of the pain will depend on skillful interpretation of the previous history, symptoms and signs.

Analgesics choice: The principle of the analgesic staircase should be used. Starting doses are shown below. It should be noted that children aged 0-1 are more sensitive to morphine than older children aged 7-15[1] It is not unusual for children aged 6 and above to require 'adult 'doses of 5-30 mg or more 4 hourly.

Table 1: **Starting doses for analgesics in children**

Drug	Frequency	0-1	2-5	6-12	13-16
Non-opioids					
Aspirin (dispersible)	4 hourly		75mg	150mg	300mg
Paracetamol(tabs, elixir)	4 hourly	60mg	120mg	250mg	500mg
Weak opioids					
Codeine(tabs, syrup)	4 hourly		0.2mg/kg	0.5mg/kg	15mg
Dihydrocodiene(elixir)	4 hourly			0.5mg/kg	30mg/kg
Strong opioids					
Morphine sulphate(soln)	4 hourly	0.15mg/kg	3mg	5mg	10mg
Diamorphine HCL(soon ,tabs)	4 hourly	0.1mg/kg	2mg	3mg	5mg
Controlled released morphine sulphate(MST tabs)	12 hourly		10mg	20mg	30mg

1. The starting doses for strong opioids assume the child was previously on a weak opioid.
2. Increased bedtime doses will usually avoid the need for 2 am doses
3. Laxative should always be prescribed prophylactically.
4. A routine antiemetic is not needed. If nausea or vomiting occur on an opioid use haloperidol.
5. Controlled –release morphine (MST) 5 mg tablets are available on a named patient basis.
6. As with adults there are indications for nepenthe or the brompton mixture.
7. There can be no indications for using other opioids.
8. Children aged 0-1 who are inadequately controlled on paracetamol can be switched directly to oral morphine at the doses shown.

DRUG PRESENTATION AND ROUTES OF ADMINISTRATION

Constant care and a little imagination are essential when selecting appropriate routes of administration. Contrary to manufacture's belief, children often prefer tables to sickly-sweat syrups and elixirs. The taste of solutions and soluble tablets can be improved if mixed with a fizzy drink or fruit juice. Sublingual preparations are not usually well tolerated and are impractical for young children .the rectal route provides effective and rapid absorption .Subcutaneous infusions using portable, battery –driven pump can also be used.

Co analgesic

NSAIDs and corticosteroid have the indications for pain relief as in adults. Typical doses are as follows

Co-analgesia in children

Drugs	Frequency 0-1	2-5	6-12	13-16
NSAIDs Aspirin Naproxen	4 hourly 12hourly	75 mg -	150mg 10mg/kg	300mg 250mg
Corticosteroids Dexamethasone (low dose) Dexamethasone (high dose)	Mane Mane and lunch time	0.5-1mg 2 mg	1-2mg 3mg	2-4mg 4-16mg

Steroid –induced Cushing's can be severe in children and doses must be reduced to the minimum required to control symptoms.

Constipation

Co-danthramer can be made more palatable in a milk shake or by adding fizzy fruit juice. Alternatives are mixing the contents of a co-danthramer capsule with ice-cream, or fruit flavored co-danthramer ice-lollies. Co-danthrusate capsules or senna are solid alternatives, but their relative potencies must be taken into account .Docusate (tablets or syrup) is a weak contact laxative which offers a milder alternative in children.

Bronchial secretions

As in adults this can be eased with Hyoscine hydrobromide

Table 2: Hyoscine hydrobromide in children

Drugs	Frequency	0-1	2-5	6-12	13-16
Hyoscine hydro bromide	2 hourly PRN	15mcg/kg	150mcg	300mcg	30-600mcg

Nausea and vomiting

Table 3: Antiemetics choices and doses are as follows

Drug	Frequency	0-1	2-5	6-12	13-16
Acting on CTZ Haloperidol(tabs, elixir)	12 hrly	25mcg/kg	200mcg	400mcg	1.5 mg
Acting on vomiting center Cyclizine(tabs,inj,suppos)	8 hrly	1mg/kg	12.5 mg	25 mg	50 mg
Acting on upper gut Domperidone(tabs,susp) Domperidone(suppos)	8 hrly 8 hrly	0.1 mg/kg 0.2 mg/kg	1 mg 3 mg	5 mg 15 mg	10 mg 30 mg

1. Low doses of Cyclizine need to be given parenterally.the via a continuous sc infusion pump.
2. Chlorpromazine is an alternative if greater sedation is required.
3. Metoclopramide is not recommended because of increase risk of extra pyramidal side effects in children.

Agitation

When a calm reassuring environment is insufficient to settle a child, psycho tropic **drugs, may** be necessary. Physical causes of agitation such as pain must be excluded if possible. Drug choices and doses are as follows.

Table 4: Drugs for agitation

Drugs	Frequency	0-1	2-5	6-12	13-16
haloperidol (tabs,inj,elixir)	12 hrly	25 mcg/kg	200 mcg	400 mcg	1.5 mg
diazepam (tabs,elixir,suppos,inj)	nocte	0.2 mg/kg	2-4 mg	5-10 mg	5-40 mg
chlorpromazine (tabs,syrup,suppos)	8 hrly	0.5 mg/kg	5-10 mg	10-25 mg	25-100 mg

Initial doses may have to be repeated until the child settles haloperidol is the least sedative of choice Diazepam if given rectally, the sodium solution is absorbed more rapidly than the suppositories.repeated use of this Inj. Locally may cause rectal irritation. Diazepam can accumulate and the consequent drowsiness can be mistakenly attributed to cancer.

ELDERLY CANCER PATIENTS

Pain considerations in elderly patients [2].

1. Elderly patients often suffer multiple chronic, painful illness and take multiple medications e.g. for ischemic heart disease, diabetes, etc. They are at greater risk for drug-drug and drug- disease interactions.
2. Pain assessment present unique problems in elderly since these patients may exhibit physiological, psychological and cultural changes associated with pain.
3. Physicians and elderly patients consider pain to be a normal part of aging. There is a belief that pain can not be relieve and elderly patients are stoic in reporting.]
4. Age nee not alter pain thresholds or tolerance. The similarities of pain experience between elderly and younger patients are far more common than are the differences.
5. Cognitive impairment, delirium and dementia are serious barriers to assessing pain in the elderly. Sensory problems such as visual and hearing changes may also interfere with the use of some of the pain assessment scales. However the clinicians should be able to obtain an accurate self report of pain from most patients.
6. NSAIDs can be used safely in elderly patients, but their use requires vigilance for side effects especially gastric and renal toxicity. Opioids are safe & effective when used appropriately in elderly patients; however elderly patients are more sensitive to analgesic effects of opiate drugs, experience higher peak effect and longer duration of pain relief. (Acute pain management. Operative procedures, USA)

Analgesics may be given safely to geriatric patients, although adjustments of doses are usually required e.g. plasma levels of Tricyclic antidepressants are usually higher for a given dose in older as compared to younger patients. I.m. morphine produces longer duration of analgesia in older patients, in part related to prolonged elimination from blood in the elderly[3]. In addition, elderly as well as younger patients with central nervous system disease may be more sensitive to opioids. So the titration of analgesic dose to a given response is even more critical in such patients.

The age does not decrease pain perception & sensitivity in the elderly, although emotional suffering related to pain may be less in older patients. The psychosocial factors affecting pain treatment are[2]

Dementia or memory impairment in the elderly leads to cognitive impairment, are unable to attend OPD alone and require special considerations for assessment and treatment

There is a significant social, psychological & physical activity limitation in the old patients

The rule for pharmacological interventions in the elderly is to start low & go slow in view of various diseases existing, or drug interactions. A nurse assisted PCA is effective with none cognitively impaired patients.

Involvement of family and friends in the treatment of old patients helps in treatment compliance and psychosocial problems, especially when there are a cognitive impairment & daily activity limitations.

REFERENCES:
1. Dahlstorm, Dohle B. Morphine kinetics in children. Clinical Pharm. And Therapeutics.1979; 26(3):354-365.
2. Harkins SW, Price D et al. Geriatric pain. In: Textbook of pain. Wall PD& Melzack R (Eds), 3rd Edition, Churchill Livingstone, Edinburgh, 1994; 769-783.
3. Kaiko RF, Wallelnstein SZ, Rogers AG et al. Narcotics in the elderly. Med. Clinic North America 1982; 66: 1079-1089.

CHAPTER 39.

Cancer therapeutics

As a patient becomes semiconscious due to the cancer, prescribing requirements will change.

The oral route becomes impractical and the need for some drugs will change or cease.

RATIONALIZING DRUGS IN THE LAST DAYS AND HOURS

Table 1: Prescribing in the last hours or days

Drug	Suggested change	Consider
Analgesics Paracetamol, aspirin,, Weak opioids Strong opioids	Stop Diamorphine sc 5-10mg 4 hrly diamorphine sc 4 hrly at equivalent do dose	Diamorphine sc 2.5mg PRN. Sc infusion of Diamorphine.
NSAID'S Eg.flurbiprofen	Stop	Diamorphine sc 2.5mg PRN
Corticosteroids Eg.dexamethasone	Stop	-
Laxatives Eg.co-danthramer	Stop	-
Anti emetics Haloperidol Cyclizine Metoclopramide	Continue by sc Injection or infusion -do- -do-	Prochlorperazine pr Cyclizine PR Chlorpromazine PR Domperidone PR
Psychotropic drugs Temazepam, Nitrazepam, Diazepam Haloperidol Chlorpromazine Antidepressants	Diazepam PR Cont.by sc injection Or infusion. Chlorpromazine PR Stop	Chlorpromazine PR Diazepam PR -do- -
Anticonvulsants	Diazepam PR 5-10 Mg 4-8hrly.	-
Anti infective	Stop	Alternative treatment For bronchial secretion
Cardiovascular Anti arrhythmic Diuretics	Stop Stop	- -
Other drugs Bronchodilators Insulin, Hypoglycemics Iron and vitamins	Stop Stop Stop	Hyoscine sc 0.4-0.8 mg 8th hourly

SUBCUTANEOUS INFUSION PUMPS
Should parenteral administration be necessary, repeated injections can be distressing. To the patient, nurse and family, and difficult to organize in the home continuous sc
Infusion is a suitable alternative.

Drugs: diamorphine, morphine sulfate. Hyoscine and Metoclopramide can be used safely.
cyclizine and methotrimeperazine occasionally cause local irritation. Chlorpromezine
Prochlorperazine and diazepam are too irritant and should never be used in an S.C. infusion pump.

DRUG INTERACTIONS

There are many such drug interactions but those below are probably of most importance to patients

Table 2: Drug interactions with advanced cancer

Drug affected	Interacting drug(s)	Effect
Analgesics		
paracetamol, aspirin	metoclopramide	Raised peak blood Levels
diamorphine	pentazocine	Reduced analgesia
	CNS sedatives	Increased risk of Sedation.
Steroids		
corticosteroids	Loop diuretics, thiazides, phenytoin, carbamazepine	Hypokalemia
	aminoglutethemide	Decreased effect of steroids
dexamethasone		Decreased effect
Anti emetics		
chlorpromazine	propranolol	Increased blood Levels
	antacids	Decreased Absorption
cyclizine		
phenothiazines	phenothiazines, tricyclics.	Increased anti cholinergic side effects
metoclopramide	Anti-cholinergic Drugs with anti cholinergic effects (tricyclics,cpz)	antagonism of Metoclopramide stimulation of upper gut
	opioids	increase in peak blood level of opioids
	haloperidol	extra pyramidal Side effects.
Anticonvulsants		
carbamazepine	dextro-propozyphene, cimetidine	Potentiation.
phenytoin	cimetidine, co trimoxazole, diazepam.	Potentiation.
CNS sedatives		
diazepam	cimetidine	Increased blood Levels
chlormethiazole	cimetidine	Potentiation.
Cardio vascular Drugs		
digoxin	bumetanide, furosemide, thiazides	Increased toxicity Due to potassium depletion
	cholestyramine	Decreased Absorption
bumetanide furosemide	corticosteroids indomethacin	Antagonism due to Fluid retention

beta blockers	corticosteroids NSAIDs	Hypokalemia Reduced anti hypertensive effects
Blood iron(oral)	Antacids, tetracycline	Decreased absorption
Anti-infective ketoconazole metronidazole	Antacids, anti cholinergic, Cimetidine Alcohol	Decreased absorption disulfiram reaction

Table 3: Common drug doses and side effects

Drug	Dosage	Side effects
acyclovir	P.O. 200mg 6hrly (for 5 days)	Rashes, transient rise in urea/creat
amitriptyline	P.O. 50-150 mg nocte	Sedation, dry mouth, constipation
aspirin	P.O. 600mg 4 hrly	GI irritation hypersensitivity
baclofen	P.O. 5-30mg 8 hrly after food	Drowsiness, fatigue, confusion hypotension, nausea
benzydamine	As a rinse or gargle 15 ml 2hrly	Local numbness
bethanechol	10-30 mg 8th hrly	Nausea vomiting, sweating, blurred vision, colic, Bradycardia
bisacodyl	P.O./P.R.10 mg after food	Colic.local rectal irritation
bumetanide	P.O. 1mg daily in morning	Polyurea+ loss
buprenorphine	S.L. 1-2 tablets 6-8 hrly	Nausea vomiting
chlorpromazine	P.O. 25-100 mg 4-8 .Hrly P.R. 100 mg 6th hrly	Extra pyramidal symptoms, anti cholinergic effects, hypotension (rare jaundice)
cholestyramine	P.O. 4g in water 6 th hrly	Constipation, anorexia, nausea, Colic rashes.
cimetidine	P.O. 400 mg bd or 800 mg nocte	Confusion, reduced hepatic metabolism
co danthromer	P.O. 10 ml syrup- 10 ml forte syrup bd	Colic perianal rash
co danthrusate	P.O. 1 nocte to 3- 8th hrly	Colic perianal rash
cyclizine	P.O. 50mg 4-8 hrly	Dry mouth, drowsiness, head ache
dantrolene	P.O. 25mg daily upto 100 mg 6th hrly	Weakness.fatigue,nausea, vomiting

		Drowsiness
dexamethasone	Low dose P.O. 2-4mg daily (low dose 12-15mg) no later than 6pm	Obesity.moonface candidiasis
diazepam	P.O. 5-20mg at night	Drowsiness confusion ,poor Co ordination, subjective change in voice
diflunisal	250-500mg bd with food	Nausea ,constipation, Colic, diarrhea
dihydrocodiene	30-60mg 4-6 hrly	Constipation ,vomiting
dimethicone	As asilone 10ml 4-6 hrly	-
distigmine	5-20mg before break fast	Gi irritation ,salivation
docusate sodium	100-200mg 8 hrly	Diarrhea ,colic
domperidone	P.O. 10mg 8hrly/pr 60mg 8hrly	Galactorrhoea ,Gynaeco mastia (long term)
flurbiprofen	P.O. 50-100mg bd	Gi irritation ,hypersensitivity
frusemide	P.O. 50-80mg mane	Polyurea , k+loss,rashes
haloperidol	P.O. 1.5mg-10mg nocte	Extra pyramidal symptoms
hyoscine hydro bromide	S.L/P.O. 0.3-0.8mg 6-8hrly	Drowsiness, dry mouth, blurred Vision ,ileus ,constipation, difficulty micturating
ketoconazole	P.O. 200mg mane For 1 wk	Nausea,constipation,rashses, Itching
loperamide	2-4mg PRN(max 16mg daily)	Nausea ,dizziness, dry mouth
metoclopramide	S.C/P.O. 10mg 4-8hrly	Extra pyramidal effects,sedation,diarrhea, Dizziness
mianserin	P.O. 30-90mg nocte	Mild anticholinergic effects
morphine	Median=20mg 4hrly	Nausea, vomiting, constipation
nystatin	P.O. 100,000units 4hrly	-
paracetamol	P.O. 0.5-1gm 4-6hrly	Rare-skin rashes
phenoxybenzamine	P.O. 10mg nocte	Tachycardia, postural hypotension Dizziness, lassitude
prochlorperazine	P.O. 5-10mg 8hrly/im 12.5mg6hrly	Drowsiness, dry mouth
propantheline	P.O. 15-3omg8hrly	Anticholinergic effects
spironolactone.the	100-200mg mane	Gi irritation, high k+, Gynaeco mastia
temazepam	P.O. 10-60mg nocte	Morning drowsiness
tetracycline (intrapleural)	500mg in 20mls 0.5% bupivacaine	Transient local pain, pyrexia

REFERENCES:

1. Wall PD & Melzack R. Textbook of pain. 4th edition. Churchil-Livingstone, Edinburgh, 2001; 1018-1019.
2. Kumar Pramod. A Hand Book of Management of pain and related symptoms in cancer, New Delhi, Samvedana, 2003.
3. Kumar Pramod. Terminal cancer care. 2nd Ed New Delhi Modern publishers, 2005.
4. Kumar Pramod-Textbook of Pain, 2nd Ed, CBS Pub New Delhi 2008.

CHAPTER 40.

PROTOCOL FOR MALIGNANT PAIN THERAPY

TREATMENT OF CANCER PAIN
Unrelieved pain causes suferring, anger, anxiety, fear, depression and suicidal tendencies. Relief ensures good quality of life.

BASIC PRINCIPLES AND APPROACH TO CANCER PAIN MANAGEMENT
By modifying the source of pain by treating the cancer: surgery, radiation bone
Metastases, chemotherapy
By altering the central perception of pain: analgesics, anti depressants, anxiolytics
By interfering with nociceptive transmission within the CNS: neuraxial analgesia
Neuroablation
Psychological care
Alternative pain management strategies: acupuncture, TENS.
Immobilization: rest, cervical collar.

Assessment of cancer pain:
Comprehensive assessment is required.
- Type
- Intensity
- Pain source.
- Psychological factors.
- Assessment of treatment/pain relief.

WHO ANALGESIC LADDER: (Revised in 1996)
Simple and effective method for controlling cancer pain by oral administration of analgesics including oral morphine,
Effective pain relief is achieved in 75-90% of patients.
Alternative methods.-11%
Freedom from pain
Strong opioid
Non-opioid
Severe pain 3
Adjuvant
Mild opioid+/- NSAIDs
Moderate pain 2
NSAIDs
Mild pain 1

ORAL OPIOID THERAPY
First line approach for patients with moderate to severe pain
Principles of drug therapy for cancer pain
By the mouth
By the clock
By the ladder
For the individual
Attention to detail is vital.
Dose titration = right dose=adequate pain relief with minimal side effects

Transdermal fentanyl (duragesic patch) provides continuous transdermal delivery pf fentanyl for 72 hrs. First line modality for moderate to severe pain.

Adjuvant drugs-tricyclics steroids (plexopathy pain) anxiolytics
Laxatives are almost always necessary with opioids.more than 50%need antiemetics

HOME CARE SERVICES:
Terminal patients
Predominant complain pain

Oral NSAIDs, tramadol:
Oral morphine
- Usual dose 50-100 mg per day.
- Rare cases 250 mg per day
- Nutritional supplementation
- Psychological support.

Drawbacks
- Retrospective
- Assessment of pain and pain relief according to pain score is not available.
- Accessible only to patients residing in Delhi

Direct drug delivery systems
Neuraxial drug delivery
Intra spinal opioid therapy

Contraindications
Thrombocytopenia
Coagulopathy
If these are present, pca with IV or sc morphine is used.

Peripheral nerve blocks
When the drugs are ineffective, nerve blocks provide effective pain relief.
Experts in nerve blocks are few and far between.

Aids -x-ray, imaging aids, CT scan.
- nerve stimulators, special electrodes, needles.
- requires hospital admission.

Training needs:
- Convince medical authorities,
- Provide adequate facility for training
- Provides platform for interaction.
- Knowledge database.

Advantages
- Effective & long lasting
- Reduces frequent visits to doctors
- Good quality of pain relief
- 50-80% patients may benefit.

Nerve blocks
1. L.A = lignocaine, bupivacaine Reduced concentrations-lignocaine 0.5%, bupivacaine 0.25%
2, Diagnostic- somatic or visceral, autonomic
3. Side effects assessment-fall in blood pressure, reduced sensation

4. To determine efficacy of neurolytic blocks.
5. Pain relief outlasts its pharmacologic action
6. disadvantages-pneumothorax, hemorrhage, infections
7. Use steroid + L.A. reduces swelling around tumour for weeks.
8. Catheters=spinal, epidural produces symptom relief for weeks.

Neurolytic blocks
Useful in terminal cancer patients
Advantage for Indian patient (rural areas)
Economically poor background
Cost effective
Longer duration of pain relief (4-6 weeks)
Stay at home
E.g. subarachnoid chemical neurolysis for gynecological and rectal malignancies.
Success rate 80%

Neurolytic agents used
- Absolute alcohol-painful, intense, recurrence
- Phenol 5-10%, biphasic, painless
- Chlorocresol
- Ammonium sulphate

Neurolytic blockade of peripheral nerves
- Use when other therapies
- Fail
- Ineffective
- Poorly tolerated
- Clinically inappropriate

Side effects
- Neuritis
- Recurrence- alcohol months
- In partial/complete denervation further chemical damage to nerve
- Dysaesthetic (neuropathic pain)

Peripheral nerve blocks
- Trigeminal
- Stellate
- Glossopharyngeal
- Intercostal
- Celiac plexus
- Hypogastric plexus

Regional neurolytic blocks
1. No neuropathic pain
2. When more extensive block needed
    - extensive growth of tumour
    - Increase in pain
3. Easy access of spinal, epidural routes

Subarachnoid neurolytic blocks
Indications- cancer of cranial nerves
- Tumour involves somatic nerves
 (Breast, abdominal wall, abdominal viscera, pelvis)

Hypobaric absolute alcohol
- Patient positioned with involved dermatomes in upper portions
- Proper positioning of operative table
- Appropriate padding
- Stability of patient position
- Needles inserted at appropriate level
- 0.10 to 0.25 ml injected at appropriate level

Leave patients for 20 minutes to consolidate block

Hyperbaric subarachnoid neurolytic block
- Phenol in 10% glycerin, prepared fresh
- Wide bored 18-21 G needles used for phenol
- Patient position- affected position downwards.
- 0.5 ml aliquots of phenol for each segment

Benzocaine
- Highly lipid soluble local analgesic
- Satisfactory analgesia
- Motor blockade, bladder/bowel dysfunction

Epidural neurolytic block
- 5-10% phenol in saline
- Used in bilateral pain.
- No motor blockade
- Useful for limb plexus block
- Slight nerve deficits
- Side effects- neuritis
  - Excessive spread
  - Accidental subarachnoid injection

Complication of S.A and epidural neurolysis
- Less pain n relief after satisfactory block
- Unplanned sensory motor deficit
- Weakness, numbness, incontinence, neuropathic pain.

Celiac plexus block
Indications-pain due to ca pancreas, git

Disadvantages
Blocks may have to be repeated after 6-8 weeks
Possibility of muscle paresis
Need of CT scans or C arm image intensifier?
Trained personal to perform the block

Neuroxial administration of narcotics and NSAIDs
- Using catheter delivery systems
- Home care possible
- Morphine side effects: pruritis, urinary retention, Respiratory depression, nausea, vomiting, delirium
- L.A side effects: weakness, numbness, fall in B.P
- Steroids in inflammatory neuropathy in epidural space
- Clonidine 2 adrenergic agonist
- Benzodiazepine in a stimulation

- NMDA antagonists
- Ion channel blocks
- NSAIDs
- Cholinesterase inhibitors

Neurosurgical ablation
- In terminal cancer with short life expectancy
- Dorsal rhizotomy-no long term effect
- Interrupt lateral spin thalamic tract of spinal chord
- 95% success rate initially,>.1yr – 25%
- N0 analgesia in cervical, upper thoracic
- Mortality 1% unilateral, 10% bilateral

Dorsal route entry zone lesioning
For refractory de afferentation pain
E.g. nerve plexus avulsion

Deep brain stimulation
- Neurosurgical implantation of electrodes
- Pain relief 30%-60%
- In peri aqueductal, peri ventricular gray matter.
- Sensory thalamus in de afferentiation pain

Radio frequency ablation
First line of treatment in chronic malignant pain syndrome
Expensive equipment required
Skilled radiologist required
Effective method of pain relief, lesion is selective, controllable
Low incidence of morbidity and mortality

Neurolytic surgical procedures
- Cryo lesioning
- Thermo coagulation of Gasserian ganglion
- Low complication, better pain relief,
- >75% success rate >9 months
- Pituitary ablation (side effect- diabetes insipid us).

REFERENCES:
1. Kumar Pramod. A Hand Book of Management of pain and related symptoms in cancer, New Delhi, Samvedana, 2003.
2. Kumar Pramod. Terminal cancer care. 2nd Ed New Delhi Modern publishers, 2005.
3. Kumar Pramod-Textbook of Pain, 2nd Ed, CBS Pub New Delhi 2008.

Annexure I

ASA Practice Guidelines for Acute Pain Management in the Perioperative Setting
An Updated Report by the American Society of Anesthesiologists Task Force on Acute Pain Management

Recommendations

I. Institutional Policies and Procedures for Providing Perioperative Pain Management

- Anesthesiologists offering perioperative analgesia services should provide, in collaboration with other healthcare professionals as appropriate, ongoing education and training to ensure that hospital personnel are knowledgeable and skilled with regard to the effective and safe use of the available treatment options within the institution. Educational content should range from basic bedside pain assessment to sophisticated pain management techniques (e.g. Anesthesiology 2012; 116:248 –73 255 Practice Guidelines epidural analgesia, PCA, and various regional anesthesia techniques) and nonpharmacologic techniques (e.g., relaxation, Imagery, hypnotic methods). For optimal pain management, ongoing education and training
- are essential for new personnel, to maintain skills, and whenever therapeutic approaches are modified.
- Anesthesiologists and other healthcare providers should use standardized, validated instruments to facilitate the regular evaluation and documentation of pain intensity, the effects of pain therapy, and side effects caused by the therapy.
- Anesthesiologists responsible for perioperative analgesia should be available at all times to consult with ward nurses, surgeons, or other involved physicians. They should assist in evaluating patients who are experiencing problems with any aspect of perioperative pain relief.
- Anesthesiologists providing perioperative analgesia services should do so within the framework of an Acute Pain Service. They should participate in developing standardized institutional policies and procedures.

II. Preoperative Evaluation of the Patient

- A directed pain history, a directed physical examination, and a pain control plan should be included in the anesthetic preoperative evaluation.

III. Preoperative Preparation of the Patient

- Patient preparation for perioperative pain management should include appropriate adjustments or continuation of medications to avert an abstinence syndrome, treatment of preexistent pain, or preoperative initiation of therapy for postoperative pain management.
- Anesthesiologists offering perioperative analgesia services should provide, in collaboration with others as appropriate, patient and family education regarding their important roles in achieving comfort, reporting pain, and in proper use of the recommended analgesic methods. Common misconceptions that overestimate the risk of adverse effects and addiction should be dispelled. Patient education for optimal use of PCA and other sophisticated methods, such as patient-controlled epidural analgesia, might include discussion of these analgesic methods at the time of the preanesthetic evaluation, brochures and videotapes to educate patients about therapeutic options, and discussion at the bedside during postoperative visits. Such education may also include instruction in behavioural modalities for control of pain and anxiety.

IV. Perioperative Techniques for Pain Management

- Anesthesiologists who manage perioperative pain should use therapeutic options such as epidural or intrathecal opioids, systemic opioid PCA, and regional techniques after thoughtfully considering the risks and benefits for the individual patient. These modalities should be used in preference to intramuscular opioids ordered "as needed."

- The therapy selected should reflect the individual anesthesiologist's expertise, as well as the capacity for safe application of the modality in each practice setting. This capacity includes the ability to recognize and treat adverse effects that emerge after initiation of therapy.
- Special caution should be taken when continuous infusion modalities are used because drug accumulation may contribute to adverse events.

V. Multimodal Techniques for Pain Management
- Whenever possible, anesthesiologists should use multimodal pain management therapy. Unless contraindicated, patients should receive an around the-clock regimen of NSAIDs, COXIBs, or acetaminophen. Regional blockade with local anesthetics should be considered.
- Dosing regimens should be administered to optimize efficacy while minimizing the risk of adverse events.
- The choice of medication, dose, route, and duration of therapy should be individualized.

VI. Patient Subpopulations
- Pediatric patients Aggressive and proactive pain management is necessary to overcome the historic undertreatment of pain in children. Perioperative care for children undergoing painful procedures or surgery requires developmentally appropriate pain assessment and therapy. Analgesic therapy should depend upon age, weight, and comorbidity, and unless contraindicated should involve a multimodal approach. Behavioral techniques, especially important in addressing the emotional component of pain, should be applied whenever feasible. Sedative, analgesic, and local anesthetics are all important components of appropriate analgesic regimens for painful procedures. Because many analgesic medications are synergistic with sedating agents, it is imperative that appropriate monitoring be used during the procedure and recovery.
- Geriatric patients Pain assessment and therapy should be integrated into the perioperative care of geriatric patients. Pain assessment tools appropriate to a patient's cognitive abilities should be used. Extensive and proactive evaluation and questioning may be necessary to overcome barriers that hinder communication regarding unrelieved pain. Anesthesiologists should recognize that geriatric patients may respond differently than younger patients to pain and analgesic medications, often because of comorbidity. Vigilant dose titration is necessary to ensure adequate treatment while avoiding adverse effects such as somnolence in this vulnerable group, who are often taking other medications (including alternative and complementary agents).
- Other subpopulations Anesthesiologists should recognize that patients who are critically ill, cognitively impaired, or have communication difficulties may require additional interventions to ensure optimal perioperative pain management. Anesthesiologists should consider a therapeutic trial of an analgesic in patients with increased blood pressure and heart rate or agitated behavior when causes other than pain have been excluded.

Appendix 2: Methods and Analyses

A. State of the Literature
For these updated Guidelines, a review of studies used in the development of the original Guidelines was combined with studies published subsequent to approval of the original Guidelines in 2003.* The scientific assessment of these Guidelines was based on evidence linkages or statements regarding potential

Annexure II

ASA Practice Guidelines for Chronic Pain Management
An Updated Report by the American Society of Anesthesiologists Task Force on Chronic Pain Management and the American Society of Regional Anesthesia and Pain Medicine

I. Patient Evaluation

All patients presenting with chronic pain should have a documented history and physical examination and an assessment that ultimately supports a chosen treatment strategy.

History:

- A pain history should include a general medical history with emphasis on the chronology and symptomatology of the presenting complaints.
- A history of current illness should include information about the onset, quality, intensity, distribution, duration, course, and sensory and affective components of the pain and details about exacerbating and relieving factors.
- Additional symptoms (e.g., motor, sensory, and autonomic changes) should be noted.
- Information regarding previous diagnostic tests, results of previous therapies, and current therapies should be reviewed by the physician.
- In addition to a history of current illness, the history should include (1) a review of available records, (2) medical history, (3) surgical history, (4) social history including substance use or misuse, (5) family history, (6) history of allergies, (7) current medications including use or misuse, and (8) review of systems. (9) The causes as well as the effects of pain (e.g., physical deconditioning, change in occupational status, and psychosocial dysfunction) and the impacts of previous treatment (s) should be evaluated and documented. Practice Guidelines Anesthesiology, V 112 • No 4 • April 2010 Practice Guidelines.

Physical examination:

The physical examination should include an appropriately directed neurologic and musculoskeletal evaluation, with attention to other systems as indicated. Psychosocial evaluation: The psychosocial evaluation should include information about the presence of psychologic symptoms (e.g., anxiety, depression, or anger), psychiatric disorders, personality traits or states, and coping mechanisms.

- An assessment should be made of the impact of chronic pain on a patient's ability to perform activities of daily living.
- An evaluation of the influence of pain and treatment on mood, ability to sleep, addictive or aberrant behavior, and interpersonal relationships should be performed.
- Evidence of family, vocational, or legal issues and involvement of rehabilitation agencies should be noted.
- The expectations of the patient, significant others, employer, attorney, and other agencies may also be considered. Interventional diagnostic procedures: Appropriate diagnostic procedures may be conducted as part of a patient's evaluation, based on a patient's clinical presentation.
- The choice of an interventional diagnostic procedure (e.g., selective nerve root blocks, medial branch blocks, facet joint injections, sacroiliac joint injections, and provocative discography) should be based on the patient's specific history and physical examination and anticipated course of treatment.
- Interventional diagnostic procedures should be performed with appropriate image guidance.
- Diagnostic medical branch blocks or facet joint injections may be considered for patients with suspected facet-mediated pain to screen for subsequent therapeutic procedures.
- Diagnostic sacroiliac joint injections or lateral branch blocks may be considered for the evaluation of patients with suspected sacroiliac joint pain.
- Diagnostic selective nerve root blocks may be considered to further evaluate the anatomic level of radicular pain.

- The use of sympathetic blocks may be considered to support the diagnosis of sympathetically maintained pain.
- They should not be used to predict the outcome of surgical, chemical, or radiofrequency sympathectomy.
- Peripheral blocks may be considered to assist in the diagnosis of pain in a specific peripheral nerve distribution.
- Provocative discography may be considered for the evaluation of selected patients with suspected discogenic pain.
- Provocative discography should not be used for the routine evaluation of the patient with chronic nonspecific back pain. Findings from the patient history, physical examination, and diagnostic evaluation should be combined to provide the foundation for an individualized treatment plan focused on the optimization of the risk– benefit ratio with an appropriate progression of treatment from a lesser to greater degree of invasiveness. Whenever possible, direct and ongoing contact should be made and maintained with the other physicians caring for the patient to ensure optimal care management.

II. Multimodal or Multidisciplinary Interventions

Multimodal interventions should be part of a treatment strategy for patients with chronic pain. A long-term approach that includes periodic follow-up evaluations should be developed and implemented as part of the overall treatment strategy. When available, multidisciplinary programs may be used.

III. Single Modality Interventions

Ablative techniques (other treatment modalities should be attempted before consideration of the use of ablative techniques): Chemical denervation (e.g., alcohol, phenol, or high concentration local anesthetics) should not be used in the routine care of patients with chronic noncancer pain. Cryoablation may be used in the care of selected patients (e.g., postthoracotomy pain syndrome, low back pain [medial branch], and peripheral nerve pain).
Thermal intradiscal procedures: IDET may be considered for young, active patients with early single-level degenerative disc disease with well-maintained disc height.

Radiofrequency ablation:

- Conventional (e.g., 80°C) or thermal (e.g., 67°C) radiofrequency ablation of the medial branch nerves to the facet joint should be performed for low back (medial branch) pain when previous diagnostic or therapeutic injections of the joint or medial branch nerve have provided temporary relief.
- Conventional radiofrequency ablation may be performed for neck pain.
- Water-cooled radiofrequency ablation may be used for chronic sacroiliac joint pain.
- Conventional or other thermal radiofrequency ablation of the dorsal root ganglion should not be routinely used for the treatment of lumbar radicular pain. Acupuncture: Acupuncture may be considered as an adjuvant to conventional therapy (e.g., drugs, physical therapy, and exercise) in the treatment of nonspecific, noninflammatory low back pain.

Blocks:

Joint blocks:

- Intraarticular facet joint injections may be used for the symptomatic relief of facet-mediated pain.
- Sacroiliac joint injections may be considered for the symptomatic relief of sacroiliac joint pain.

Nerve and nerve root blocks:

- Celiac plexus blocks using local anesthetics with or without steroids may be used for the treatment of pain secondary to chronic pancreatitis.

- Lumbar sympathetic blocks or stellate ganglion blocks may be used as components of the multimodal treatment of CRPS if used in the presence of consistent improvement and increasing duration of pain relief.
- Sympathetic nerve blocks should not be used for the longterm treatment of non-CRPS neuropathic pain.
- Medial branch blocks may be used for the treatment of facet-mediated spine pain.
- Peripheral somatic nerve blocks should not be used for long-term treatment of chronic pain.

Electrical nerve stimulation:

Neuromodulation with electrical stimulus:

- Subcutaneous peripheral nerve stimulation: Subcutaneous peripheral nerve stimulation may be used in the multimodal treatment of patients with painful peripheral nerve injuries who have not responded to other therapies.
- Spinal cord stimulation: Spinal cord stimulation may be used in the multimodal treatment of persistent radicular pain in patients who have not responded to other therapies.

Spinal cord stimulation may also be considered for other selected patients (e.g., CRPS, peripheral neuropathic pain, peripheral vascular disease, and postherpetic neuralgia).

Shared decision making regarding spinal cord stimulation should include a specific discussion of potential complications associated with spinal cord stimulator placement.

A spinal cord stimulation trial should be performed before considering permanent implantation of a stimulation device.

TENS:
- TENS should be used as part of a multimodal approach to pain management for patients with chronic back pain and may be used for other pain conditions (e.g., neck and phantom limb pain).

Epidural steroids with or without local anesthetics:
Epidural steroid injections with or without local anesthetics may be used as part of a multimodal treatment regimen to provide pain relief in selected patients with radicular pain or radiculopathy.
- Shared decision making regarding epidural steroid injections should include a specific discussion of potential complications, particularly with regard to the transforaminal approach.
- Transforaminal epidural injections should be performed with appropriate image guidance to confirm correct needle position and spread of contrast before injecting a therapeutic substance
- Image guidance may be considered for interlaminar epidural injections to confirm correct needle position and spread of contrast before injecting a therapeutic substance

Intrathecal drug therapies:

Neurolytic blocks: Intrathecal neurolytic blocks should not be performed in the routine management of patients with noncancer pain.

Intrathecal nonopioid injections:
- Intrathecal preservative-free steroid injections may be used for the relief of intractable postherpetic neuralgia nonresponsive to previous therapies.
- Ziconotide infusion may be used in the treatment of a select subset of patients with refractory chronic pain.

Intrathecal opioid injections: Intrathecal opioid injection or infusion may be used for neuropathic pain patients.

- Shared decision-making regarding intrathecal opioid injection or infusion should include a specific discussion of potential complications.
- Neuraxial opioid trials should be performed before considering permanent implantation of intrathecal drug delivery systems.

Minimally invasive spinal procedures: Minimally invasive spinal procedures (e.g., vertebroplasty) may be used for the treatment of pain related to vertebral compression fractures.

Pharmacologic management:

Anticonvulsants: Anticonvulsants (e.g., _-2-delta calciumchannel antagonists, sodium-channel antagonists, and membrane- stabilizing drugs) should be used as part of a multimodal strategy for patients with neuropathic pain.

Antidepressants:
- Tricyclic antidepressants should be used as part of a multimodal strategy for patients with chronic pain.
- Serotonin–norepinephrine reuptake inhibitors should be used as part of a multimodal strategy for a variety of chronic pain patients.
- Selective serotonin reuptake inhibitors may be considered specifically for patients with diabetic neuropathy.

Other drugs:
- As part of a multimodal pain management strategy, extended- release oral opioids should be used for neuropathic or back pain patients, and transdermal, sublingual, and immediate-release oral opioids may be used.
- For selected patients, ionotropic NMDA receptor antagonists (e.g., neuropathic pain), NSAIDs (e.g., back pain), and topical agents (e.g., peripheral neuropathic pain) may be used, benzodiazepines and skeletal muscle relaxants may be considered.

A strategy for monitoring and managing side effects, adverse effects, and compliance should be considered for all patients undergoing any long-term pharmacologic therapy.

Physical or restorative therapy:

Physical or restorative therapy may be used as part of a multimodal strategy for patients with low back pain.

Physical or restorative therapy may be considered for other chronic pain conditions.

Psychological treatment:

Cognitive behavioral therapy, biofeedback, or relaxation training:

These interventions may be used as part of a multimodal strategy for patients with low back pain, as well as for other chronic pain conditions.

Supportive psychotherapy, group therapy, or counseling: These interventions may be considered as part of a multimodal strategy for chronic pain management.

Trigger point injections: These injections may be considered for treatment of myofascial pain as part of a multimodal approach to pain management.

Appendix: Methods and Analyses

A. State of the Literature

For these Guidelines, a literature review was used in combination with opinions obtained from expert consultants and other sources (e.g., ASA members, ASRA members, open forums, and Internet postings). Both the literature review and opinion data were based on evidence linkages or statements regarding potential relationships between clinical interventions and outcomes.
Practice Guidelines

Anesthesiology, V 112 • No 4 • April 2010 Practice Guidelines listed below were examined to assess their impact on a variety of outcomes related to chronic noncancer pain.

I. Patient evaluation:

 1. Medical records review or patient condition
 2. Physical examination
 3. Psychological and behavioral evaluation
 4. Interventional diagnostic procedures

Diagnostic facet joint block
Diagnostic sacroiliac joint block
Diagnostic nerve block (e.g., peripheral or sympathetic, medial branch, celiac plexus, and hypogastric).
Provocative discography

II. Multimodal or multidisciplinary pain management programs (e.g., pain centers vs. single discipline care)

III. Single Modality Interventions

Ablative techniques:
Chemical denervation
Cryoneurolysis or cryoablation
Thermal intradiscal procedures (intervertebral disc annuloplasty [IDET], transdiscal biaculoplasty)
 1. Conventional or thermal radiofrequency ablation (facet joint, sacroiliac joint, dorsal root ganglion)
 2. Acupuncture
 3. Blocks:

Joint blocks
Facet joint injections
Sacroiliac joint injections
Nerve or nerve root blocks
Celiac plexus blocks
Lumbar sympathetic blocks or lumbar paravertebral sympathectomy
Medial branch blocks
Peripheral nerve blocks
Stellate ganglion blocks or cervical paravertebral sympathectomy

 4. Botox
 5. Electrical nerve stimulation:

Peripheral nerve stimulation
Spinal cord or dorsal column stimulation

TENS
 6. Epidural steroids:

Interlaminar steroids versus placebo Interlaminar steroids with local anesthetics versus without local anesthetics Transforaminal steroids versus placebo Transforaminal steroids with local anesthetics versus without local anesthetics
 7. Intrathecal drug therapies

Intrathecal neurolytic blocks
Intrathecal nonopioid injection (e.g., ziconotide, clonidine, or local anesthetics)
Intrathecal opioid injection

8. Minimally invasive spinal procedures
Kyphoplasty (percutaneous, glue, and balloon) Vertebroplasty Percutaneous disc decompression

9. Pharmacologic interventions Anticonvulsants
Alpha-2-delta calcium channel antagonists
Sodium channel blockers
Membrane-stabilizing drugs
Antidepressants
Tricyclic antidepressants
Selective serotonin–norepinephrine reuptake inhibitors
Selective serotonin reuptake inhibitors
Benzodiazepines
NMDA receptor antagonists
NSAIDs
Opioid therapy
Sustained or controlled-release opioids
Tramadol
Skeletal muscle relaxants
Topical agents
Capsaicin
Lidocaine
Ketamine

10. Physical or restorative therapy
11. Psychologic treatment or counselling Cognitive behavioral therapy, biofeedback, or relaxation training Supportive psychotherapy or group therapy
12. Trigger point injections.

www.ingramcontent.com/pod-product-compliance
Lightning Source LLC
Chambersburg PA
CBHW062319220526
45469CB00008B/2559